Color Atlas and Text of

SMALL ANIMAL UROLOGY

Peter Holt
BVMS, PhD, CBiol, MIBiol, DiplECVS, FRCVS
Department of Clinical Veterinary Science
Division of Companion Animals (Surgery)
University of Bristol

Mosby-Wolfe

London Baltimore Bogotá Boston Buenos Aires Caracas Carlsbad, CA Chicago Madrid Mexico City Milan Naples, FL New York Philadelphia St. Louis Sydney Tokyo Toronto Wiesbaden

Project Manager: Anton Lawrencepulle
Cover Design: Pete Wilder
Illustration: Jenni Miller
Production: Michael Heath
Index: Jill Halliday
Publisher: Jane Hunter

Published in 1994 by Mosby-Wolfe, an imprint of Times Mirror International Publishers Limited

Printed by Grafos S. A. Arte sobre papel, Barcelona, Spain.

ISBN 0 7234 1817 9

For full details of all Times Mirror International Publishers Limited titles, please write to Times Mirror International Publishers Limited, Lynton House, 7–12 Tavistock Square, London WC1H 9LB, England.

A CIP catalogue record for this book is available from the British Library.

Contents

Preface

'Learn from the mistakes of others; you may not live long enough to make them all yourself.' (Coats, 1988)

In 1973, Osborne, Low and Finco wrote the first authoritative text on small animal urology. Since then, although urological disorders are included in general veterinary medical or surgical texts, there have been few specialized books on small animal urology. With the exception of the fine text by Elizabeth Stone and Jeanne Barsanti (1992), this is particularly true of urological surgery

The author is consulted by an average of five veterinary surgeons daily for advice on small animal urological cases. By far the commonest enquiries are those relating to diagnosis and surgical treatment. Many veterinary surgeons request advice on how to proceed further with diagnostic investigations in animals with urological signs. Others find difficulty in performing urological surgical techniques and the author is frequently telephoned by colleagues in practice who have embarked on attempts to perform urological surgery only to find that "it looks nothing like the picture in the book!" The reason for this last statement is that most surgical texts illustrate procedures by means of line drawings, usually of surgery on normal organs. In clinical practice, however, one is rarely operating on a normal organ and although line drawings are helpful, they may also be a poor reflection of the actual situation which will be encountered.

A less-frequent but difficult situation is where an attempt has been made at an unfamiliar urological technique and a serious error made. Whereas this may reflect on the abilities of the veterinary surgeon concerned, it may also be associated with the fact that few texts point out potential problems and how to avoid them.

This colour atlas is intended primarily for the small animal veterinary surgeon in general practice, although it is hoped that it will also be of value to veterinary undergraduates, residents, interns, house surgeons, veterinary nurses and veterinary or medical researchers in urology. Thus, it is assumed that the reader is a competent veterinary surgeon, able to interpret clinical, laboratory and radiographic findings, aware of aseptic surgical techniques and capable of performing surgical approaches to the abdominal viscera. The atlas will concentrate, therefore, on the methodology of diagnostic techniques relevant to small animal urological disorders and on related surgical procedures.

In the first part of the book, urological investigative procedures are described, with greater emphasis given to those which are more readily available for use in general practice. Particular attention is given to radiographic techniques since these are essential in the investigation of animals with urological disorders and the facilities required are available in most practices. The remainder of the book is centred around descriptions of urological surgical techniques. The indications for each technique are illustrated and potential problems (and their avoidance) discussed. The techniques themselves are illustrated in colour and supplemented by black and white radiographs, line drawings and tables. The illustrations are of procedures on actual clinical cases, not normal animals or cadavers. Any illustrations of normal animals are intended only for comparison with the abnormal situation and are acknowledged as such. For this reason, the technique of nephrotomy is illustrated using line drawings only as, at the time of writing (and for the reasons given in Chapter 4), it is five years since the author last performed this technique and he has no suitable photographs.

The material which is presented in this atlas is based entirely on the author's experience, both in general veterinary practice and in a busy University Veterinary Surgery Department dealing with referred cases. Inevitably, other veterinary urologists may have different views on methods of diagnosis and treatment to those which are presented in this book. However, the descriptions of the diagnostic and surgical techniques which follow are those which have worked best for the author.

Peter E. Holt

Acknowledgements

My interest in veterinary urology began in general practice but was really stimulated when I took up a lectureship in the Department of Veterinary Surgery at Bristol University. I consider myself extremely fortunate to have had as my mentors Professor Harold Pearson and Dr Christine Gibbs and I will always be grateful for their advice and encouragement.

Most of the photographs used in this book were taken by Mr J. Conibear and Mr M. Parsons. I sincerely hope that I have done justice to their photographic skills.

A number of friends and colleagues gave freely of their advice and expertise and it is a pleasure to thank the following: the radiographers, anaesthetists, house surgeons, residents and nurses who helped to investigate, treat and care for the cases used to illustrate this book; Professor Harold Pearson for permission to use two of his illustrations (**4.83a** and **b**); Dr G. R. Pearson for cytological photography and advice; Mr A. Skuse for advice on the staining of cytology specimens; Dr F. Barr for assistance with ultrasonographic illustrations and advice. I also wish to thank Jenni Miller who was responsible for the line-drawings.

I am grateful to the Editors of the following journals for permission to reproduce illustrations which have been previously published: *In Practice* (**1.2, 2.13, 2.14, 2.57, 2.59, 3.4, 3.15, 3.20, 4.2, 4.97, 4.99, 4.113, 4.146, 4.169, 4.181, 4.186, 5.27, 5.39, 5.42a**); *The Journal of Small Animal Practice* (**2.33b, 2.35, 2.43, 2.44, 2.45, 3.17, 3.31b, 4.160–4.168**); *Research in Veterinary Science* (**3.30, 3.31a**); *Waltham International Focus* (**1.8, 3.16, 3.36, 4.77, 4.84, 4.107, 4.138, 4.143b, 4.171, 4.172, 4.174a, 5.26**).

Finally, I wish to thank my wife Sylvia and son Andrew for their patience and understanding during my prolonged affair with the word processor.

This is for my family

Dedicated to the memory of my father, Eric R. Holt, whose enthusiasm for my work remains a constant source of encouragement to me.

1 Clinical Assessment

This chapter gives a brief account of the clinical assessment of small animals presented with signs of urological disease.

Most animals with urological presenting signs can be divided into those presenting primarily with dysuria, haematuria, urinary incontinence or frequency/urgency. The conditions leading to these signs are listed in **Tables 1.1–1.5**.

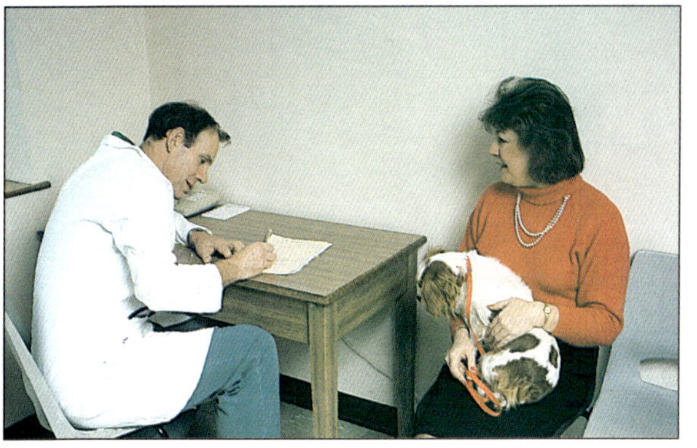

1.1 A good history is essential. In many animals with urological signs, especially incontinent dogs and cats, there may be few or no detectable abnormalities on clinical examination but a good history will usually suggest which part of the urinary tract merits more detailed ancillary investigations.

The clinical assessment of animals with these signs can be divided into history-taking and clinical examination for the purposes of description but these two activities are closely interrelated; further interrogation of the owner may be suggested by clinical findings whereas the history may point to a particular type of examination.

Table 1.1. Dysuria.

Urethral calculus
Prostatic disease
Bladder neck neoplasia
Urethral neoplasia
Urethral trauma
Urethritis
Urethral stricture
Neurogenic dysuria
Bladder displacement/entrapment
External pressure on bladder neck/urethra

Table 1.2. Haematuria.

Urinary tract infection
Urolithiasis
Prostatic disorders
Urinary tract neoplasia
Urinary tract trauma
Idiopathic renal haemorrhage
Bleeding/clotting disorders

Table 1.3. Congenital urinary incontinence.

Ureteral ectopia
Urethral sphincter mechanism incompetence
Pervious urachus
Bladder hypoplasia
Intersexuality
Congenital neurological abnormalities

Table 1.4. Acquired urinary incontinence.

Urethral sphincter mechanism incompetence
Prostatic disease
Bladder/urethral neoplasia
Uretero- or vesicovaginal fistula
Detrusor instability
Paradoxical overflow incontinence (e.g. urolithiasis)
Neurological abnormalities

Table 1.5. Frequency/urgency (pollakiuria).

Cystitis/urethritis
Cystolithiasis
Bladder/urethral neoplasia
Prostatic disease
Bladder hypoplasia/detrusor instability
Lower urinary tract trauma

As well as the breed, sex and age of the animal, the presence or absence and, where relevant, frequency and severity of the following should be determined:

- Entire or neutered animal.
- Anorexia/inappetance.
- Polydypsia/polyuria.
- Dysuria (differentiate from faecal tenesmus or urinary tenesmus with the bladder empty).
- Anuria.
- Oliguria.
- Nocturia.
- Urinary incontinence (differentiate from inappropiate micturition – e.g. behavioural or the untrained puppy).
- Urinary frequency/urgency (pollakiuria).
- Haematuria (differentiate from haemoglobinuria and determine the phase of urination during which most blood is present – in male dogs with prostatic disease, the first part of the stream may be most bloody, bladder urothelial tumours often bleed towards the end of micturition and the urine is usually equally bloody throughout micturition in cases of renal haemorrhage; however, these are not hard and fast rules).
- Pyuria (determine if a purulent urethral discharge is also present – e.g. the dog with prostatic abscessation).
- Urethral discharge (differentiate from preputial or vaginal discharge and urinary incontinence: determine nature of discharge).
- Oversexuality (in males).
- Vulval/preputial licking.
- Neurological signs.

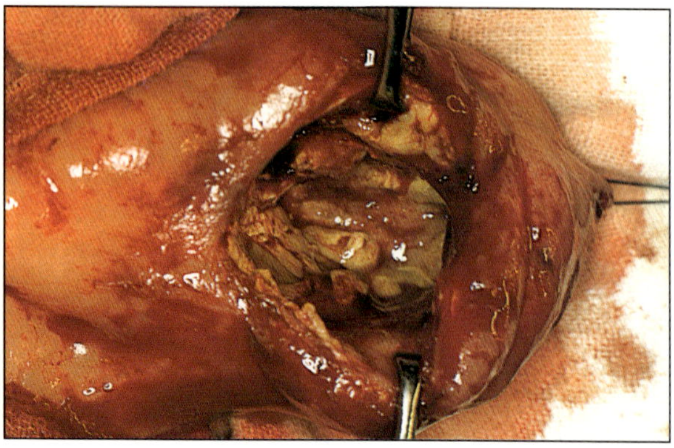

1.2 A detailed clinical examination in animals with obstructive dysuria is less of a priority than relief of the dysuria. Prolonged bladder distension may result in bladder wall ischaemia. Initially, this affects the urothelium which may become necrotic and slough, as illustrated in a dog five days after acute dysuria. Sloughed urothelium may be a further cause of obstructive dysuria. If acute bladder distension is prolonged, the ischaemia may involve all layers of the bladder wall and the result may be a bladder which is a non-functional fibrotic sac. In addition, bladder nerve stretching, demyelination and breakdown of tight junctions may occur, resulting in neurogenic dysuria following relief of the obstruction. Dysuria should be relieved by catheterization or cystocentesis (see Chapter 3).

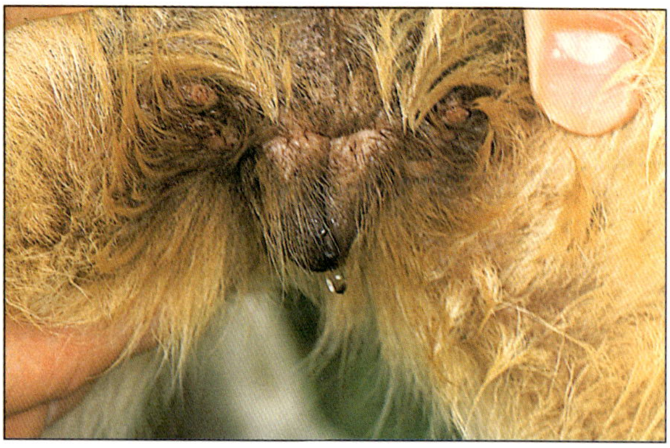

1.3 Urinary incontinence. A continuous dripping incontinence in a juvenile animal may suggest ureteral ectopia but it can also be associated with uretero- or vesicovaginal fistula and paradoxical overflow incontinence associated with obstructive or neurogenic dysuria.

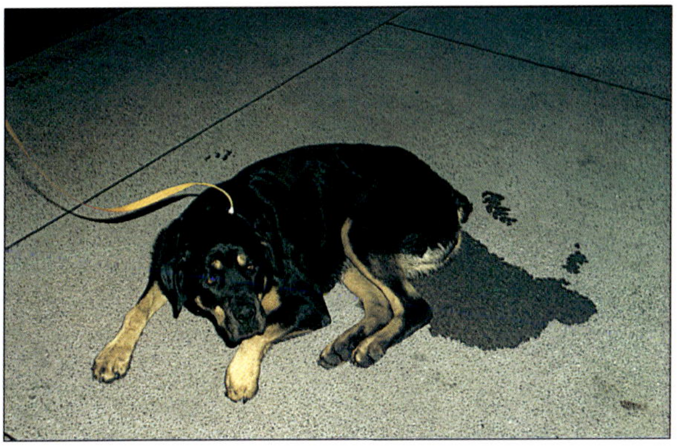

1.4 Intermittent, more copious incontinence which occurs predominantly during recumbency is suggestive of urethral sphincter mechanism incompetence. However, this sign is not pathognomonic and clinical, contrast radiographic and laboratory examinations are required to make an accurate diagnosis.

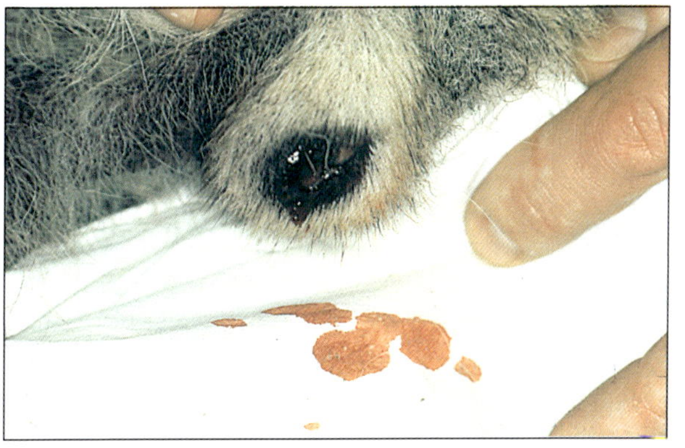

1.5 A bloody urethral discharge in male dogs is sometimes mistaken by the owners for haematuria or incontinence of bloody urine. A good history should differentiate these and clinical examination will exclude lesions of the prepuce and/or penis as the source of haemorrhage. If the urine is said to be clear of or to contain much less blood, such a discharge suggests prostatic or urethral disease. Bleeding in this dog originated from the prostate gland.

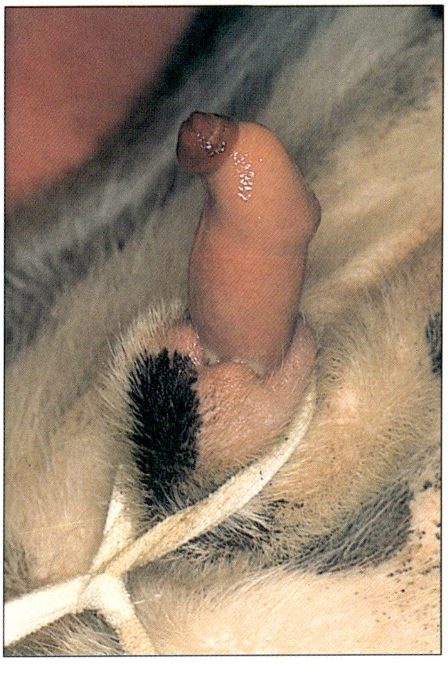

1.6 A bloody preputial discharge may be due to a preputial or penile lesion. In the case of this Bulldog, a urethral prolapse was the source of the haemorrhage.

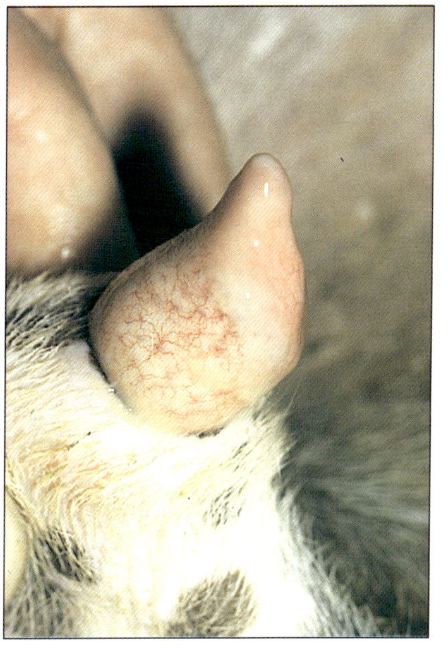

1.7 Clinical examination revealed that the purulent discharge in this dog was urethral rather than preputial in origin. Cytological and bacteriological examinations of the discharge should be performed to confirm its nature, obtain antibiotic sensitivities and look for the presence of malignant cells. This Boxer had a prostatic abscess.

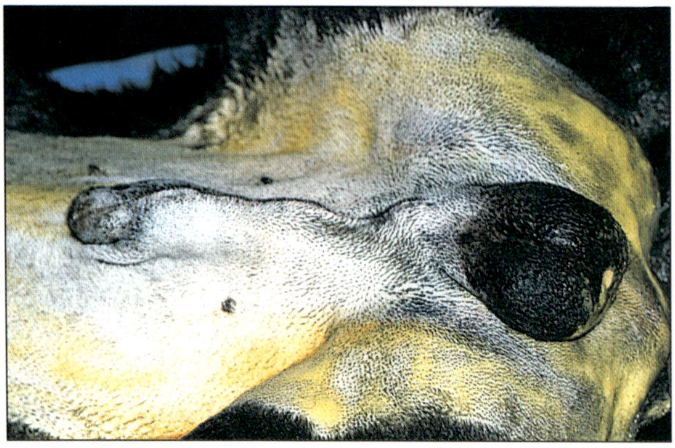

1.8 The urethra should be palpated for abnormal masses. This dysuric German shepherd had a firm mass at the caudal end of the os penis (just cranial to the scrotum). Masses in this region may be large urethral calculi but these are not always palpable. This dog had a tumour of the os penis (a chondrosarcoma). Its treatment is illustrated later (see **4.115–4.126**).

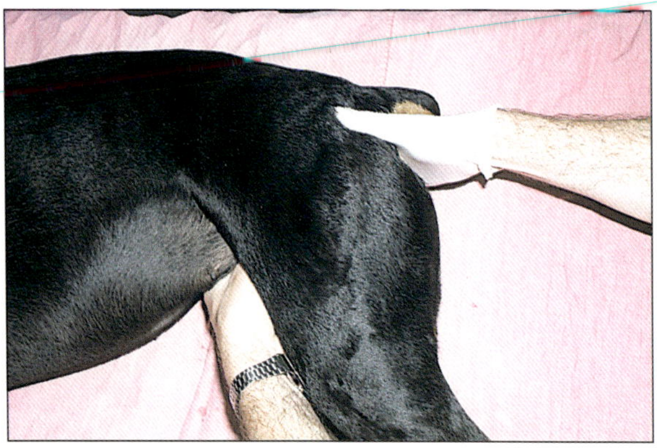

1.9 In male dogs, the prostate is best examined by a combination of abdominal and rectal palpations. In the case of a right-handed person, the left hand is used to push the prostate caudodorsally onto the right-hand index finger which is in the rectum. If the animal is recumbent, palpation is easier in right lateral recumbency (as shown) for a right-handed person. Left-handed clinicians should reverse this advice. The prostate is examined for size, symmetry, texture and pain; the value of the findings in differential diagnosis is summarized in **Table 1.6**.

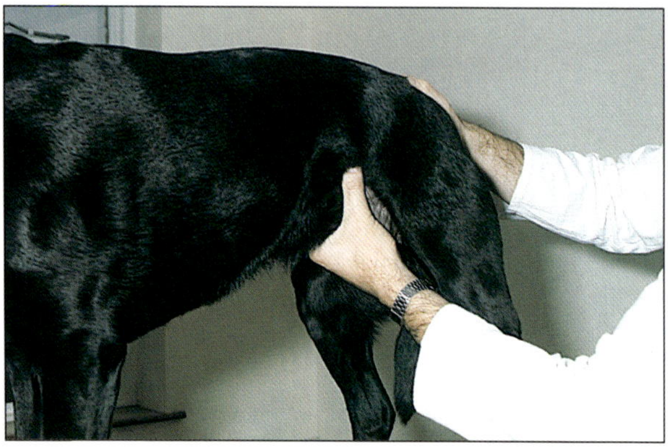

1.10 In the author's view, bladder palpation is best performed with one hand (unless the size of the animal or bladder makes this impossible). The size, degree of turgidity, thickness of bladder wall and presence of abnormal masses should be determined. The detection of crepitation suggests the presence of multiple cystoliths or bladder wall mineralization.

1.11 Bladder wall thickness can be assessed (as long as the bladder is not distended with urine) between the thumb and fingers as the (doubled) bladder wall is pinched between them.

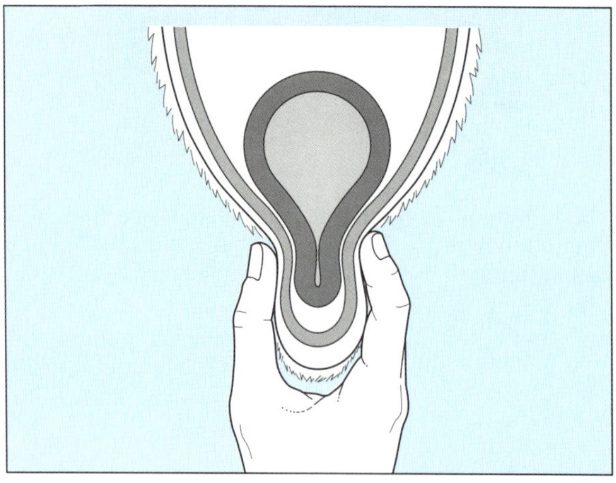

Table 1.6. Differential clinical findings in prostatic disease.

	Enlarged	*Symmetrical*	*Painful*	*Firm (FM)/ Fluctuant (FL)*	*Urethral discharge*
Hyperplasia/ Metaplasia	+	+	–	FM	± (semen)
Prostatitis	±	+	+	FM	± (blood, pus)
Abscessation	+	–	+	FL	± (pus)
Cysts	+	–	–	FL	–
Neoplasia	±	±	+	FM	–
Idiopathic haemorrhage	–	+	–	FM	+ (blood)

The pelvic urethra can be palpated *per rectum* in males and females and examination of the female urethra can be performed *per vaginam* in large bitches. In male and female cats, only external and rectal palpations are practicable and rectal examination of this species usually requires sedation or general anaesthesia.

The kidney position, size, texture and shape should be assessed. In the author's experience, renal pain is difficult to assess in small animals. Dogs and cats with renal lesions which one would expect to be painful frequently show no signs of pain whereas spinal pain in animals is sometimes misdiagnosed as renal pain.

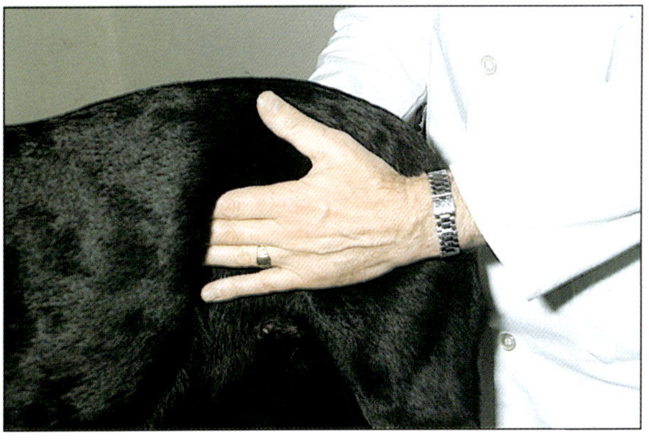

1.12 The kidneys can be palpated in the craniodorsal part of the abdomen. If the animal is sufficiently relaxed, it is possible to palpate deep to the costal arch, as illustrated. This may be necessary to locate the right kidney which is more cranial than the left.

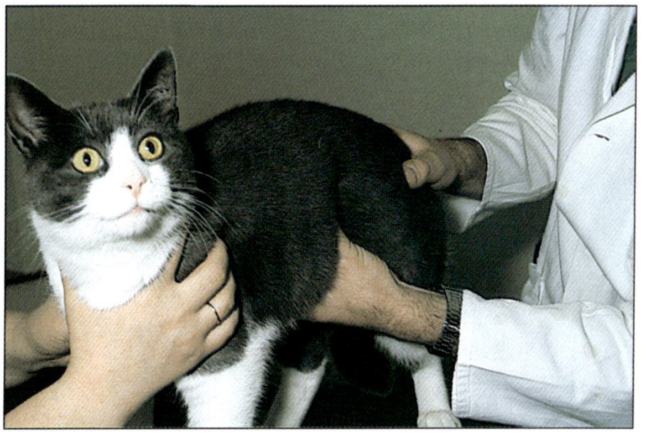

1.13 The kidneys of cats are more easily located than those of dogs and, in cats and small dogs, may be palpated using one hand.

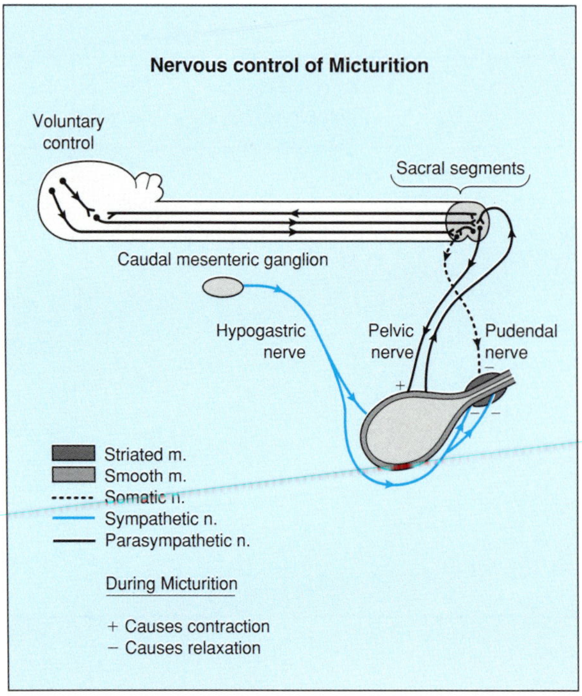

1.14 Micturition and urinary continence control depend upon complex neuromuscular activity and co-ordination. Most clinicians are familiar with the animal with thoracolumbar spinal disease which develops urinary retention as part of a more widespread problem, but neurogenic urological problems can occur without overt neurological limb abnormalities. This is particulary true if the sacral segments of the spinal cord or their nerve roots are affected. If so, much of the nerve supply to hind limb musculature may be intact (as it originates from caudal lumbar spinal cord segments and is cranial to the lesion) and the animal may show little, if any, hind limb gait abnormalities. However, evidence of cauda equina disease should be detectable – i.e. bladder and possibly rectal paralysis, tail paresis or paralysis and perineal skin desensitization.

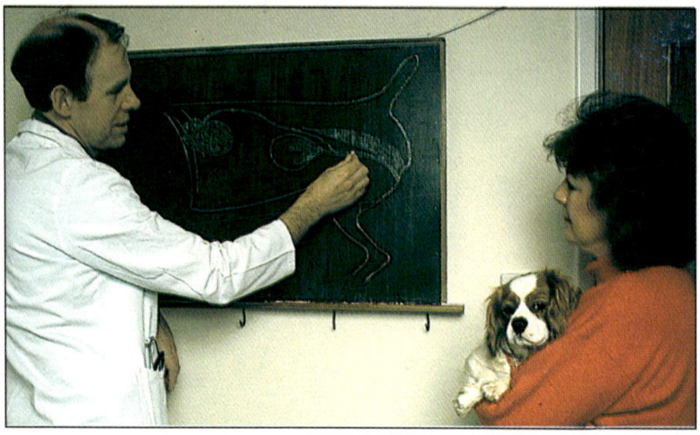

1.15 A blackboard or wipe-clean board is a useful addition to the consulting room. It greatly facilitates explanations of possible diagnoses, further investigative procedures, potential treatments and complications to the owner of the animal.

2 Radiographic Investigations

Radiographic investigations are frequently required in the differential diagnosis of conditions leading to urological presenting signs in small animals. Plain abdominal radiographs are mandatory and thoracic radiography should not be neglected in cases of suspected malignancy (to examine for the presence of pulmonary metastases). In the majority of cases, plain radiographs alone are insufficient for diagnostic purposes and contrast radiographs are required.

In this chapter, intravenous urography, vagino-urethrography, urethrography and cystography will be described as these are the commonest techniques employed in urological cases and are applicable in general practice. The descriptions will concentrate on indications, techniques and problems in technique and interpretation and how to avoid them. No details of radiographic exposure will be given as these will vary considerably depending on the equipment available to the reader. In addition, a reasonable level of radiographic competence by the reader is assumed.

It is vital that all radiographs are taken when the animal is still. This is particularly important when examining the kidneys, which move caudally and cranially during inspiration and expiration, respectively, due to diaphragmatic movements. Radiographic exposures should therefore be made immediately after expiration, during the respiratory pause when the animal is still. The exception is thoracic radiography, which is usually performed at full inspiration.

Plain films

Indications

- Urolithiasis.
- Determination of organ size, shape and position.
- Evidence of local or distant tumour metastases.
- As control films, prior to contrast radiography.

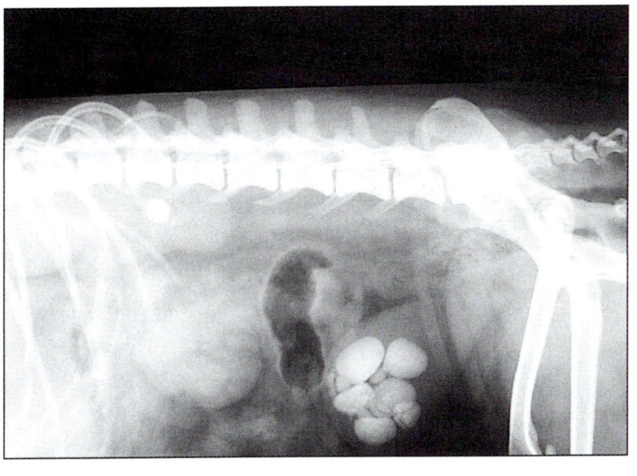

2.1 Bladder calculi can usually be seen on plain films. Radiographs should be made when the bladder is full of urine, rather than empty, as the calculi will then be more apparent. Non-radio-opaque calculi can be demonstrated by double contrast cystography but, somewhat surprisingly, are not well outlined by pneumocystography alone. If plain radiographs are not made before positive contrast radiographic techniques, vesical calculi may be obscured by the contrast medium and remain undetected. This Cavalier King Charles spaniel also has a renal calculus (see also **4.29**).

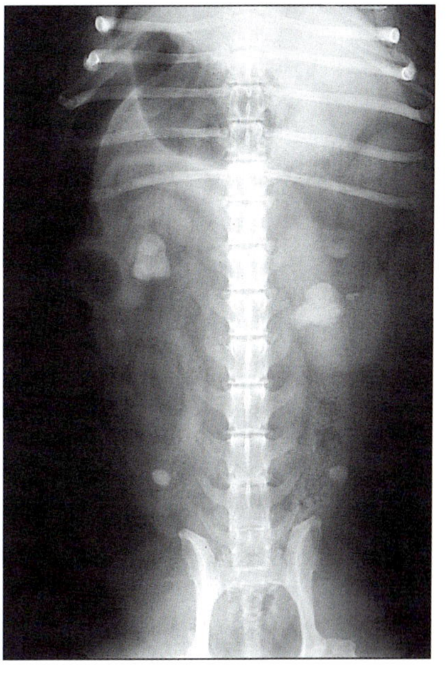

2.2 Renal calculi are also easily seen on plain ventrodorsal radiographs. However, care should be taken in bitches not to confuse large nipples with renal calculi.

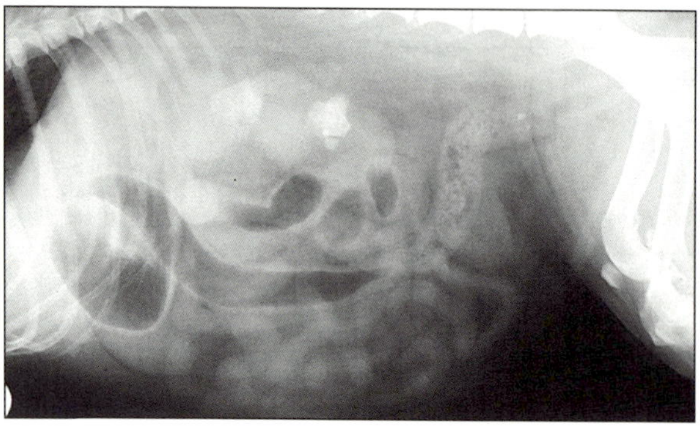

2.3 Lateral abdominal radiography will distinguish between large nipples and renal calculi. The nipples will now be on the ventral abdominal wall whereas the calculus or calculi will still be in the region of the renal pelvis/pelves in the craniodorsal abdomen.

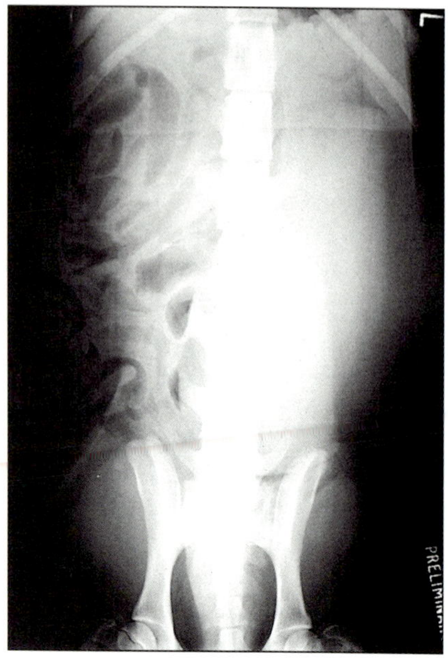

2.4 The size, shape and position of urinary tract organs can sometimes be seen in plain films. In many cases, however, contrast radiographic techniques are required to distinguish more accurately urinary tract organs from surrounding soft tissues. In addition, although this dog appears to have an enlarged left kidney in this plain ventrodorsal abdominal radiograph, additional techniques (intravenous urography, ultrasonography, urine laboratory examinations) are required before the reason for the enlargement can be determined (see **2.16, 2.17**).

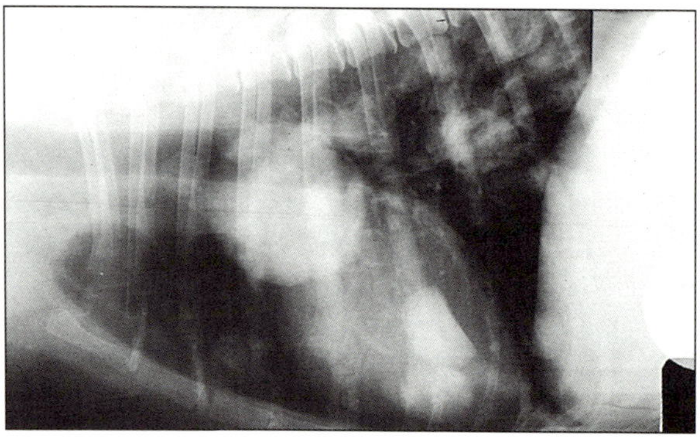

2.5 Thoracic radiography should always be performed in cases of possible urinary tract malignancy. This aged Miniature poodle was treated by castration and oestrogens for 12 months for benign prostatic enlargement. On presentation, the dog screamed during any attempt to examine or handle it. The reason for the pain is apparent in the next two illustrations but a simple thoracic radiograph would have demonstrated that this was not a benign condition.

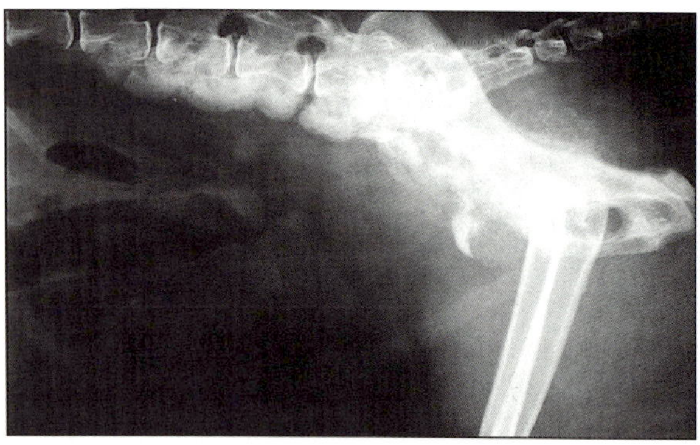

2.6 A plain lateral caudal abdominal radiograph of the dog in 2.5. The periosteal bone reactions on the pelvis and sublumbar/sacral vertebrae are highly suggestive of intrapelvic malignancy (in this case, prostatic carcinoma) but are frequently not neoplastic themselves.

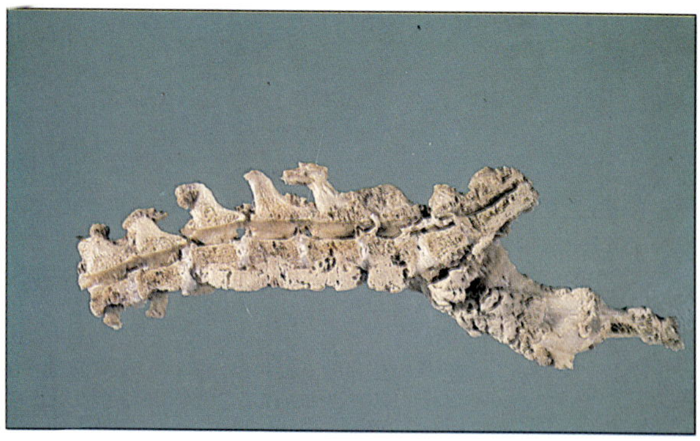

2.7 *Post mortem* specimen from the dog in 2.5 and 2.6. The periosteal bone reactions can be seen. A metastasis from the prostatic carcinoma is present in the body of the sixth lumbar vertebra.

2.8

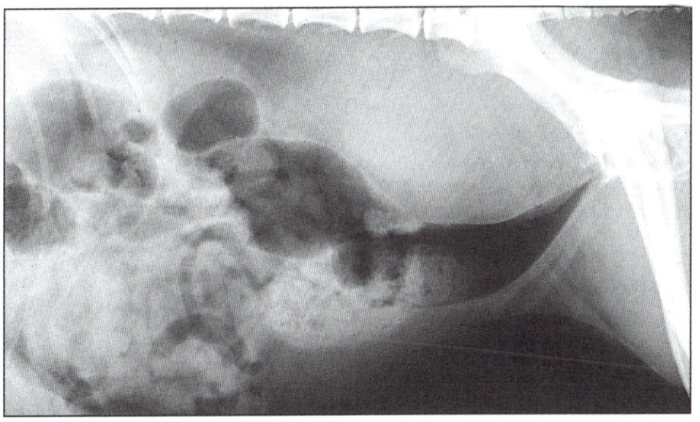

2.8 In cases of suspected malignancy, the soft tissues ventral to the caudal lumbar and sacral vertebrae should be examined for evidence of sublumbar/iliac lymph node enlargement, suggesting lymphatic spread. In some instances, the enlargement of the sublumbar lymph nodes may be responsible for the urological signs. Dysuria and dyschezia in this dog are due to external pressure on the bladder neck/proximal urethra and rectum by a neoplastic sublumbar lymph node (lymphosarcoma).

Techniques

The positioning techniques for radiography of urinary tract organs are illustrated in the section on contrast radiographic procedures (see **2.20–2.28**). Thoracic and distal male canine urethral radiography are illustrated below.

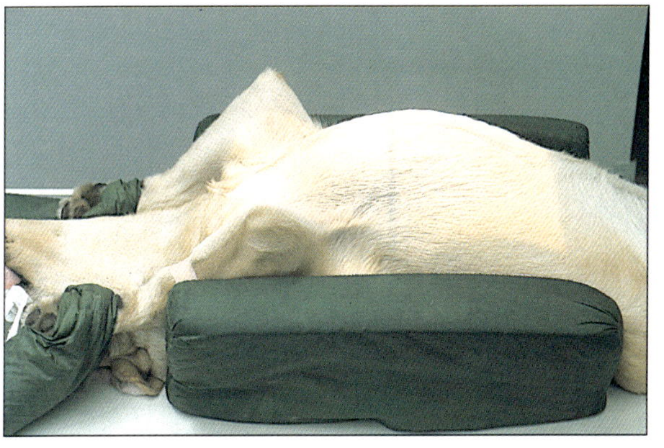

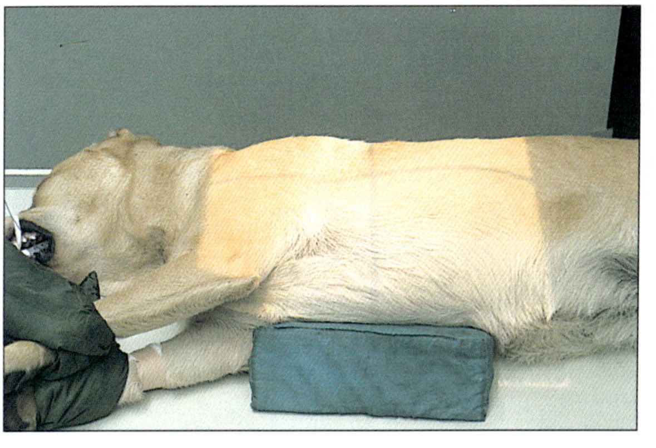

2.9 Thoracic radiographs should be made at full inspiration as this improves the radiographic contrast between pulmonary masses and surrounding air. In anaesthetized animals, this is achieved by forcibly inflating the lungs via the endotracheal tube. **(top)** For ventrodorsal radiography, the animal is supported in a sponge (or other radiolucent) cradle. The forelimbs are extended using sandbags and the X-ray beam is centred mid-way along the sternum. **(bottom)** During lateral thoracic radiography, the forelimbs are again extended and the sternum is elevated to the level of the vertebral column with a radiolucent wedge. The X-ray beam is centred at the levels of the caudal edge of the scapula and just over a third of the way up the thoracic wall from the sternum. Lateral thoracic radiographs are usually adequate for the diagnosis of pulmonary metastases.

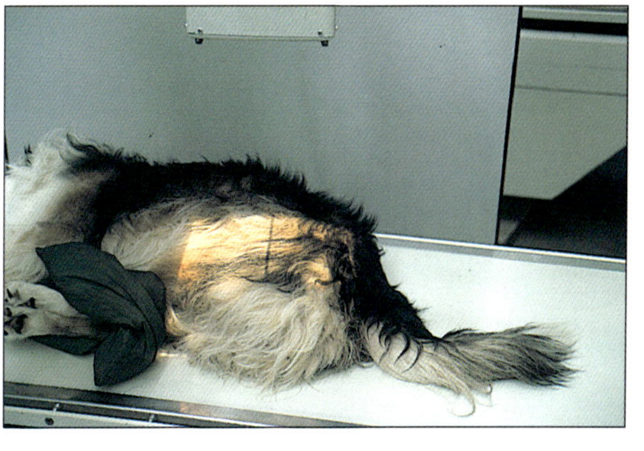

2.10 The penile and ischial urethra in the male dog is best radiographed with the hind limbs flexed cranially using sandbags and the X-ray beam centred on the penile/ischial urethra. In this way, the stifle joints and/or femurs are not superimposed on the caudal penile urethra (see **2.13, 2.14**).

Problems

Many problems are due to incorrect radiographic exposure or positioning. The latter is described further below and time spent on obtaining correct exposures is never wasted. Other problems are associated with the presence of overlying viscera or abnormal, but clinically insignificant, tissues.

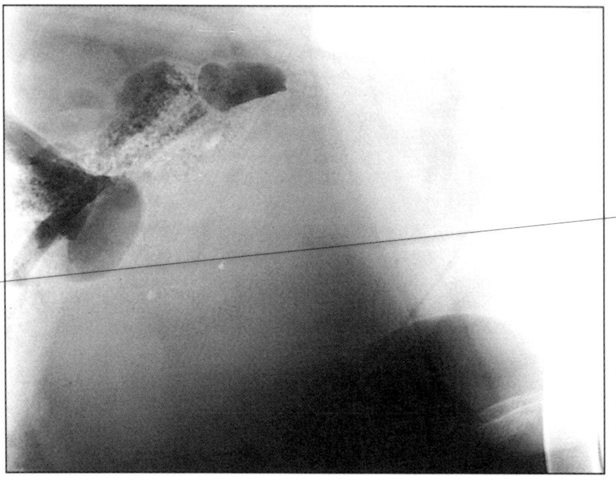

2.11 Care should be taken in interpretation when other viscera overlie urinary tract organs. The problem of nipples being misdiagnosed as renal calculi has already been mentioned (**2.2, 2.3**). In this illustration, mineralized material in overlying bowel may be confused with vesical calculi; a radiograph made in the other plane (in this case, a ventrodorsal radiograph) would clarify the situation.

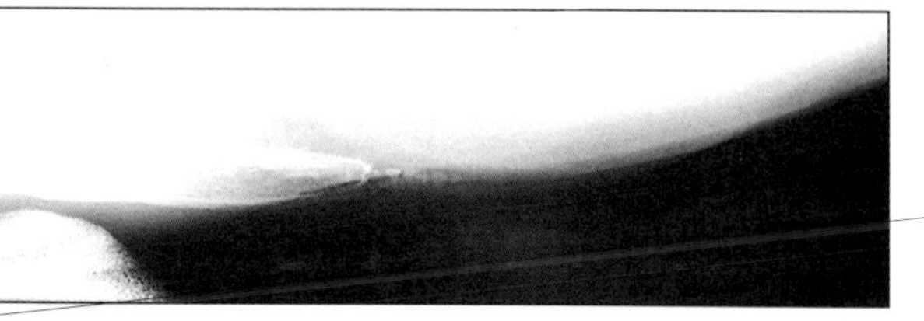

2.12 Bony reactions or separate centres of ossification of the caudal os penis may be mistaken for urethral calculi in dysuric animals but are of no clinical significance. (See also 'Catheterization'.) In fact, these are dorsal to the urethra itself and, in case of doubt, this will be apparent if a retrograde positive contrast urethrogram is performed.

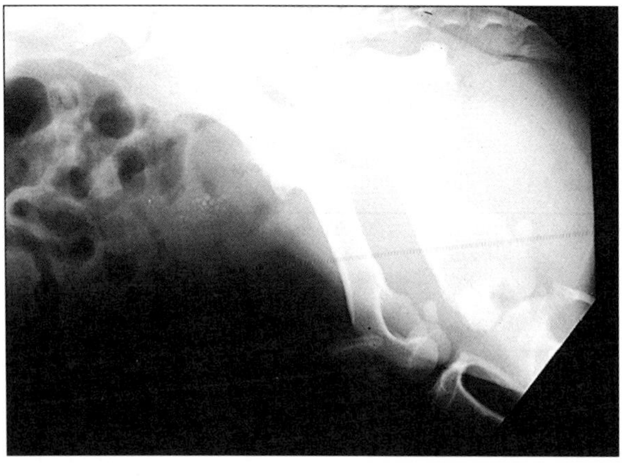

2.13 Urethral calculi proximal to the caudal os penis may be obscured by the stifle joints when the dog is positioned with the hind limbs extended for caudal abdominal radiography. (See **2.28.**) However, this position is useful for demonstrating the vesical calculi which are usually also present.

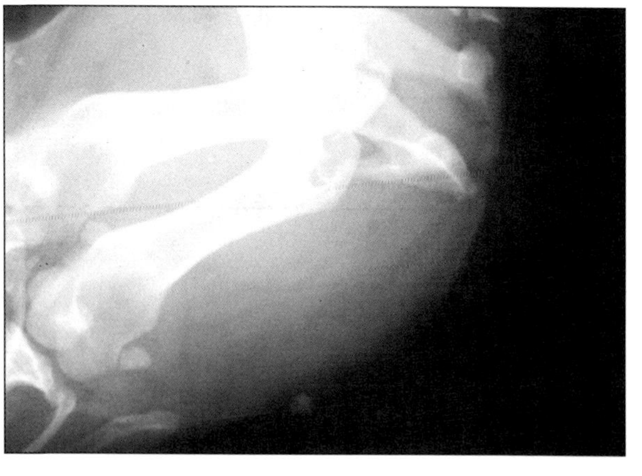

2.14 The problems are overcome by repeating the radiograph with the legs flexed forward and the X-ray beam centred on the ischial and penile urethra. (See **2.10.**) The urethral calculus responsible for the dysuria can now be seen.

Intravenous urography (IVU)

Indications

- Urinary incontinence.
- Suspected renal or ureteral lesions.
- Suspected lesions of the bladder trigone.
- An abdominal mass in an otherwise healthy animal.

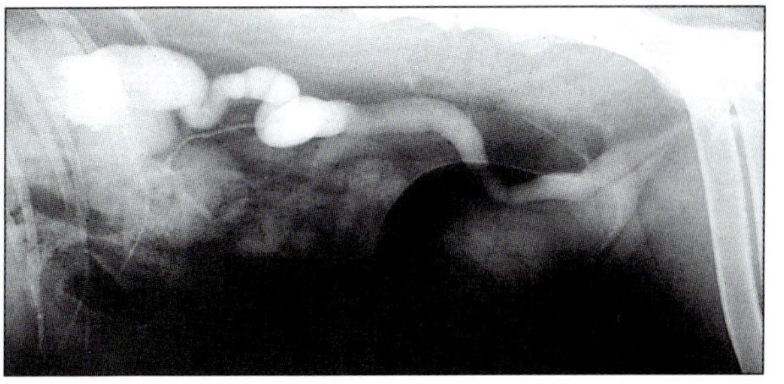

2.15 Intravenous urography is mandatory in cases of urinary incontinence. In this example, a dilated ectopic ureter is demonstrated terminating beyond the bladder neck (retrograde contrast techniques are frequently required, however, to identify the exact site of the ectopic opening).

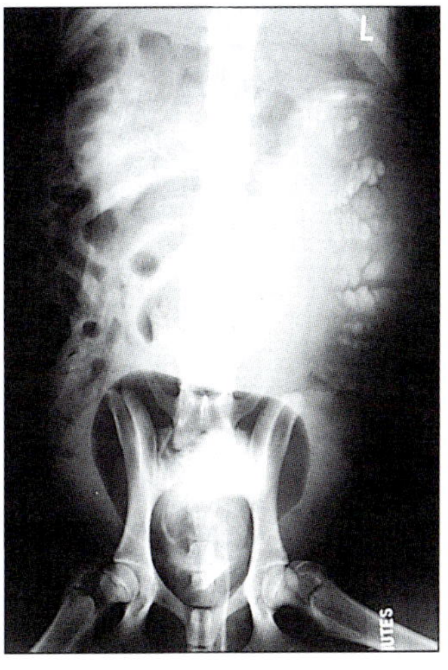

2.16 Gross renal lesions are usually demonstrated by intravenous urography. Hydronephrosis may result in bizarre radiographs, as illustrated in this juvenile male Golden retriever with ureteral ectopia, hydro-ureter and hydronephrosis (this is the same dog as shown in **2.4**).

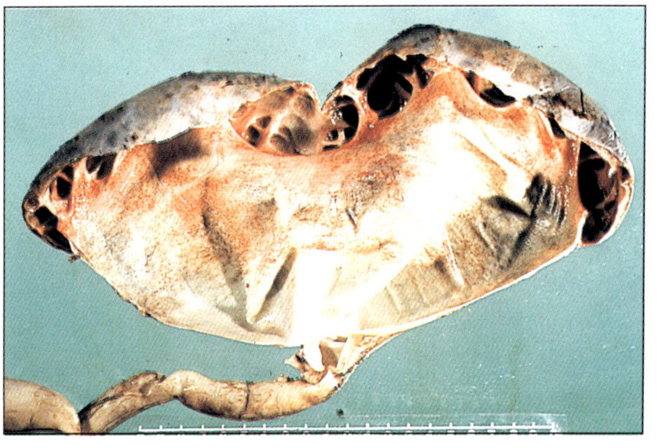

2.17 The reason for the bizarre appearance can be seen in this specimen of the excised kidney and ureter. The contrast medium accumulates in the dependant pockets of the hydronephrotic kidney cavity. It is always surprising that there is any significant excretion of contrast medium at all in cases such as this in which there is only a thin layer of renal tissue remaining.

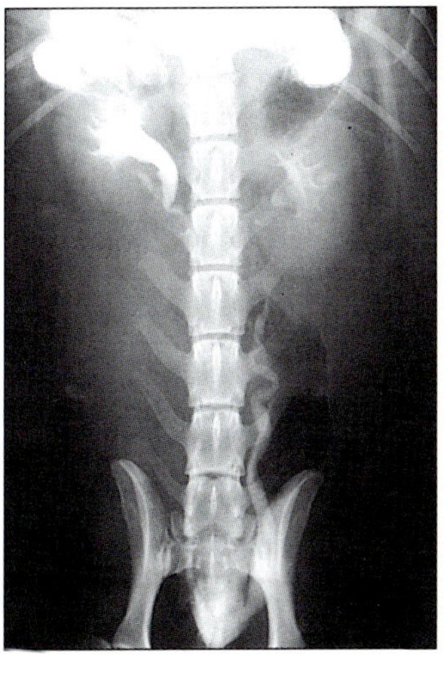

2.18 Ureteral lesions are rare but rupture of the proximal right ureter following ureterolithiasis is demonstrated by intravenous urography in this Golden retriever. (The radio-density in the cranial abdomen is barium, administered by mouth to investigate the presenting sign of vomiting.) The ureteral calculus responsible for the rupture is now obscured by the contrast medium in the proximal ureter, underlining the need for plain radiographs before administration of contrast medium.

2.19 Intravenous urography may prevent unnecessary surgery. In this German shepherd dog, a mass was palpated in the caudal abdomen during a routine examination. Intravenous urography demonstrates that this is an ectopic kidney (arrowed), which is of no clinical significance.

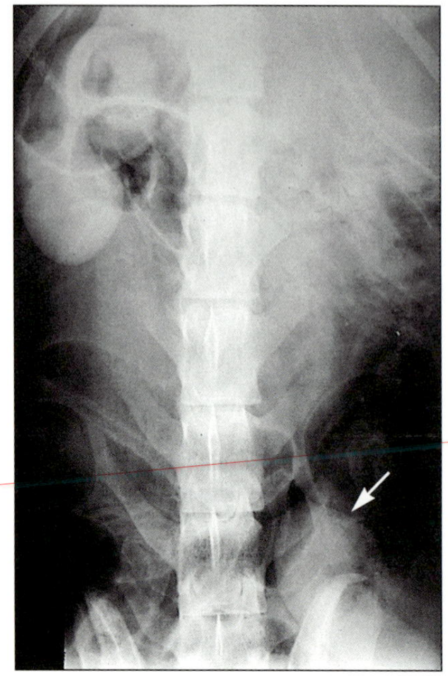

Technique

It is important that the gastro-intestinal tract is empty as the presence of ingesta makes radiographic interpretation difficult. This state is achieved by the use of enemata. Soapy water enemas are not suitable, as the edges of bubbles in the large bowel may be confused with ureters.

Proprietary enemas usually work well and the author routinely uses Fletchers Phosphate enemas (Pharmax) in medium- and large-sized dogs and Micralax enemas (Evans) in toy breeds and cats. A third of a phosphate enema (7–8 ml) is sufficient for a medium-sized dog, half an enema (10 ml) for a large breed and a full enema (20 ml) for giant breeds. The enema can be given at the time of premedication and the dog then walked or allowed the use of an enclosed run.

Intravenous urography is usually performed under general anaesthesia except in debilitated patients.

As with all contrast radiographic techniques, plain radiographs should be made of the area of interest before contrast medium is used.

The radiographic timings and positionings illustrated below are for a standard intravenous urogram but some flexibility is necessary, as dictated by the radiological features which are demonstrated. The technique is demonstrated in incontinent (but otherwise normal) bitches but is identical in cats and in both sexes.

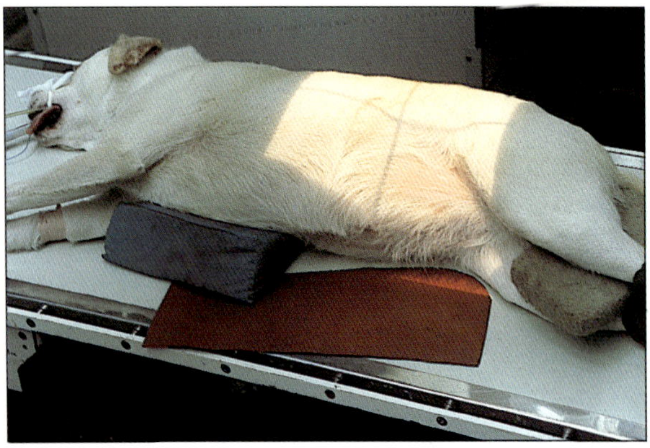

2.20 Under general anaesthesia, a plain lateral abdominal radiograph is made, centred on the sublumbar region at the level of the umbilicus. Right lateral recumbency is preferred to left lateral recumbency as this results in better separation of the kidneys on lateral radiography due to the relative mobility of the left kidney compared to the right. In addition, it is important to standardize the technique. Note the use of the sponge wedge (blue) to lift the sternum to the same level as the spine and the sponge between the hind limbs to avoid pelvic tilting. These measures are to ensure that a true lateral radiograph is made. Soft sandbags (green) are used to extend the hind legs and a piece of lead sheet (brown) absorbs X-rays ventral to the abdomen, thus reducing scattered radiation. For caudal abdominal radiography, the film should be centred as shown in **2.28**.

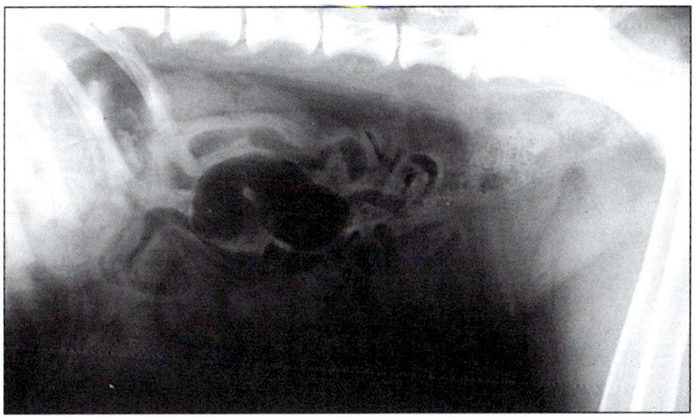

2.21 The resultant radiograph is examined for evidence of any abnormalities and can be compared with those obtained after contrast administration. It is also used to determine the efficacy of the enema; in this case, some faecal material remains in the descending colon and rectum and should be removed by lavage with saline.

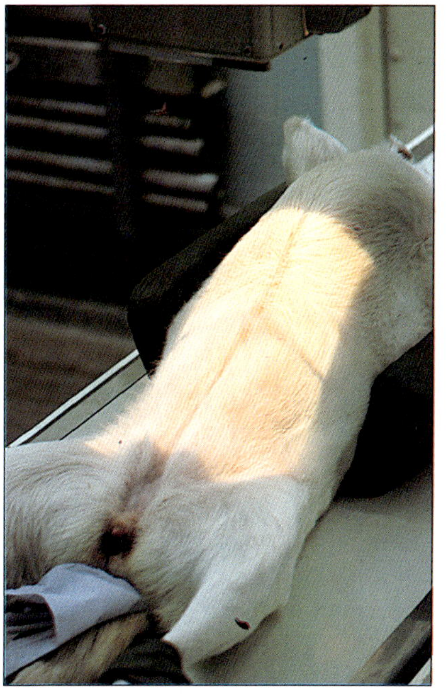

2.22 The dog is then placed in dorsal recumbency and a ventrodorsal radiograph made, again centred on the umbilicus. Note the use of a sponge cradle to support the thorax. It is not necessary to support the abdomen and so the possibility of a dirty cradle introducing artefacts on the radiograph is avoided. Soft sandbags are again used to extend the hind limbs. It is important to prevent spillage of urine onto the X-ray table or/and the animal's coat, particularly after administration of contrast medium. Spilled urine containing contrast medium will show up on subsequent radiographs and may make radiographic interpretation difficult.

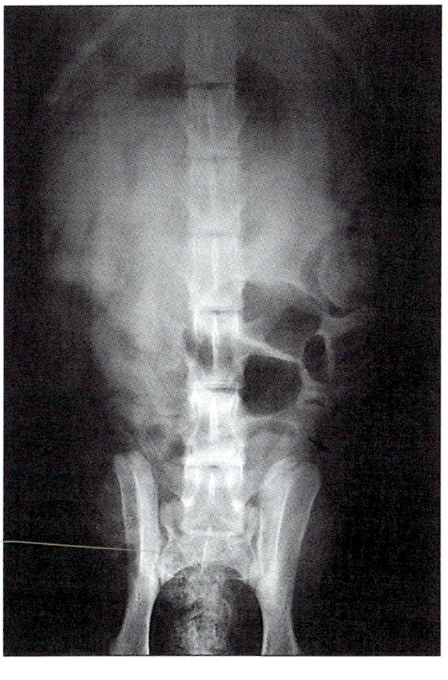

2.23 The resultant radiograph is also examined for evidence of any abnormalities (particularly of the kidneys). The kidneys, especially the right kidney, are not always visible, but if they are their position can be assessed and the centring (relative to the umbilicus) adjusted for the next film – the nephrogram.

2.24 The dog remains in dorsal recumbency and the radiographic beam is centred over the kidneys. If these are not visible on the plain ventrodorsal radiograph, the beam should be centred on a point midway between the umbilicus and the xiphisternum, as illustrated.

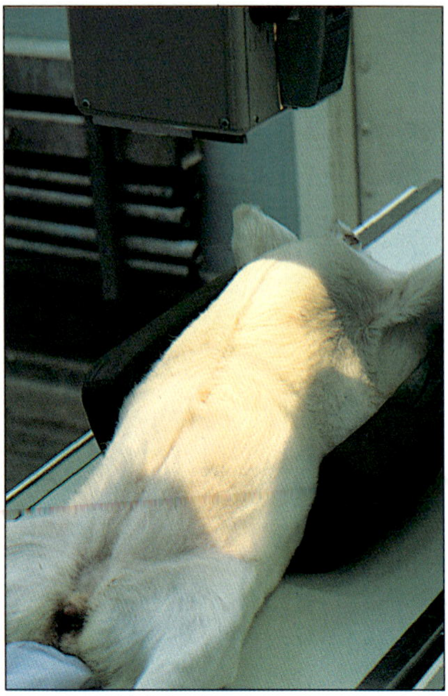

The bladder is emptied of urine (which is submitted for laboratory analysis) and a small volume of air introduced into it. It is inadvisable to overdistend the bladder during intravenous urography as the increased intravesical pressure may compress the intramural part of the ureters, making interpretation of their terminations difficult. One millilitre of air per kilogram body weight is usually sufficient.

A water-soluble, iodine-based contrast medium containing the equivalent of approximately 400 mg iodine per ml of contrast solution (e.g. 70% sodium iothalamate; Conray '420', May & Baker) is used in large dogs whereas solutions containing about 200 mg iodine per ml are suitable for cats and toy breeds of dog. A bolus of approximately 400 mg/kg of iodine equivalent (i.e. 1 ml/kg of Conray '420') is administered by rapid intravenous injection. A higher dose, 500–600 mg/kg (or approximately 1.5 ml/kg of Conray '420'), is required in dogs and cats less than 10 kg in body weight whereas animals over 60 kg do not require more than 25 g of iodine equivalent total dose (i.e. 60 ml Conray '420').

The positioning of the dog is quickly checked (and corrected if the dog has been inadvertently moved during the injection) and the radiograph made immediately. The time is noted as all further radiographic timings are relative to the time of intravenous injection.

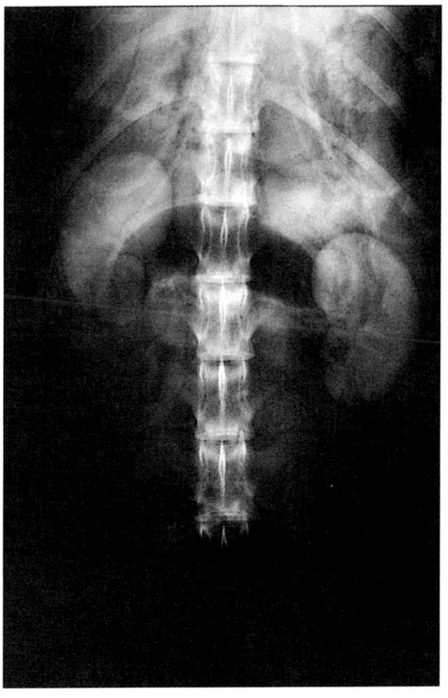

2.25 The radiograph made immediately after intravenous injection of contrast medium should result in good renal opacification, the nephrogram. Poor opacification should be interpreted as a sign of possible poor renal function and is an indication for biochemical renal function tests, if these have not already been performed. The nephrogram is examined for number of kidneys, renal position, size and shape and abnormal filling with contrast medium. If any apparent lucent areas are seen within the kidney(s), the plain radiographs should be examined to ensure that such lucency is not just due to overlying loops of gas-filled bowel.

2.26 Five minutes after administration of contrast medium, a ventrodorsal radiograph is made, centred again on the umbilicus. This should show the kidneys, renal pelves and at least the proximal ureters. The renal pelves often appear as small triangles (as illustrated) but fine, additional lines may sometimes be seen extending from the non-ureter corners of the triangle and retrograde filling of normal renal pelvic diverticula may also be observed. The author used to use compression of the caudal abdomen in the belief that this improved the radiographic evaluation of the renal pelves but no longer considers this to be necessary; with experience in interpretation, abdominal compression is not required. The ureters usually appear as broken lines. This is perfectly normal and is due to ureteral peristaltic waves which originate in the renal pelves. However, such peristalsis is often impaired in animals with ureteral disease (e.g. hydro-ureter). The five-minute radiograph, though useful for detecting renal pelvic abnormalities (dilation, abnormal masses such as calculi or tumours, pyelitis/pyelonephritis) and lesions of the ureters such as obstruction by calculi and tumours, hydro-ureter and rupture, is of little value in the diagnosis of ureteral ectopia (apart from demonstrating any associated hydro-ureter/hydronephrosis or pyelonephritis).

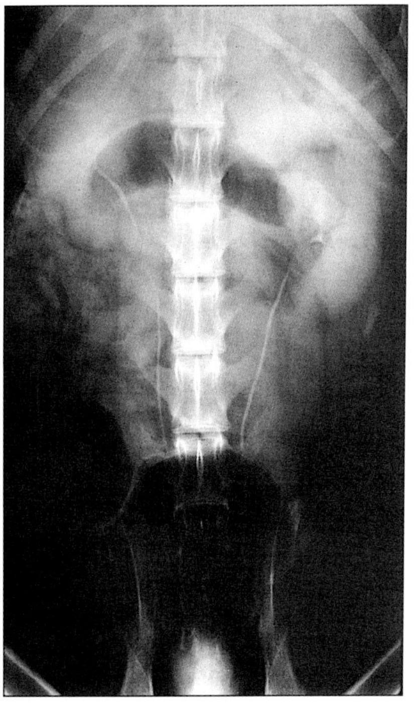

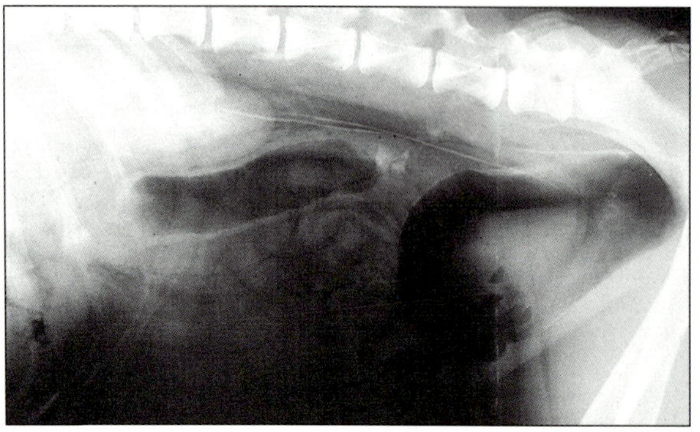

2.27 The animal is placed in right lateral recumbency and a lateral radiograph made, centred as in 2.20, 10 min after administration of contrast medium. As well as providing an alternative view of the kidneys, the distal ureters are now visible. If one is fortunate, the ureters will be seen to be emptying into the urinary bladder, as illustrated above. Although this is facilitated by the degree of contrast between the positive contrast-filled distal ureters and the air-filled bladder and also the fact that the colon and rectum are now empty of faeces, a certain amount of luck is also involved. Unless one happens to make an exposure just as a ureteral peristaltic wave propels urine through the distal ureter into the bladder, the termination of the ureter may be missed (e.g. **2.29**). The availability of radiographic screening facilities overcomes this problem; otherwise, several consecutive radiographs may have to be made before the terminations of the ureters are seen. In addition, if the bladder neck is intrapelvic, as in this bitch, it may be difficult to decide if the ureters are terminating beyond the bladder neck, hence the necessity for the next film.

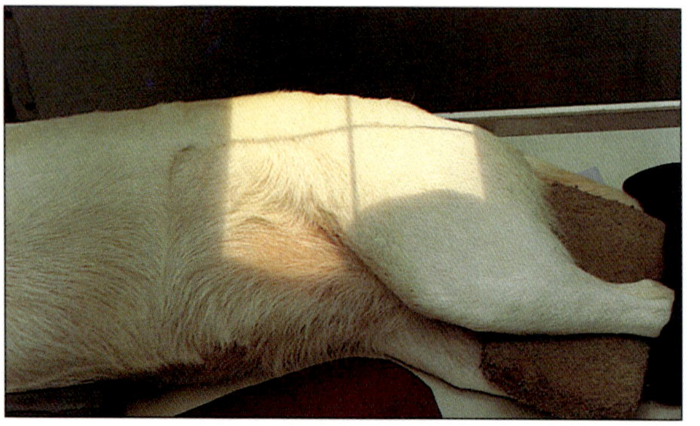

2.28 Fifteen minutes after administration of contrast medium, a right lateral radiograph is made, centred just cranial to the greater trochanter of the hip and ensuring that the perineum is included on the radiograph.

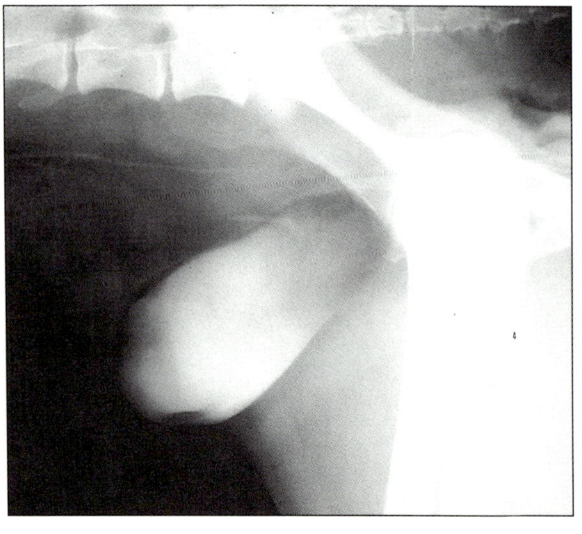

2.29 The fifteen-minute film is made mainly to examine for the location of the bladder neck and the presence of ureteral ectopia. In this animal (a different bitch from that illustrated in the previous IVU figures), one ureter can be seen to be emptying into the bladder but the termination of the other ureter is unclear. This is because the peristaltic wave in the uppermost ureter had not resulted in distal ureteral filling at the time the radiograph was made. This bitch appears to have a caudally positioned bladder neck but the pelvis is rotated and so the positioning is not truly lateral. The radiograph should be repeated with the animal positioned so that the hips are superimposed before bladder neck position is assessed. In this incontinent bitch, urine can be seen to have leaked into the vagina and vestibule but the cause of the leakage is not demonstrated on this radiograph and further investigations such as vagino-urethrography are indicated. Leakage of urine from the bladder may, however, suggest other abnormalities which require further investigations using retrograde techniques. For example, urine leaking into the urethra may demonstrate the presence of abnormal diverticula or outline radiolucent masses.

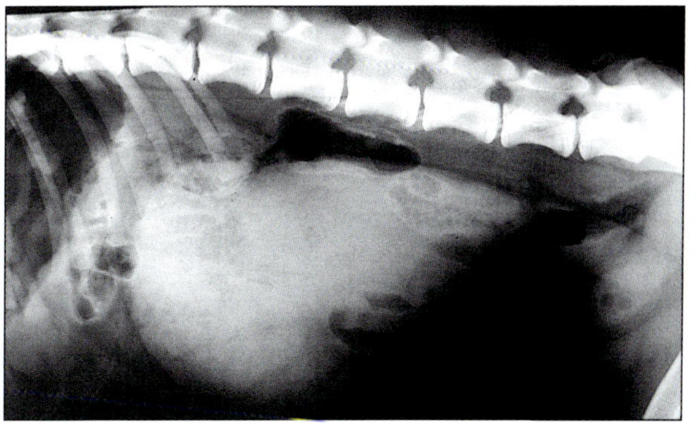

2.30 The above is usually sufficient in most animals but, in some cases, further radiographs will be required, some in different positions (e.g. oblique views). In this example, a radiograph has been made 24 hours after administration of contrast medium to show the grossly dilated ureter and kidney of the dog with hydro-ureter and hydronephrosis, illustrated previously (**2.4, 2.16, 2.17**). In such cases, poor renal excretion into a large volume of residual urine make the normal IVU timings inappropriate.

Problems

Adverse reactions to the contrast medium occur uncommonly but are described below.

In lightly anaesthetized or conscious animals, vomiting may occur immediately after administration of contrast medium. Although this is transient, it underlines the needs for adequate starvation of the animal prior to general anaesthesia, the use of an endotracheal tube during maintenance of anaesthesia and an adequate depth of anaesthesia (unless the patient is debilitated or sick).

Other adverse reactions to the contrast medium are anaphylaxis and acute renal shutdown.

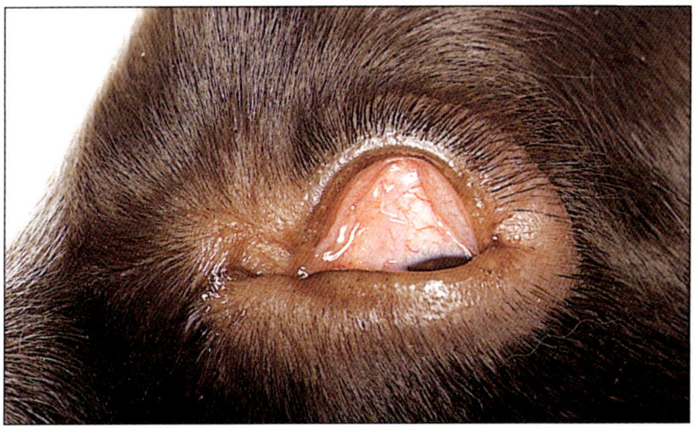

2.31 Anaphylactic reactions to contrast media can occur and were manifested in this Springer spaniel as acute palpebral oedema. Such reactions are obviously more serious if they are generalized, especially if lung oedema develops. Fortunately, they are extremely rare and if they do occur, they respond rapidly to intravenous hydrocortisone.

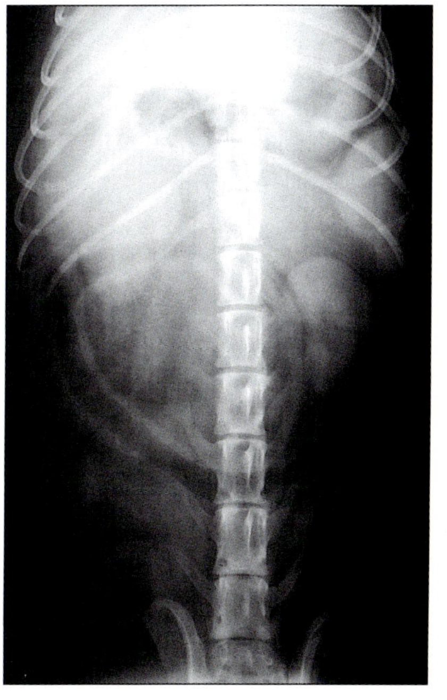

2.32 Acute renal shutdown is an unusual complication of IVU. Following administration of contrast medium, a nephrogram is obtained but the ureters fail to be opacified. The nephrogram persists with no evidence of further excretion; this is shown in the above radiograph of a Miniature poodle bitch made 20 minutes after administration of contrast medium. This condition is remedied by diuresing the animal using intravenous fluids (normal saline or glucose–saline) combined with intravenous frusemide (Lasix, Hoechst Animal Health). Recommencement of renal function, as judged by excretion of contrast medium into the renal pelves and ureters, begins usually within 15 minutes of this treatment. However, blood urea and creatinine levels are monitored over the next 24 hours to confirm that they are not elevated , or if they are that they return to normal.

Vagino-urethrography

Indications

- Vaginal abnormalities, particularly where these prevent physical examinations.
- Suspected urethral lesions.
- Dysuric female dogs and cats.

- Incontinent female dogs and cats.
- Assessment of urethral length and bladder neck position in bitches with suspected urethral sphincter mechanism incompetence.

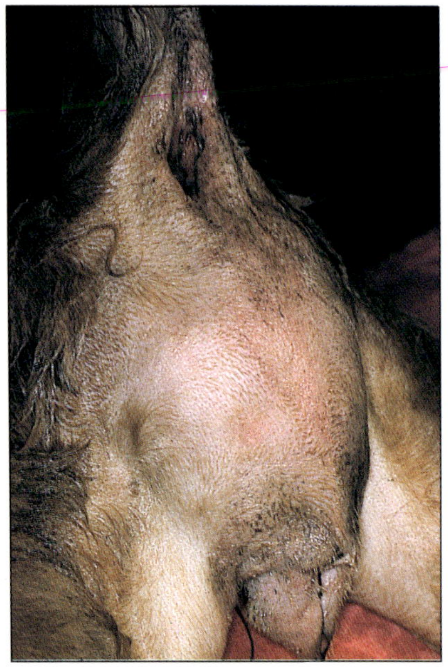

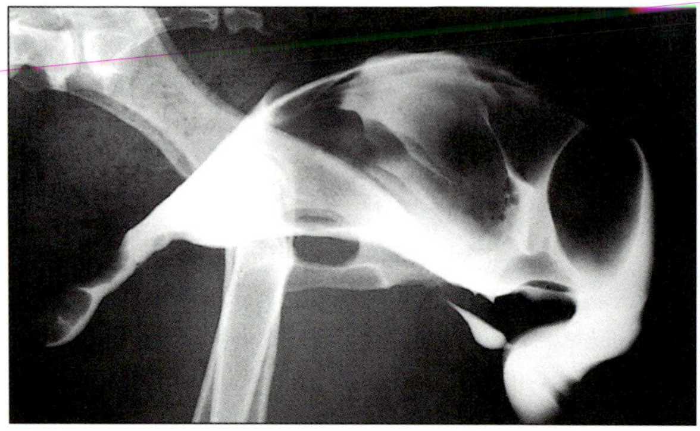

2.33 Extensive vaginal neoplasia in this bitch (left) prevented adequate digital or endoscopic examination. Vagino-urethrography **(above)** was used to determine the sites and extent of the tumours before surgical intervention. (See also **5.61.**)

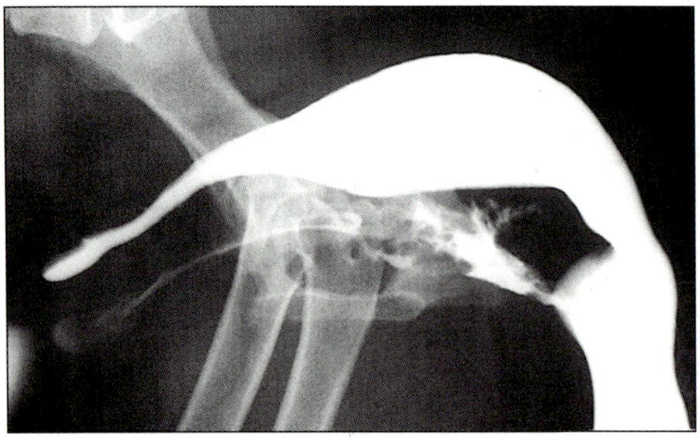

2.34 Vagino-urethrography demonstrated marked urethral irregularity in this dog with urethral malignancy. If urethrography had been performed, part of the lesion would have been obscured by the catheter used to introduce contrast medium.

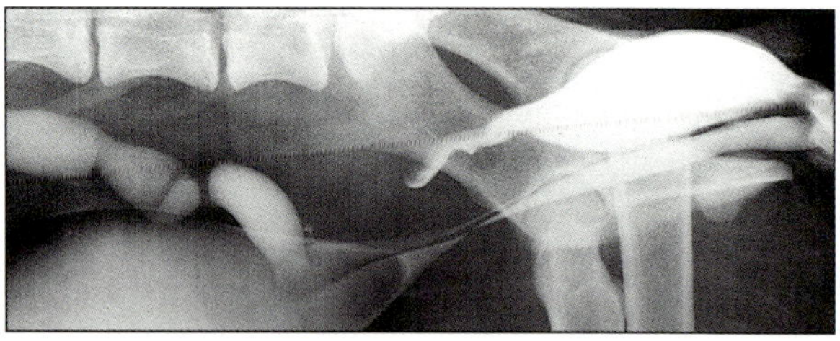

2.35 In this example, vagino-urethrography was used to demonstrate the termination of an ectopic ureter in the distal urethra. This might have been missed during urethrography if the urethral catheter cuff was obscuring the ureteral orifice. In addition, urethrography alone fails to demonstrate vaginal terminations of ectopic ureters. In incontinent bitches with a suspected diagnosis of urethral sphincter mechanism incompetence, vagino-urethrography is the preferred radiographic method of assessing urethral length and bladder neck position.

Technique

The patient should be prepared as described previously for an IVU and the bladder emptied of urine by catheterization or centesis. General anaesthesia is required for vagino-urethrography. The radiographic positioning is as illustrated in **2.28** and, as with any contrast radiographic technique, a plain film of the area should be made first. Air can be used as a contrast medium but water-soluble iodine-based positive contrast media (e.g. sodium and meglumine diatrizoate; Urografin '150', Schering) are preferable.

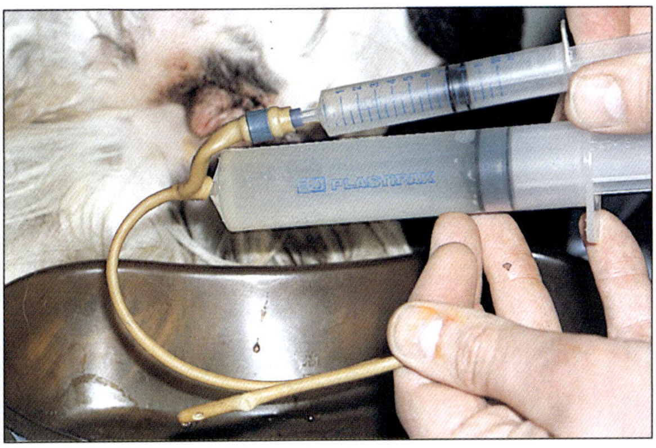

2.37 As with any retrograde radiographic contrast technique, the catheter should be filled with contrast medium before being inserted. If not, air bubbles may be introduced into the urethra and can be misdiagnosed as calculi or tumours. The Foley catheter is designed to take a wide-nozzle syringe or adaptor but this end of the catheter can be trimmed to allow a Luer syringe nozzle to be attached directly. Approximately 1 ml/kg body weight is required to fill the vagina to the point when the urethra begins to fill. This volume is larger in entire than spayed bitches and is less if the bitch is incontinent. It is also larger if the bitch is under the influence of endogenous or exogenous sex hormones, particularly oestrogens, and, in incontinent bitches, any oestrogen therapy should be discontinued for at least a month before vagino-urethrography. Unlike the situation in IVU, the contrast medium is seen undiluted on the radiograph and so a high iodine content is unnecessary. Solutions containing approximately 150 mg iodine equivalent per ml are suitable. The syringe is filled with a volume of contrast medium equivalent to 2 ml/kg body weight. The second syringe is used to inflate the Foley catheter cuff. An 8Fr catheter is suitable for cats and toy breeds of dog and 10–12Fr catheters for larger patients. In animals with short and/or narrow vaginas, especially cats, it is useful to remove the tip of the Foley catheter beyond the cuff to facilitate adequate insertion.

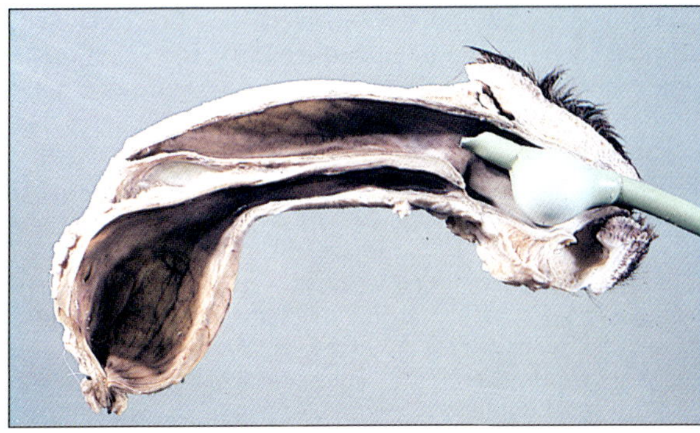

2.36 The principle of vagino-urethrography is that contrast medium is introduced into the vestibule, usually using a Foley catheter. Once the vagina is filled, contrast medium enters the urethra. The advantage of this technique over urethrography is that the whole length of the urethra is demonstrated without the presence of a catheter which might obscure or distort a lesion.

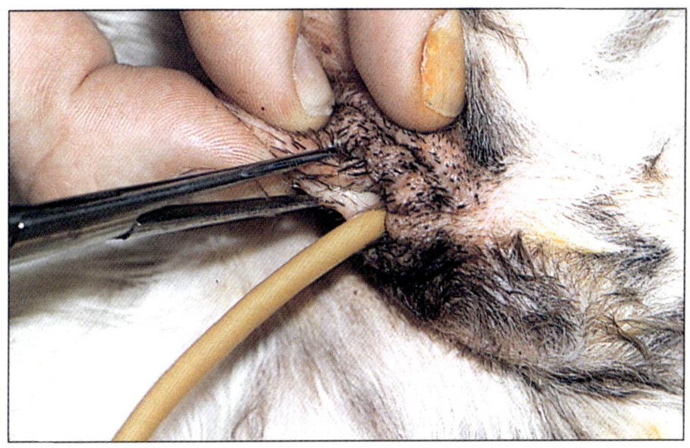

2.38 The Foley catheter cuffed tip is inserted into the vestibule and the cuff inflated. Very little air is required in the cuff of Foley catheters used in cats (0.5–1.0 ml) but the volume of air needed to inflate the cuff in dogs varies from 5 ml (5–15 kg dog) to 10 ml (15–40 kg dog). The cuff should be inflated sufficiently to prevent contrast medium escaping from the vagina, around the catheter. However, overinflation should be avoided to prevent the inflated cuff from obstructing the external urethral orifice, thus impeding flow of contrast medium. The vulva is then closed caudal to the inflated cuff to prevent the catheter leaving the vagina during filling (the inflated cuff alone is often insufficient to prevent this). The author uses two Allis tissue forceps in bitches and one in cats for this purpose. The first tissue forcep is placed just ventral to the catheter which is against the dorsal commisure of the vulval lips.

2.39 Once the second tissue forcep has been applied, contrast medium can be introduced into the vagina. The radiographic exposure is made during the injection of the last quarter of the calculated dose. If fluoroscopic screening facilities are available, the exposure is made once the urethra is adequately filled. If such facilities are not available, it is safest to inject 1 ml/kg and make an exposure during the last part of the injection. The resultant film can be examined and, if urethral filling has not occurred, may give an impression of how much more contrast medium is required. It is best to fill incrementally, exposing the film during each injection until adequate urethral filling is obtained. This is to avoid the possibility of damage to the lower urogenital tract due to overdistension or introduction of large volumes of contrast medium into ectopic ureters (in incontinent animals) with possible resultant renal pelvic damage.

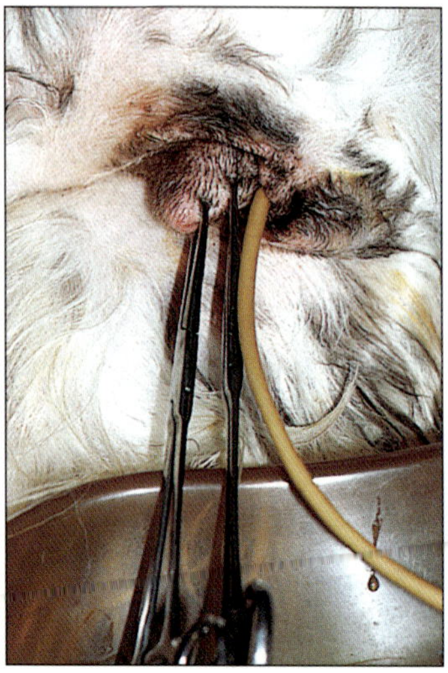

2.40 A vagino-urethrogram in a normal Standard poodle. There is often a narrowing at the junction between vestibule and vagina, just cranial to the external urethral orifice; but in approximately a quarter of bitches a stricture or perforate hymen may be detected at this site. The dorsal mid-line filling defects in the cranial vagina are normal and represent dorsal mid-line folds in the paracervical region. These are more prominent in entire bitches and in entire or neutered bitches under the influence of sex hormones, particularly oestrogens. They should not be confused with vaginal tumours. The urethra usually appears to be widest in its caudal quarter and sometimes urethral folds are delineated by the contrast medium as longitudinal striations.

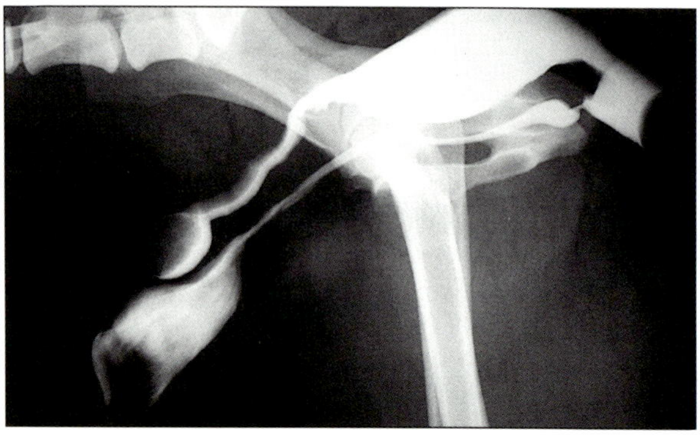

2.41 A normal feline vagino-urethrogram. Note the narrow, short vagina and the long urethra (compared to the bitch).

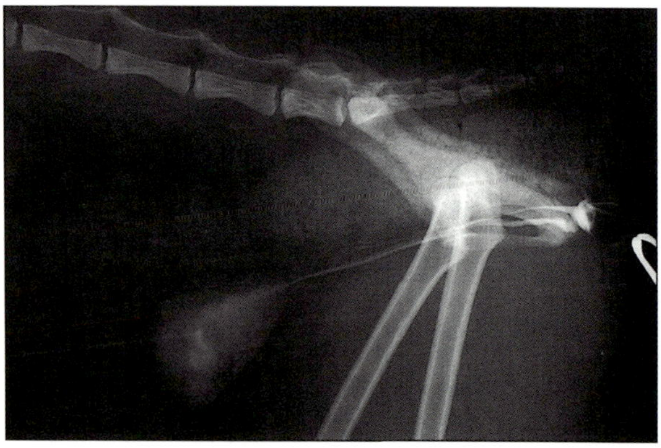

Problems

There are few problems associated with vagino-urethrography and most can be avoided using a correct technique. There is a theoretical risk of introducing vaginal and/or urethral organisms into the bladder. However, the author has used this technique on over 600 bitches, without the use of prophylactic antibiotics, and has not encountered the problem of urinary tract infection after vagino-urethrography. Vaginal rupture may occur if contrast medium cannot overflow from the vagina into the urethra but this is extremely rare.

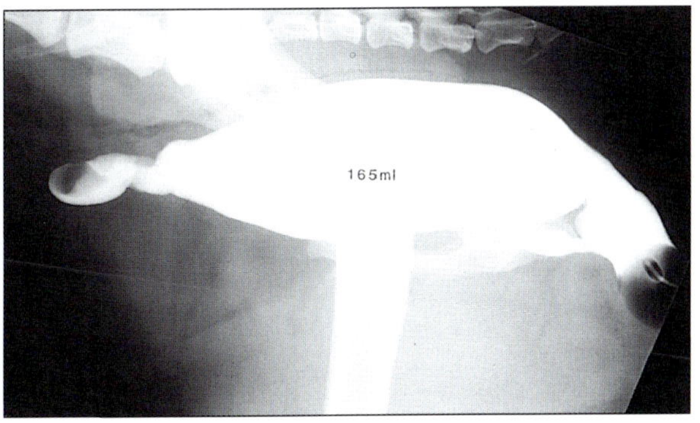

2.42 Vagino-urethrography should not be performed in bitches under the influence of endogenous or exogenous sex hormones. This is particularly true of incontinent bitches which are being treated with oestrogens. The vagina of such animals requires considerably more contrast medium to fill it. The results are that by the time the vagina is full enough for urethral filling to commence, the urethra is under pressure from the distended vagina: contrast medium cannot pass cranially down the urethra and urethral lesions may remain undetected. In addition, the abnormally distended intrapelvic vagina displaces the bladder cranially, making interpretation of bladder neck position inaccurate in bitches with suspected urethral sphincter mechanism incompetence. A distended rectum can have the same effect, underlining the need for the use of an enema before contrast radiography.

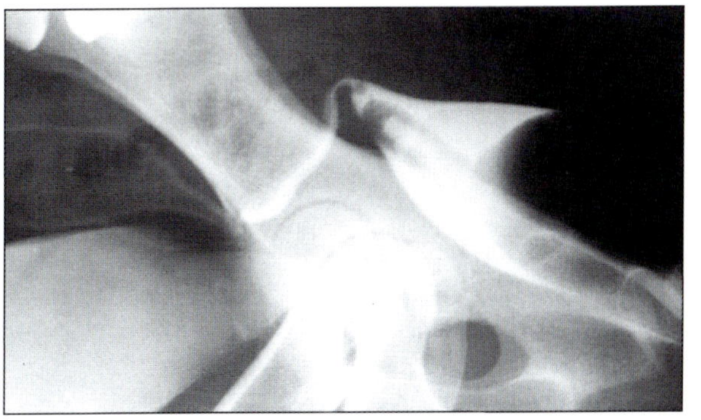

2.43 If vagino-urethrography is performed at the end of an IVU study, care should be taken not to misinterpret ureteral filling due to the IVU as that resulting from reflux of contrast medium introduced during vagino-urethrography. In this example, the distal ureter is overlying the contrast-filled cranial vagina; this may be misdiagnosed as a ureterovaginal fistula. However, apart from the fact that if such a fistula was present the distal ureter would be dilated, retrograde filling would result in denser filling of the ureter than filling due to the more diluted contrast medium of the IVU. In addition, care should be taken not to overfill the Foley catheter cuff or to insert the catheter too far into the vagina, as is the case in this illustration. The result is that the contrast medium is unable to overflow from the vagina into the urethra and thus, if sufficient contrast medium is introduced, iatrogenic vaginal rupture can occur.

2.44 It is important that the animal is adequately anaesthetized for vagino-urethrography. If it is not, contraction of the constrictor vestibuli muscles may occur, giving the appearance of a vestibulovaginal stricture, as illustrated.

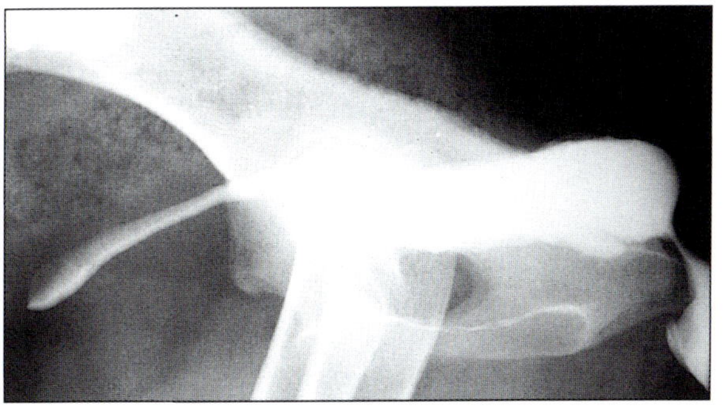

Urethrography

Indications

- Suspected urethral lesions in male dogs and cats.
- Suspected urethral lesions in female animals in which vagino-urethrography fails adequately to demonstrate the urethra.
- Dysuric animals.
- Incontinent animals.
- Animals with urethral discharges.
- Animals with suspected prostatic disease.

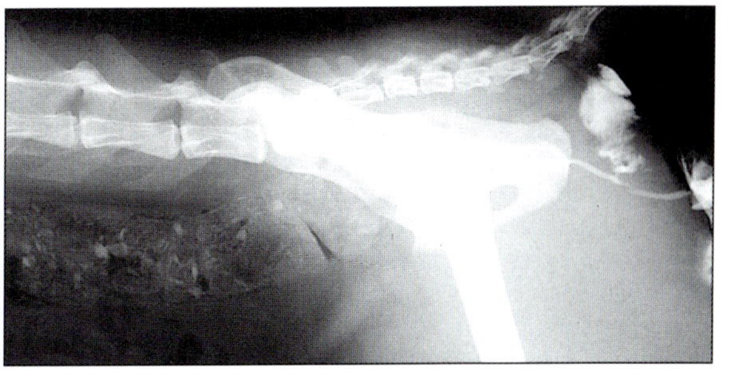

2.45 Urethral lesions are well defined by positive contrast retrograde urethrography. In this cat, the technique demonstrated accurately the site and extent of urethral rupture, essential information in deciding the best form of treatment.

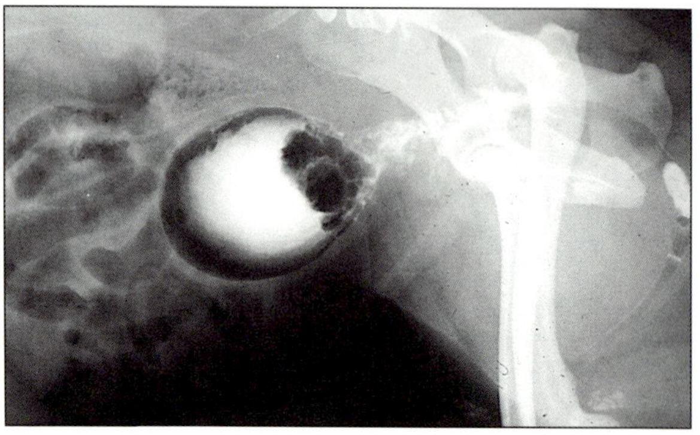

2.46 The additional time spent on contrast radiography is seldom wasted. In this dysuric Pug, a plain radiograph had demonstrated the ischial urethral calculus. This prevented the passage of a urethral catheter but a retrograde, double contrast urethrocystogram revealed that the prognosis was much worse than that associated with urolithiasis. In addition to the urethral calculus, this dog had a transitional cell carcinoma of the bladder neck extending into the pelvic urethra.

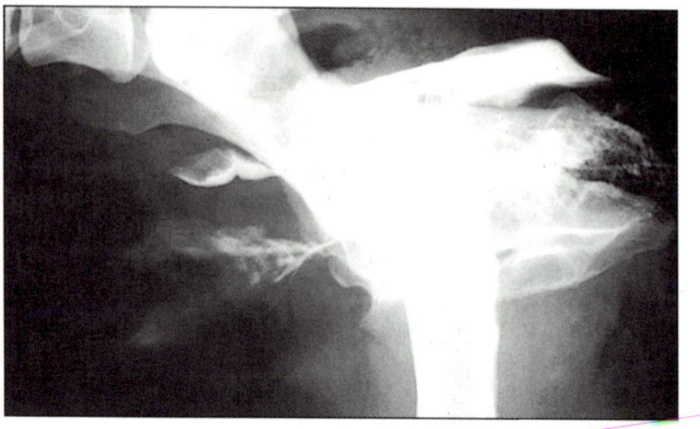

2.47 Urethrography performed in a dysuric bitch in which vagino-urethrography failed to outline the urethra (some contrast medium from the attempted vagino-urethrogram remains in the vagina). A destructive urethral carcinoma was present and became compressed by the vagina as contrast medium was introduced for vagino-urethrography, preventing urethral filling. The urethrogram demonstrates the destructive nature of the disease, although the caudal urethra is obscured by the catheter used to introduce contrast medium. In the presence of a less extensive lesion a biopsy may be required to differentiate neoplasia from urethritis (see Chapter 3), since both can have similar contrast radiographic appearances.

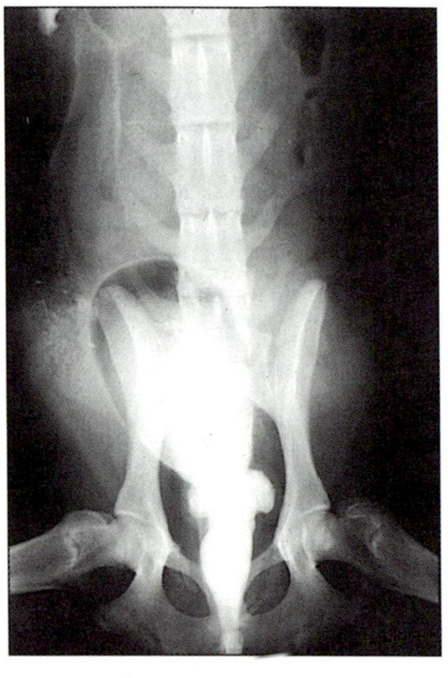

2.48 Urethrography is useful in incontinent male animals. In this example **(left)**, congenital prostatic urethral diverticula were demonstrated in an incontinent juvenile male Golden retriever. The *post mortem* appearance is shown in **(right)**.

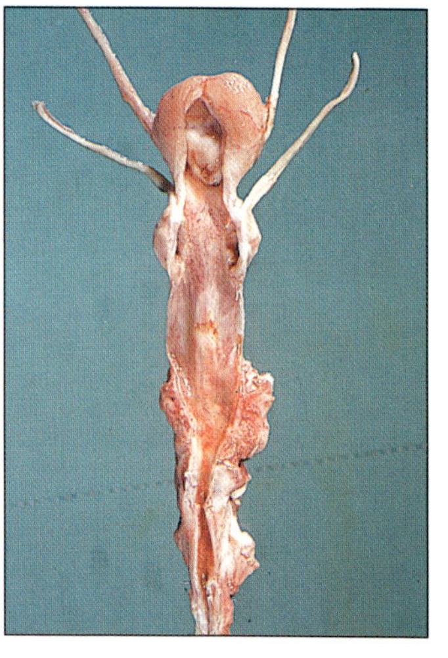

2.49 In prostatic disorders, urethrography is useful in demonstrating abnormalities of the prostatic urethra, abnormal cavities within the gland which communicate with the urethra (e.g. neoplasia, abscessation), and asymmetry of the gland. The urethra should bisect the gland on a lateral urethrogram. Asymmetry is indicative of possible neoplasia, abscessation or intraprostatic cysts. In this example, more prostatic soft-tissue density can be seen dorsal to the urethra than ventral to it, and the urethra can be seen to be stretched by the enlarged prostate gland. This Rottweiler had a large intraprostatic cyst. (See also **4.174.**)

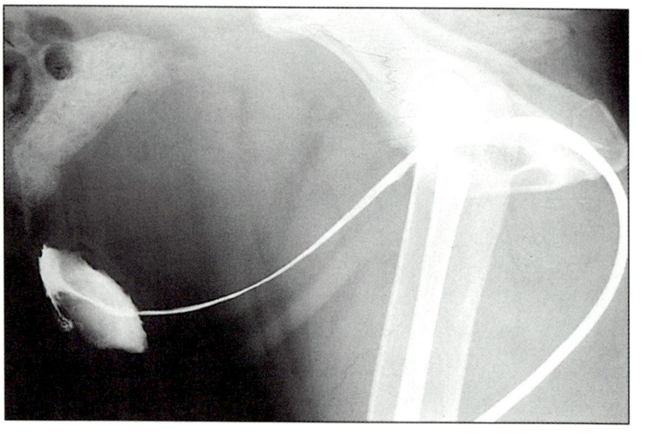

Techniques

The patient should be prepared as described above under 'Vagino-urethrography'. General anaesthesia is required for retrograde urethrography. The radiographic positioning is as illustrated in **2.28** but in male dogs an additional radiograph should be made centred over the penile/ischial urethra with the hind limbs flexed cranially (see **2.10**). As with any contrast radiographic technique, plain films of the area should be made first. Air can be used as a contrast medium but water-soluble, iodine-based positive contrast media (e.g. Urografin '150', Schering) are preferable.

The technique varies slightly between dogs and cats because of the small size of the feline urethra which does not allow the use of a Foley catheter.

If sufficient contrast medium is introduced, a urethrocystogram can be obtained (see also 'Cystography').

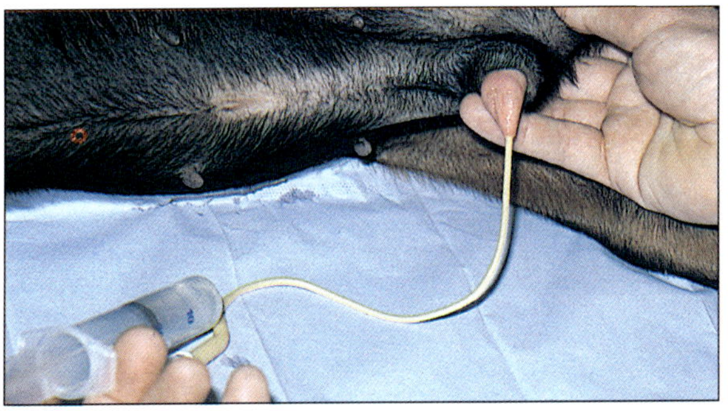

2.50 In male dogs, the tip of an 8Fr Foley catheter, which has been pre-filled with contrast medium, is inserted into the penile urethra. As in vagino-urethrography, the Foley catheter can be trimmed to allow direct insertion of the nozzle of a Luer fitting syringe. The volume of contrast medium which will be required varies from approximately 5 ml in toy dogs to 30 ml in giant breeds. The cuff of the catheter is inflated with air to prevent leakage of contrast medium from the distal urethra; approximately 1–3 ml of air is sufficient for dogs of 5–30 kg body weight.

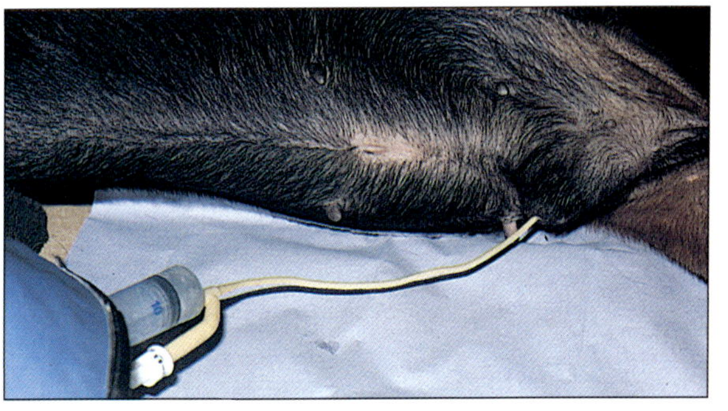

2.51 The dog is then positioned for radiography. For the pelvic and ischial urethra the position shown in **2.28** is suitable, but for suspected lesions of the penile urethra, the hind limbs should be flexed cranially, as illustrated in **2.10**, and the X-ray beam centred on the area of interest. As in vagino-urethrography, the radiograph should be made while the urethra is distended with contrast medium. This is accomplished by making the radiographic exposure as the last quarter of the estimated amount of medium is being introduced.

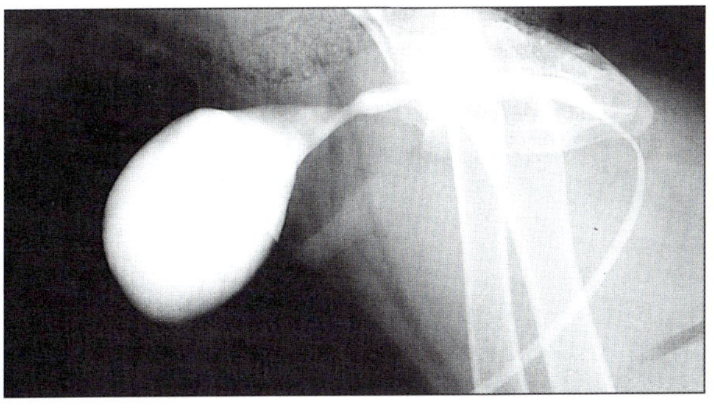

2.52 In the normal dog, the penile urethra is fairly uniform in outline and diameter but the urethra usually narrows as it passes round the ischial arch. The pelvic urethra is usually wider than the distal urethra but the appearance of the urethra as it passes through the prostate is variable: although its outline should be smooth, there is often some variation in the diameter and sometimes urethral folds can be seen as longitudinal striations in the contrast column.

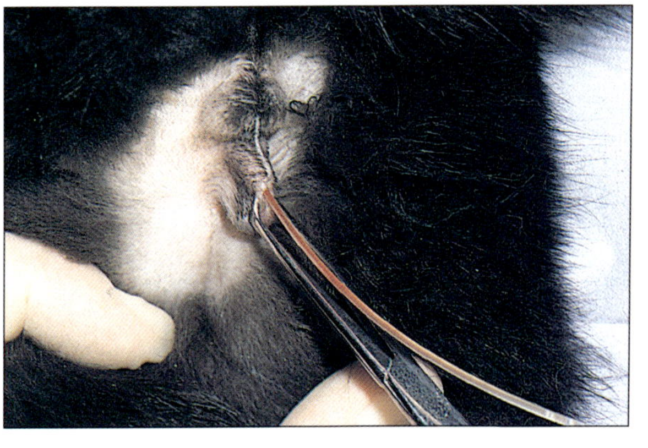

2.53 Urethrography in male cats is identical to that in dogs except that the small diameter of the urethra precludes the use of a Foley catheter. A 3 or 4Fr cat catheter is therefore inserted into the penile urethra. To prevent leakage but avoid the risk of penile trauma, the prepuce (not the penis) is occluded around the catheter using Allis tissue forceps.

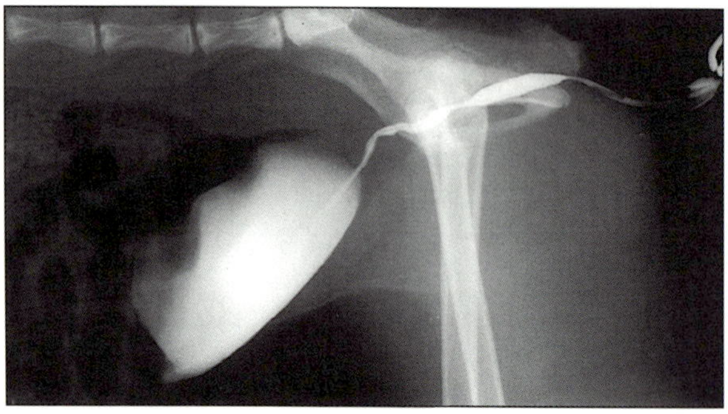

2.54 The urethrogram of a normal male cat. The penile urethra is much narrower than the membranous (pelvic) urethra.

Problems

The problem of air in the catheter being introduced with the contrast medium and air bubbles being misdiagnosed as tumours or urethral calculi have already been touched on in the preceding vagino-urethrography section.

Iatrogenic damage to the lower urinary tract is rare unless complete urethral obstruction is present or an excessive amount of contrast medium is used (see **2.59**). As with any retrograde technique, there is the potential for introducing organisms, in this case into the proximal urethra or bladder. In practice, the risk of this happening appears to be slight.

Cystography

Indications

- Location of bladder when not visible on plain radiographs.
- Suspected bladder lesions.
- Incontinent animals.
- Dysuric animals.
- Animals with haematuria.

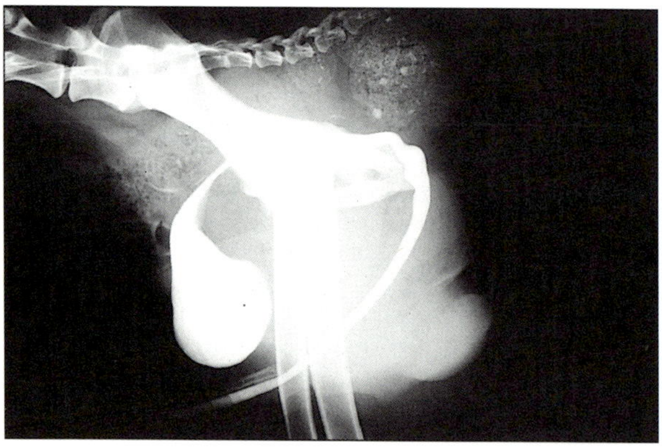

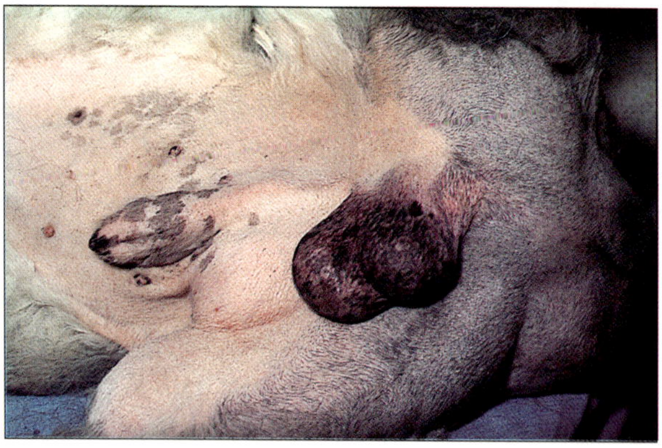

2.55 Retrograde positive contrast urethrocystography (top) in an Old English sheepdog with a bilateral perineal rupture and an inguinal hernia (bottom). The cystogram showed that the bladder, which was not visible on plain abdominal films, is in the inguinal hernia rather than the perineal rupture. In such cases, urethrocystography is preferable to cystography as, if the bladder is displaced, the urethra may be kinked and attempts to catheterize the bladder may result in iatrogenic urethral damage (see also Chapter 5).

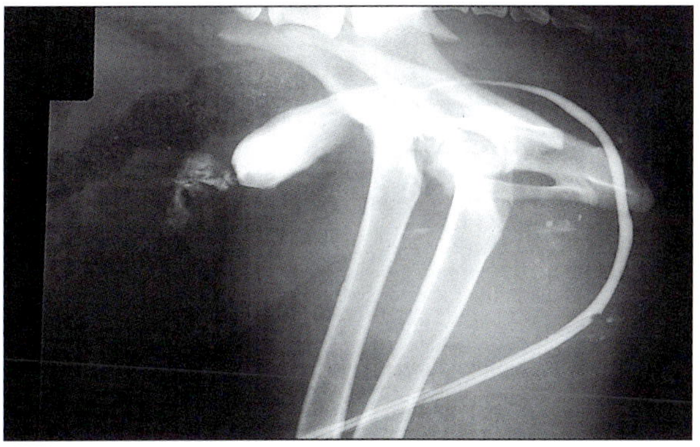

2.56 The site of bladder rupture demonstrated in a male Flat-coated retriever by retrograde positive contrast urethrocystography. (See also **3.21**). Urethrocystography is preferable to cystography alone in traumatized animals because of the possibility that the urethra may be damaged; passage of a catheter into the bladder and cystography alone would not demonstrate such damage.

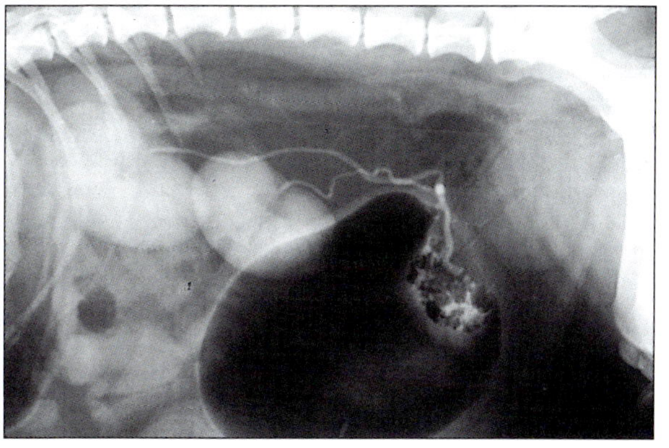

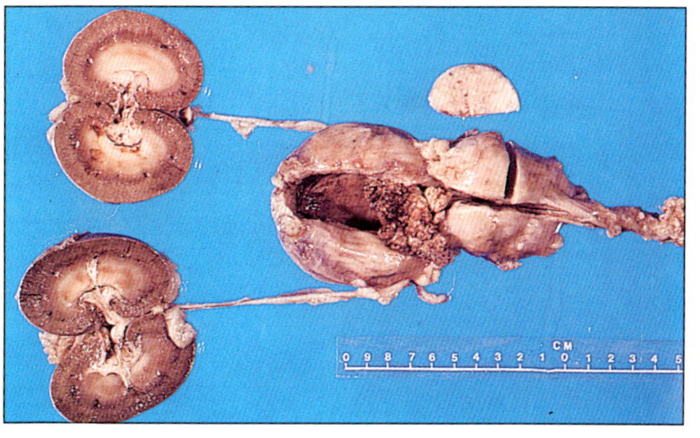

2.57 Transitional cell carcinoma of the bladder neck demonstrated by double contrast cystography in a corgi (top). An IVU was also performed to determine if there was any ureteral involvement in the neoplasia. The tumour retained positive contrast medium and was clearly outlined by the surrounding air. Although the tumour was close to the trigone, there was no evidence that the ureters or adjacent bladder wall were involved in the neoplasia, an important pre-operative consideration. Euthanasia was carried out and the post mortem appearance of the tumour can be seen **(bottom).** (This dog had an enlarged prostate due to castration and excessive treatment with oestrogens, leading to squamous metaplasia of the gland.)

Techniques

Negative, positive and double contrast techniques are applicable to the urinary bladder. Plain radiographs should be made first. It may be necessary to compare these with the cystogram(s) but, in addition, the contrast medium may obscure abnormalities such as calculi, which are usually best seen in plain radiographs.

Negative contrast medium is usually air, although other gases such as carbon dioxide can be used. In the author's experience, negative contrast cystography is of little value apart from improving radiographic contrast during IVU and demonstrating gross bladder lesions or bladder position. It is unsuitable for assessing the position of the bladder in bitches with suspected urethral sphincter mechanism incompetence as the air-filled urinary bladder tends to 'float' and, on lateral projections, often appears to be located further cranially than it actually is. This can be misleading if one is trying to determine if the bladder neck is intrapelvic or not. Negative contrast cystography is a poor technique for demonstrating subtle bladder urothelial abnormalities.

Positive contrast cystography (with the same contrast media as used in vagino-urethrography and urethrography) can demonstrate bladder ruptures and diverticula but may obscure other abnormalities such as urothelial tumours or vesical calculi.

In the author's view, the best technique is to perform retrograde positive contrast urethrography (or vagino-urethrography in female animals) and then to catheterize and empty the bladder of most of the positive contrast medium which has been introduced. The bladder is then filled with air via the same catheter to obtain a double contrast cystogram. This has the advantage that no lesions are obscured by positive contrast medium but this contrast medium adheres to bladder urothelial abnormalities and radiolucent calculi which can then be seen clearly against the surrounding negative contrast medium.

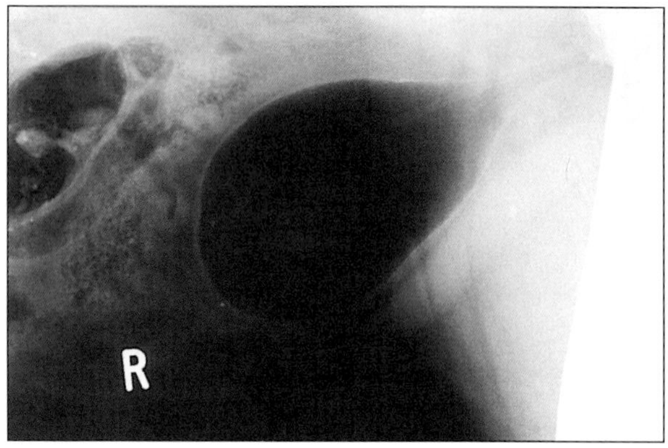

2.58 A normal double contrast cystogram. Most of the positive contrast medium which entered the bladder during urethrography has been removed (it is almost impossible to remove all of it). The bladder has then been filled with air. The volume required varies considerably and it is difficult and inadvisable to give 'dose rates'. Bladder volume varies between animals of different and even the same sizes and the volume required adequately to fill the bladder but not leading to iatrogenic bladder rupture and/or vesico-ureteral reflux has yet to be determined. The bladder should be palpated during filling and filled until it begins to feel turgid. It is best to err on the side of caution, make a radiograph and introduce more contrast medium if required. Contrast medium can be introduced via polyurethane catheters or, in bitches, using the softer Foley catheters (see 'Catheterization', Chapter 3). However, the cuff of the Foley catheter should not be inflated. The inflated cuff may obscure bladder neck lesions and make interpretation difficult. In addition, it may obstruct the ureteral orifices if overinflated and will also prevent air leaking from the bladder around the catheter. Although in some instances (e.g. the bitch with poor urethral sphincter tone) inflation of the Foley catheter cuff may be useful in allowing adequate inflation of the bladder, it also increases the risk of iatrogenic bladder rupture.

Problems

Rarely, pneumocystography has been associated with fatal air embolism; this is more likely if bladder wall damage is present. Other problems are iatrogenic bladder rupture or/and vesico-ureteral reflux and misdiagnoses of vesical calculi or bladder wall thickening when neither are present. The latter is most likely if the bladder is inadequately filled with contrast medium or if residual urine is present during pneumocystography.

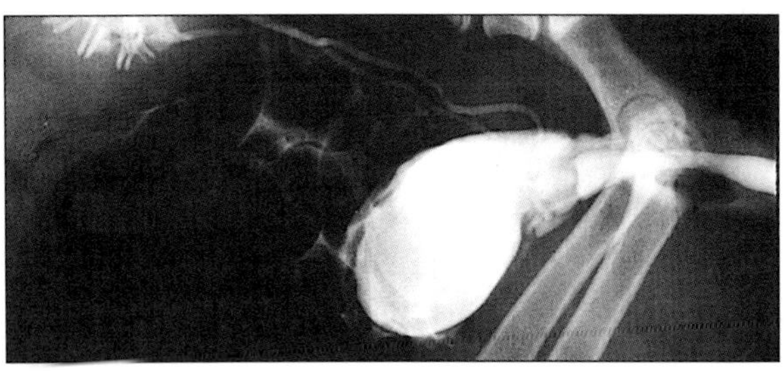

2.59 Iatrogenic bladder rupture and vesico-ureteral reflux in a West Highland White terrier puppy during retrograde positive contrast urethrocystography. Unknown to the author, this dog had bladder hypoplasia and a relatively small amount of contrast medium was required to cause the damage illustrated. This type of bladder rupture usually takes the form of several urothelial slits through which contrast medium finds its way into the peritoneal cavity: it is difficult to find the defects in the detrusor muscle through which the contrast medium has leaked and these do not usually overlie the urothelial slits. Obviously, prevention by careful cystography is best but, if iatrogenic rupture does occur, it can be treated by using an in-dwelling vesical catheter for 7–10 days until the bladder has healed.

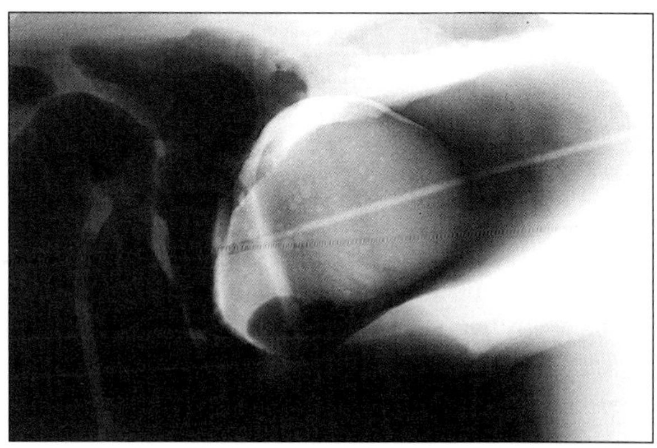

2.60 'Cerate' calculi in a dog, demonstrated by double contrast cystography. These are the result of the previous insertion of a cattle intramammary preparation into the bladder. The same artefacts can be generated by using oil-based lubricants on the urinary catheter used to introduce the contrast medium.

3 Other Diagnostic Aids

In this chapter, other aids to diagnosis in small animals with suspected urological abnormalities are presented. These include ultrasonography, urethral catheterization, fluid collection and examination, biopsy techniques, blood and urine analyses and urodynamics.

Ultrasonography

Ultrasonography has revolutionized the diagnosis of urological disorders. It is the perfect partner to good radiography as the contrast of ultrasound pictures is often best at times when radiographic contrast is reduced, for example in the presence of fluid. It is particularly useful in demonstrating abnormalities of the internal architecture of soft tissue organs and in the diagnosis and localization of collections of fluid within viscera. In the author's experience, it is especially helpful in the differentiation of prostatic disorders. This is particularly true of prostatic cysts and abscesses. Ultrasonography allows accurate localization of a lesion so that meaningful (ultrasound-guided) biopsy (e.g. **3.25**) or fluid samples can be obtained.

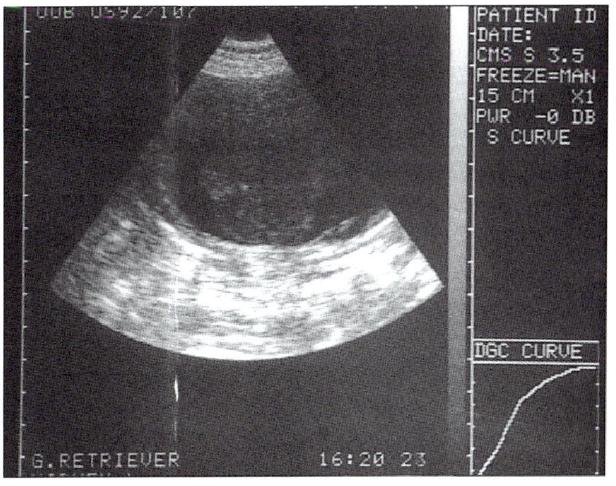

3.1 Renal tumour (embryonal nephroma; see also 4.1) demonstrated ultrasonographically in an adult Golden retriever bitch. The tumour was obstructing the renal pelvis, resulting in hydronephrosis. The accummulation of urine in the renal pelvis improves the ultrasonographic contrast, enhancing demonstration of the hilar mass.

Indications

- Any suspected abnormalities of urinary tract viscera suggested by clinical or/and radiographic investigations.

Techniques

Ultrasonographic practice and interpretation requires considerable expertise, based on experience. The would-be veterinary ultrasonographer is referred to the excellent book on the subject by Frances Barr (1990) and the descriptions which follow are merely overviews of the use of ultrasonography in the urinary tract.

In the urinary tract, real-time B mode ultrasonography is most commonly employed to examine the internal structure of the kidneys, bladder and prostate. The patient preparation is the same for all organs and involves clipping of the coat from the area to be scanned, cleaning the skin with surgical spirit to remove dirt and grease, and application of liberal quantities of commercial acoustic gel to ensure good contact between the skin and transducer.

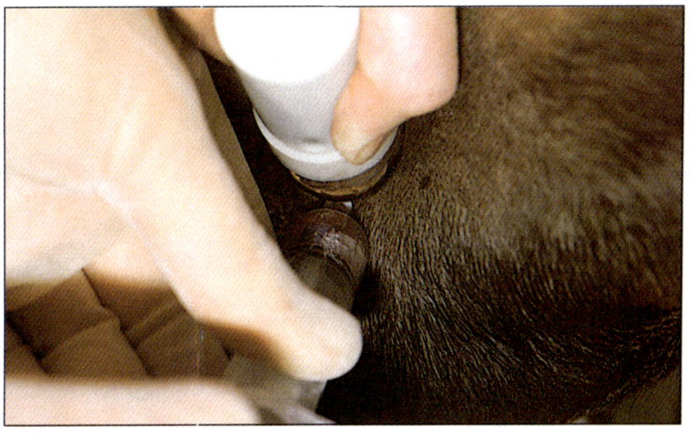

3.2 Ultrasound-guided centesis of the prostate. Ultrasonography allows needles to be inserted accurately into small intraprostatic cysts and abscesses for drainage of fluid for cytology, bacteriology, etc. It can also be used to guide biopsy needles into urinary tract organs and to ensure that the region to be biopsied is not fluid-filled (e.g. an abscess), thus reducing the risk of peritonitis.

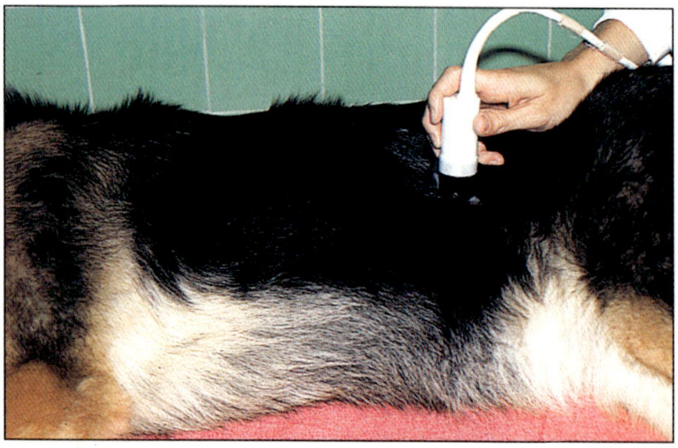

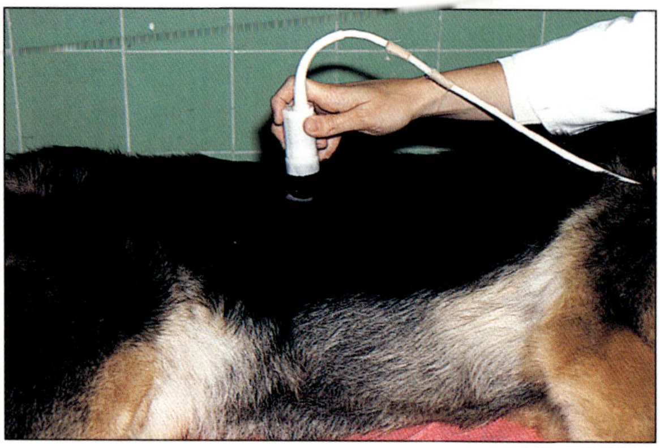

3.3 The kidneys are usually imaged from the flanks. (top) The site for the left kidney is just caudal to the last rib, ventral to the sublumbar muscles (cranial is to the left in this illustration).**(bottom)** The right kidney is further cranial and so is imaged between the last two or three ribs on the right (cranial is to the right in this illustration). However, the presence of the ribs means that acoustic shadows due to the ribs may be cast on the renal image, preventing the whole kidney from being imaged at once.

The urinary bladder and prostate are imaged from a prepubic (in the case of male dogs, parapenile) site, as used in the dog shown in **3.2**. Rectal ultrasonography of the prostate is possible in large dogs but requires a transducer specifically designed for rectal work.

Problems

There are few problems associated with ultrasonography apart from those encountered in technique and interpretation due to inexperience. The presence of the ribs can lead to difficulties imaging the right kidney and similar problems are encountered if gas-filled bowel is interspaced between the transducer and the organ being imaged.

Urethral catheterization

Indications

- To obtain urine samples for laboratory analysis.
- To relieve dysuria.
- To provide urinary by-pass (e.g. urethral injuries) or drainage (e.g. bladder paralysis).
- To detect urethral obstruction (inaccurate).
- To introduce contrast media into the urinary tract.

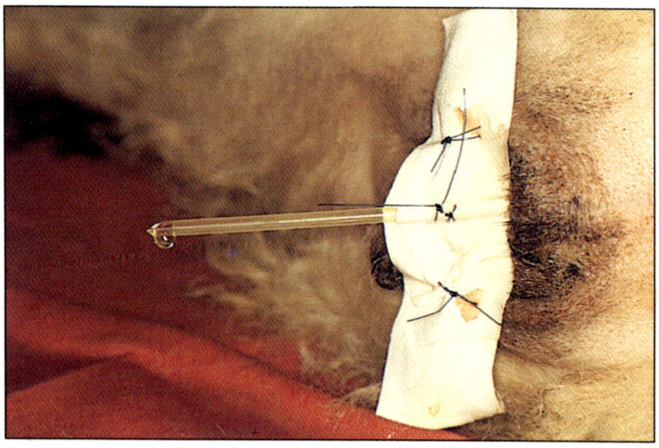

3.4 A catheter can be used to relieve dysuria temporarily, allowing the animal to recover from the systemic effects of urinary obstruction before the cause is treated. Although passage of a urethral catheter is suitable in cases of neurogenic dysuria or partial obstruction by soft tissue masses, it should be performed with care in cases of suspected urolithiasis. Attempts forcibly to pass a catheter in such cases are likely to result in iatrogenic urethral trauma (see **3.15**). Soft Foley catheters are usually unsuitable (they may be difficult to pass in animals with urethral narrowing, are too large for cats and are rarely long enough for male dogs). Foley catheters can be used in bitches without urethral obstruction (see **3.5**), but in most other animals polyurethane catheters are required for relieving dysuria. Once the bladder has been drained the catheter can be sutured *in situ* and maintained as an in-dwelling catheter until the animal is fit for elective surgery if this is necessary to treat the cause of the dysuria. In dogs, the catheter can be fixed to the perivulval (in bitches, as illustrated) or cranial preputial (in male dogs) skin using a butterfly made from adhesive tape.

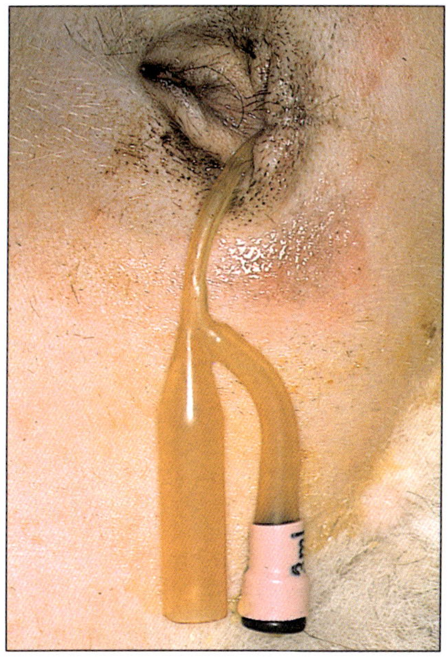

3.5 In bitches, a Foley catheter can be used as an in-dwelling catheter, provided it can be passed along the urethra. If this is not possible, a prepubic Foley catheter can be used for urinary bypass (see **4.140**). Any urine obtained should be submitted for laboratory analysis. Urine samples are useful in the differential diagnosis of the cause of dysuria (e.g. cytology in the case of suspected malignancy) and urinary tract infections are common in animals with urinary retention. However, because of the potential for introduction of urethral organisms into the bladder (and thus the urine sample), low bacterial counts in catheterized urine samples are probably insignificant and should be ignored. Ideally, in-dwelling catheters should be connected to closed urine collecting systems. Whereas this is possible in recumbent (e.g. **3.21**) or paraplegic patients using, for example, sterile intravenous drip tubing and bags, it may be impracticable in ambulatory patients and the system may have to be left open. In the author's experience, significant urinary tract infections in animals with such open systems are remarkably uncommon, although he routinely uses prophylactic antibiotics in such cases. There is some argument about the use of prophylactic antibiotics. Some authors are concerned that these may lead to proliferation of resistant organisms but this has not been the author's experience. Bacteriological cultures of urine are recommended following catheter removal.

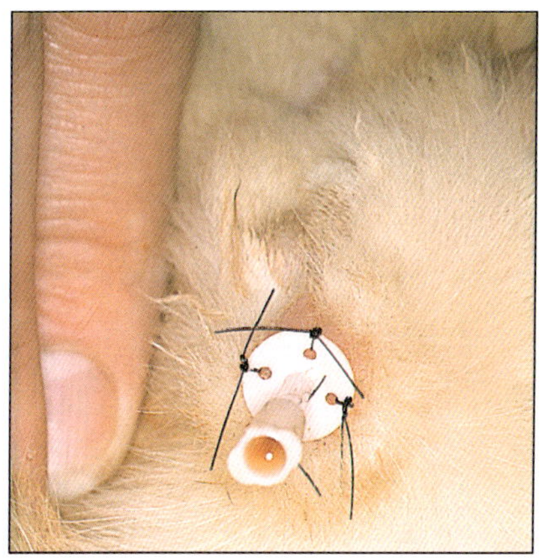

3.6 In dysuric cats, the Jackson's catheter is designed for use as an in-dwelling catheter. Once the catheter has been inserted, it is sutured to the prepuce using the holes in the catheter flange. An Elizabethan collar should be fitted to the cat as many felines are able to detach the catheter from the flange and remove it.

Techniques

The technique varies between the sexes and between dogs and cats. Most dogs can be catheterized without chemical restraint but cats, especially males, usually require sedation or anaesthesia.

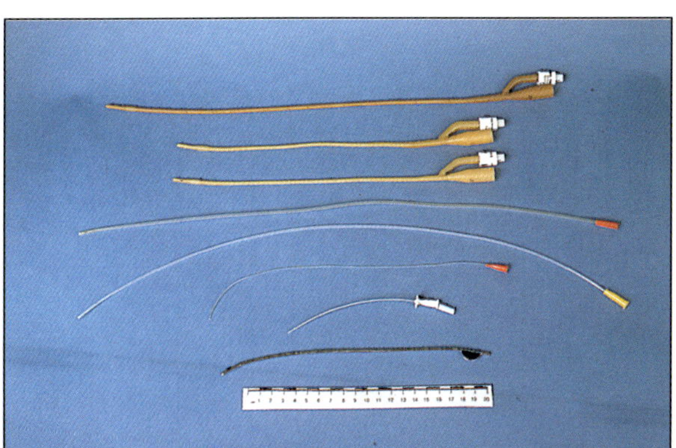

3.7 A variety of catheters are available for urethral catheterization of small animals. In general, polyurethane catheters are suitable for use in both sexes of dogs and cats. Foley catheters may be employed in bitches (but may be difficult to introduce). The catheters illustrated are, with one exception, suitable for most urological situations in small animals. These are, from top to bottom: 12Fr, 10Fr and 8Fr Foley catheters – the 12Fr and 10Fr sizes are suitable for introducing contrast medium during vagino-urethrography in medium to large bitches, the 10Fr and 8Fr sizes can be used for canine urethral catheterization and urethrography (the 10Fr in large bitches) and the 8Fr Foley catheter is suitable for vagino-urethrography in cats and toy breeds of dog. 8Fr and 6Fr polyurethane catheters – suitable for urethral catheterization in large and medium-sized male and female dogs. 3Fr and 4Fr polyurethane catheters – suitable for catheterization of small dogs (the longer catheter) and cats. The lower of the two catheters is a Jackson's catheter designed for use as an in-dwelling catheter in cats. A metal bitch catheter – metal catheters are more likely to traumatize the urethra and/or bladder and in the author's opinion should not be used.

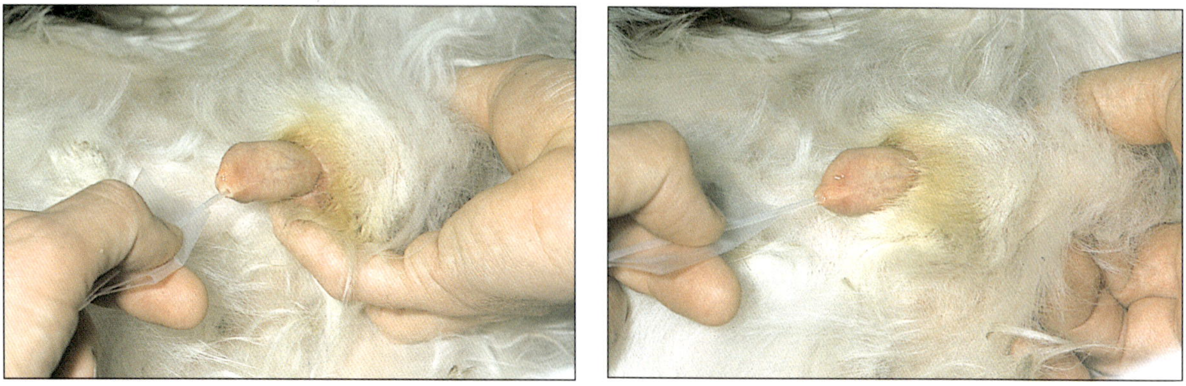

3.8 In male dogs, the caudal os penis is grasped with one hand and the other hand used to retract the prepuce caudally, exposing the glans penis. One of the fingers of the hand holding the penis (the little finger, in this case) is looped dorsal to the retracted prepuce and used to keep the glans exposed whilst the catheter is inserted **(left)**. Catheters should be lubricated with water-soluble jelly (e.g. K-Y Lubricating Jelly, Johnson and Johnson) and inserted into the urethra under aseptic conditions. The use of oil-based lubricants is inadvisable, particularly if contrast radiography is to be performed (see **2.60**). The catheter should be handled through its sterile polythene bag (as illustrated) or a sterile surgical glove should be worn on the hand used to insert the catheter. Once the catheter has been inserted to the level of the caudal os penis, the grip of the hand holding the penis is relaxed slightly during further passage of the catheter (this hand may be kinking the urethra, making catheter passage more difficult), as shown in **(right)**. Passage of the catheter is discontinued as soon as the catheter tip enters the bladder and urine appears at the catheter hub.

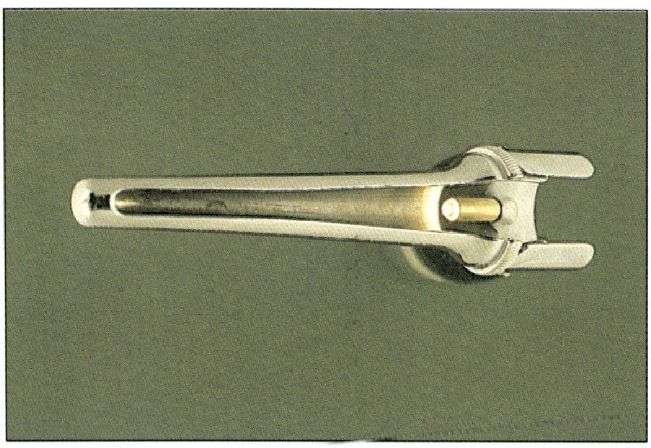

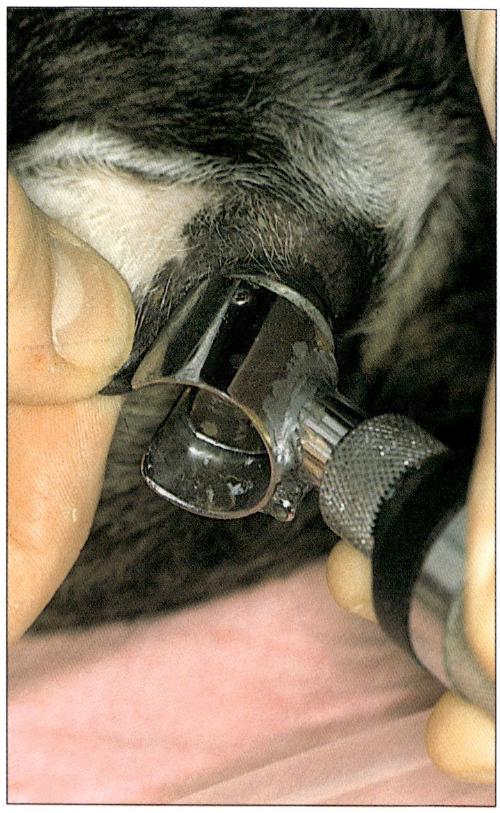

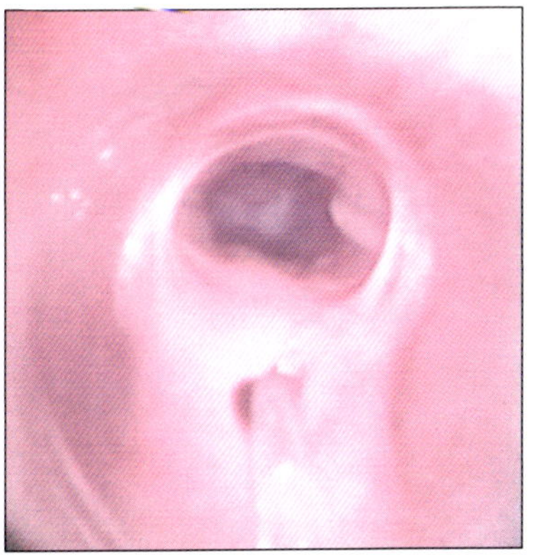

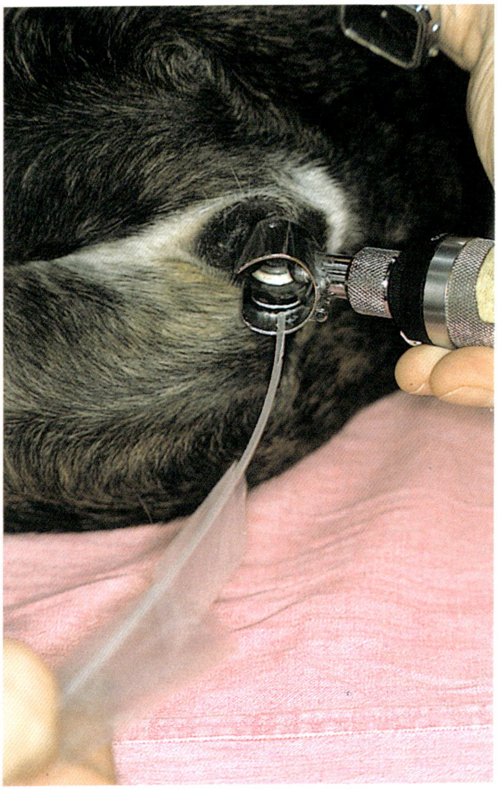

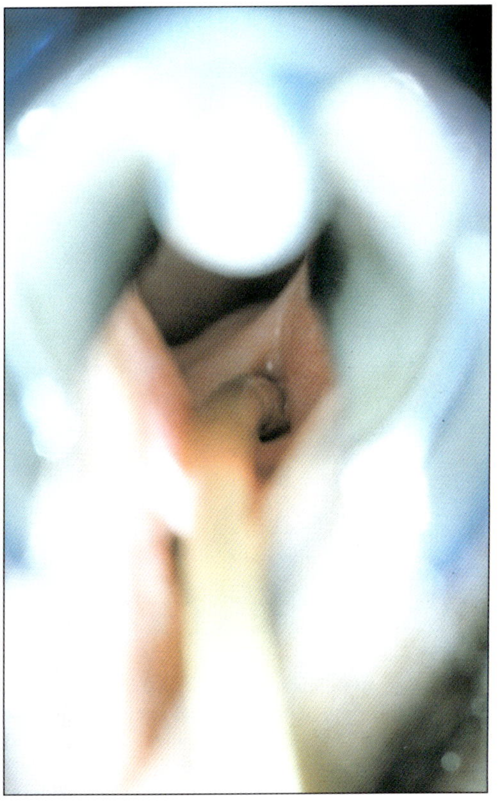

3.9 A variety of vaginal specula are available to facilitate passage of a urinary catheter in bitches (e.g. Kilians, Sims and McIntyre specula). The speculum viewed from above in **(lower left, page 36)** is designed with an open slit which is apposed to the vaginal floor. The speculum is inserted into the vagina, slit side ventrally as shown in **(lower right, page 36)** (taking care to avoid the clitoral fossa), and the raised external urethral orifice identified on the floor of the cranial vestibule, at its junction with the vagina. This can be seen in the endoscopic view **(top),** in which a catheter has been placed into the urethra, cranial to which the vaginal opening can be seen through the vestibulovaginal junction. The bitch can be positioned in dorsal or lateral recumbency for catheterization. If the dorsal recumbent position is used, the hind limbs should be flexed; if difficulty is encountered in locating the external urethral orifice with the bitch in this position, catheterization in right lateral recumbency (if one is right-handed; left lateral recumbency if left-handed) should be attempted as this is frequently easier. Location of the external urethral orifice and passage of the catheter is often facilitated if an assistant pulls the ventral vulva caudally **(lower right, page 36)**. This has the effect of flattening the vestibular floor which is advantageous, – particularly if there are vestibular and vaginal mucosal folds (these are more pronounced in some breeds – e.g. bulldogs – or in bitches under the influence of endogenous or exogenous sex hormones). The catheter is then inserted into the urethra aseptically **(left)** and advanced until urine just begins to flow. The view through the speculum of the catheterized external urethral orifice is shown in **(right)**.

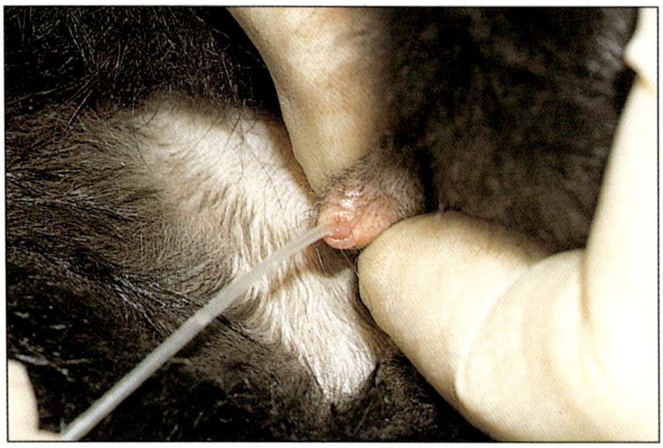

3.10 In male cats, the thumb and index finger of the left hand (if one is right-handed) are used to push the prepuce cranially and expose the glans penis. The catheter tip is inserted into the penile urethra. Further attempts at passage at this stage are inadvisable; the left-hand fingers almost invariable kink the urethra, making further passage difficult and increasing the risk of iatrogenic urethral trauma.

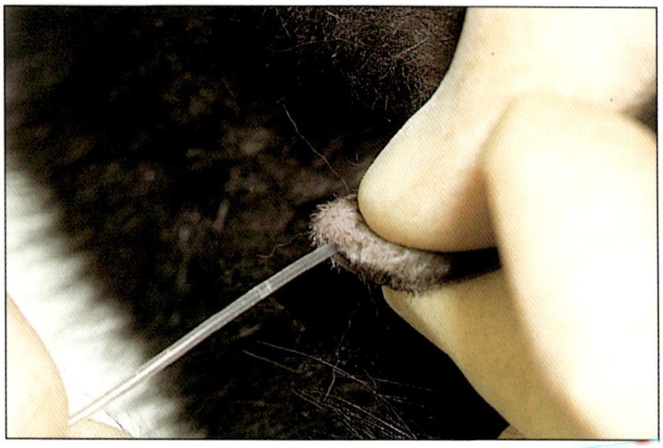

3.11 Further passage of the catheter is accomplished by gripping the prepuce with the left hand and pulling it caudally. This has the effect of aligning the penile and membranous urethrae and usually the catheter can now be passed without difficulty.

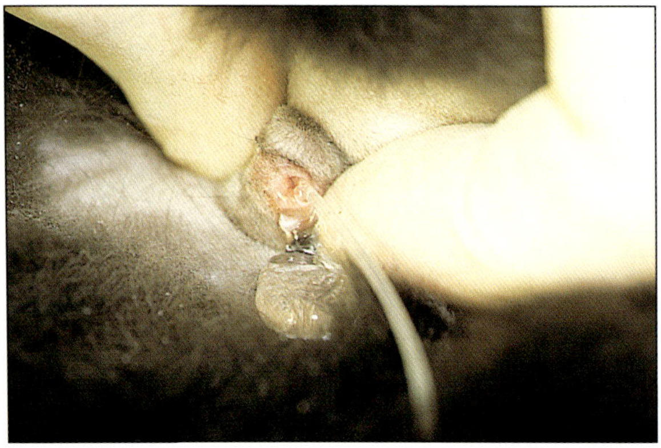

3.12 In obstructed male cats, urinary catheters are not suitable for flushing calculus material from the penile urethra. It is not usually possible to introduce the catheter so that both side holes are within the penile urethra. Thus, any flushing liquids merely pass out of the catheter side hole outside the urethra, as illustrated, and fail to dislodge calculus material.

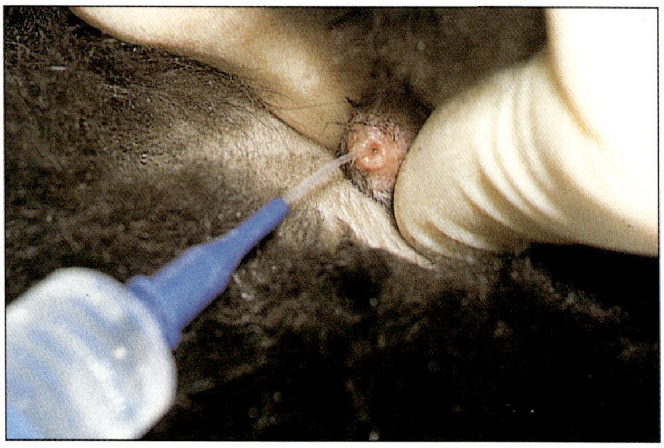

3.13 Initially, it is better to use a lacrymal cannula to flush the obstructed feline penile urethra. Before doing so, however, it is important that the bladder is emptied of urine by cystocentesis (see below). As well as being part of the pre-operative management of obstructed animals, this will ensure that the flushing fluids are not working against a high intravesical pressure. Once the penile urethra has been cleared, a cat catheter can then be passed, used to flush remaining calculi from the membranous urethra and maintained as an in-dwelling catheter to allow the animal to recover from the effects of the obstruction and to introduce calculus dissolution or flushing fluids into the bladder. In the author's view, it is the flushing itself which dislodges the calculus material from the urethra rather than any dissolution by the flushing solution. He therefore prefers to use sterile normal saline to other proprietary solutions such as Walpole's solution which may irritate an already-inflamed urethra and worsen urethritis.

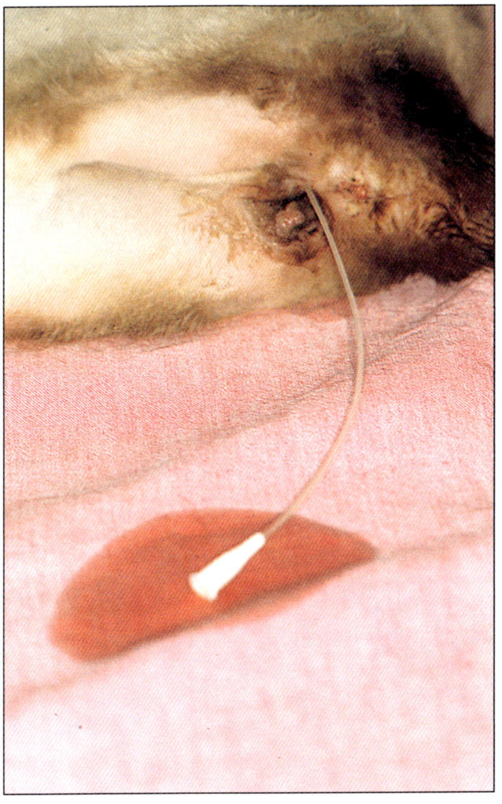

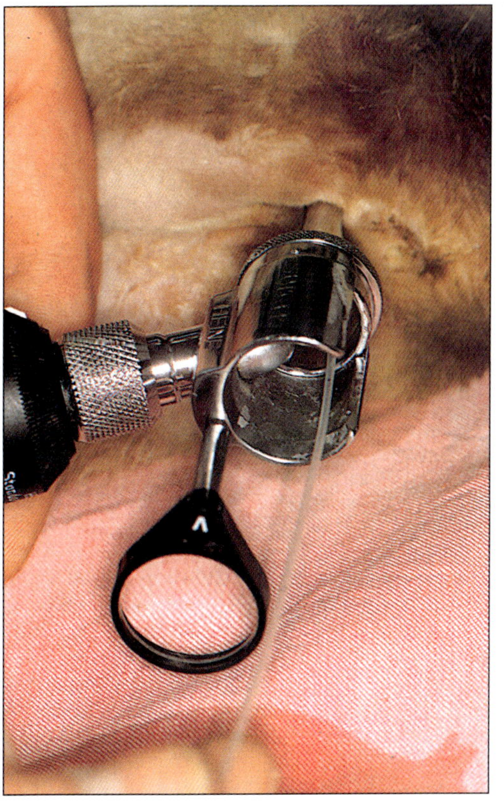

3.14 Female cats can often be catheterized 'blind'. Unlike the situation in the bitch, the feline external urethral orifice is not raised on a papilla but is a mid-line apparture on the vaginal floor. A catheter placed in the mid-line on the vestibular floor and passed cranially will often enter the urethra **(left)**. If not, an auroscope makes a useful vaginoscope for female cats, through whose external urethral orifice, once identified, a catheter can be passed **(right)**. Note: the skin discoloration to the right of the vulva in this Siamese cat was due to scalding with urine – the animal was being investigated for urinary incontinence and proved to have bilateral ureteral ectopia).

Problems

Urethral catheterization is associated with two main problems, both of which can be overcome by attention to technique. These are introduction of organisms into and iatrogenic trauma to the lower urinary tract.

If catheterized urine is to be examined for the presence of blood, the urine should be allowed to flow freely into the sample bottle. Attempts to increase urine flow down the catheter by bladder compression or syringe suction on the catheter may result in iatrogenic haematuria.

During bladder compression the catheter tip may be rubbed against the bladder urothelium, and if suction is applied to the catheter,then bladder urothelium may be sucked into the side holes of the catheter (see 'Biopsy Techniques' below).

Both problems may result in a diagnosis of haematuria in the sample obtained, whereas the animal may have had no haematuria before catheterization. For this reason some authors prefer cystocentesis, but this can also lead to iatrogenic haematuria.

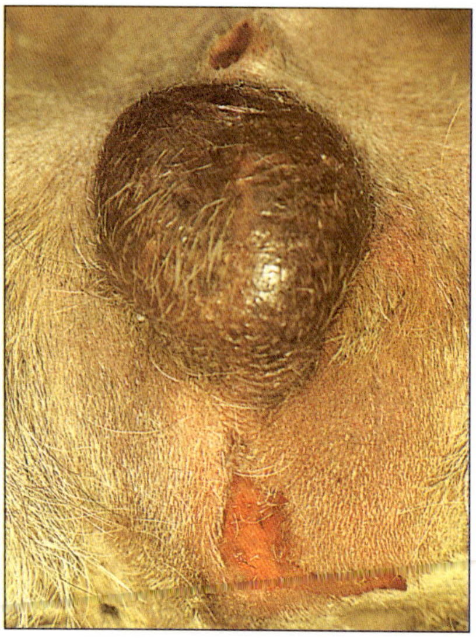

3.15 Ischial urethral abscess, draining through the perineum, due to previous attempts to catheterize a dysuric male dog with urolithiasis. This could have been avoided by attention to aseptic technique and avoidance of excessive pressure during attempts to pass the catheter. If a catheter cannot be passed easily, attempts to pass it should be abandoned and the reason for the apparent urethral obstruction ascertained. Bony reactions on the caudal os penis (see **2.12**) or a tortuous groove of the os penis may prevent passage of a urinary catheter and feel like an obstruction due to a urethral calculus. In fact, they are of no clinical significance but underline the inadvisability of using a urinary catheter to detect urethral obstruction. If in doubt, urethrography should be performed.

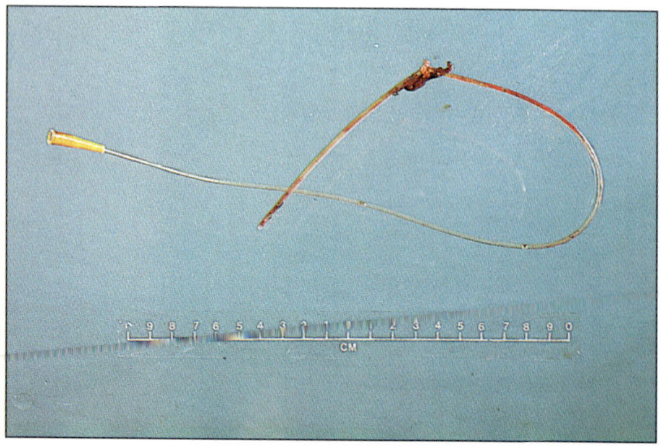

3.16 If the catheter is introduced too far, it may follow the contour of the bladder wall and begin to exit into the proximal urethra alongside itself. Even worse, it may form a knot inside the bladder. Under these circumstances, the catheter may be very difficult or even impossible to remove via the urethra. The catheter illustrated was passed too far into a dog's bladder via a perineal urethrostomy and became knotted. Fortunately, because of the urethrostomy, it could be removed via the urethra but this resulted in urethral damage and haemorrhage, as can be seen from the blood clots attached to the catheter.

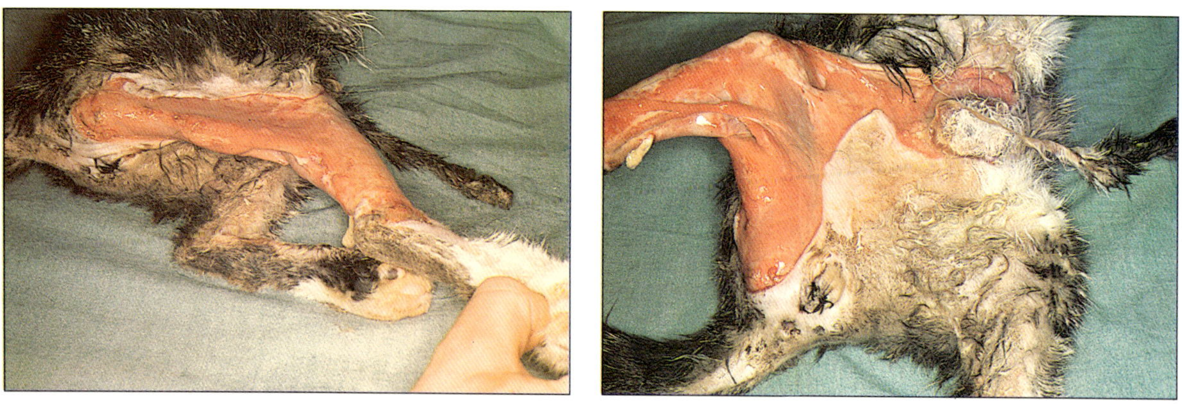

3.17 Unless severely debilitated, cats should never be catheterized without adequate chemical restraint. The skin loss from the lateral **(left)** and medial **(right)** aspects of this cat's hind leg was due to the effect of subcutaneous urine after urethral rupture. The rupture was iatrogenic, resulting from attempts to catheterize the cat in a conscious state after it had become dysuric (due to urethritis) two days after perineal urethrostomy.

3.18 Urine for laboratory analysis (particularly if haematuria is suspected) should be allowed to flow passively from the catheter. Manual compression of the bladder with the catheter *in situ* or suction on the catheter may result in iatrogenic haematuria, which in turn may lead to misinterpretation of the laboratory results.

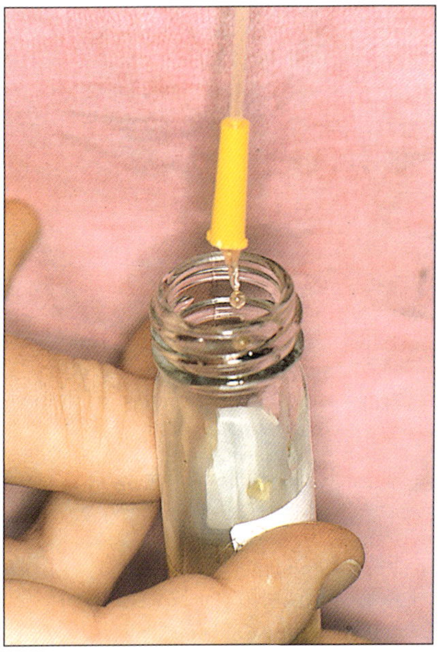

Centesis

Indications

- Collection of fluids for laboratory examination.
- Drainage of fluids from the abdomen or urinary tract organs.

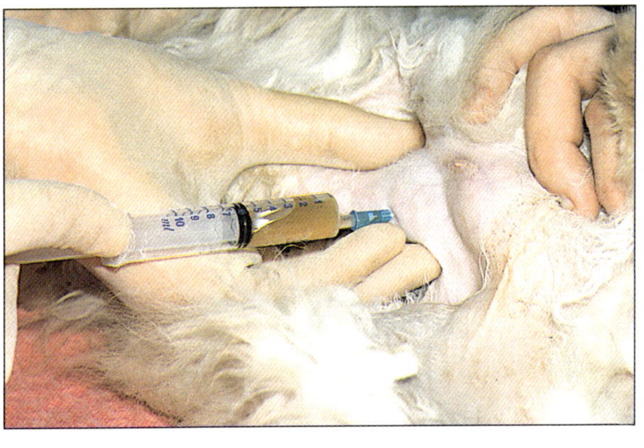

3.19 Centesis can be used to obtain samples for laboratory examinations. In this example, urine was being obtained from a sick, aged cat for bacteriology. This avoids the need for sedation or anaesthesia for catheterization and, in the view of many veterinary urologists, is the preferred method of obtaining urine samples for bacteriological examinations.

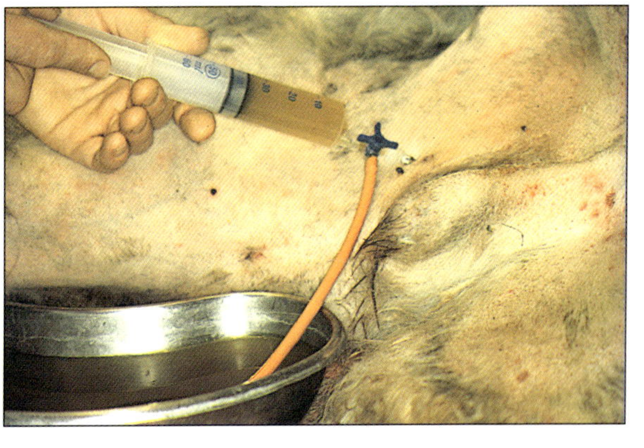

3.20 In this dysuric dog, cystocentesis was being used as an emergency procedure to drain the urinary bladder. (See also **5.38.**) In addition to bladder drainage, the metabolic consequences of the dysuria should be corrected; these measures take priority over determination of the cause of the dysuria.

Techniques

The technique varies slightly depending on the site of the fluid; centesis of the abdomen, urinary bladder and prostate gland is described. In all cases, attention should be paid to aseptic and atraumatic technique.

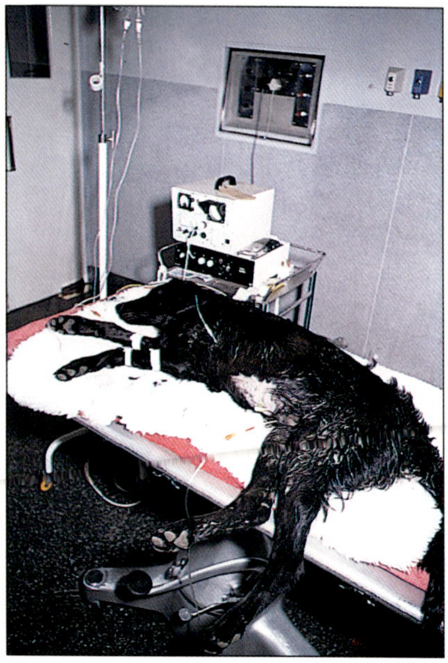

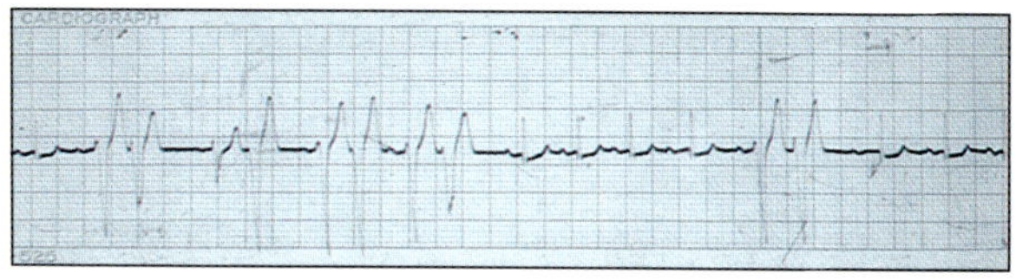

3.21 For abdominocentesis, the author's preferred site is just caudal to the umbilicus. Attempts to drain abdominal fluid from sites cranial to the umbilicus usually fail because the end of the draining needle or catheter becomes obstructed by falsiform fat. Fenestrated abdominal drains can be used, but if these are not readily available large bore (14–18 g) over-the-needle cannulae are suitable for abdominocentesis. The bladder can be drained via a prepubic, median (female animals and male cats) or paramedian (male dogs) site with the needle angled caudally towards the bladder neck (see **3.19**). For bladder emptying, the needle should be inserted into the caudal bladder; otherwise, as the bladder empties it may retract caudally off the needle. A fine (21–25 g) needle should be used to reduce the possibility of urine leakage from the bladder puncture site. Cystocentesis is easy to perform if the bladder is palpable but may be difficult if the bladder is empty and/or caudally positioned, as it may be in cases of bladder rupture and in incontinent bitches. The Flat-coated retriever shown in **(top right)** had a ruptured bladder; the urethrocystogram is illustrated in **2.56**. The dog was not sedated but rather was collapsed due to the metabolic consequences of uroperitoneum – i.e. hyperkalaemia, acidosis and azotaemia. The effects of the acidosis and hyperkalaemia on the heart can be appreciated from the ECG **(lower right)**. An over-the-needle intravenous cannula had been inserted just caudal to the umbilicus and was used both to drain urine from – and to introduce dialysing fluids into – the peritoneal cavity. In this example, abdominocentesis was used (along with intravenous fluid therapy and the insertion of an in-dwelling urethral catheter) to relieve the uroperitoneum and its metabolic consequences. Although syringe suction may speed the rate of fluid removal, it is frequently counterproductive as omentum or other abdominal viscera may be sucked onto the end of the drain/catheter, preventing the exit of fluids. It is often better to allow the fluid to drain passively through the drain/catheter.

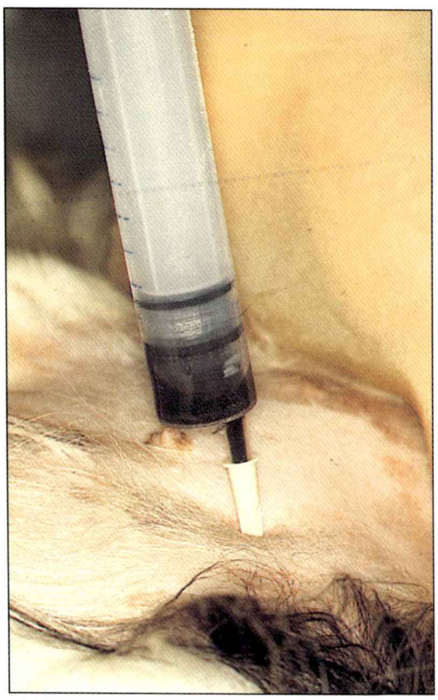

3.22 Large prostatic cysts or abscesses can be drained by centesis. (See also **3.26, 4.170 and 4.173.**) As well as providing fluid for laboratory examinations, such drainage may also be used as a first aid measure to relieve dysuria and reduce toxaemia (in the case of abscesses), thus allowing the animal to be stabilised before any surgery is performed. The site for centesis is chosen by palpation of the location of the fluid-filled cyst or abscess, although small lesions can be more accurately located using ultrasound (see **3.2**).

Problems

Potential problems include introduction of infection into the area from which fluid is being removed, leakage of fluid from a viscus into the surrounding tissues or peritoneum and iatrogenic visceral trauma. The risk of these complications can be minimized by aseptic, atraumatic technique and the use of the smallest needle/cannula compatible with the fluid to be removed. For example, urine can be drained from the bladder using fine needles (21–23 g), whereas a larger bore may be necessary to remove thick, viscous pus from a prostatic abscess or adequately to drain fluid from the abdomen.

Cytology

Indications

- In urology, mainly to differentiate inflammatory and malignant conditions.

Techniques

Cytological examinations can be performed on cellular material in fluids such as urine, ascitic fluid or prostatic secretions, on that obtained by urethral washings, and on samples obtained from brushings during endoscopy of the lower urinary tract.

Several smears of the sample should be made onto microscope slides. The retrieval of cells is higher if the smears are made of the material at the bottom of the container after standing or if a Cytospin/Cytoslide system (Shandon Scientific) is used. The slides are then air-dried and, in most practice situations, packaged according to Post Office regulations and forwarded to a diagnostic laboratory. If such a laboratory is not available and/or a veterinary surgeon with an interest or training in pathology is employed within the practice, the slides may be stained and examined immediately.

A number of staining techniques can be used for cytology but Rapid Haematoxylin and Eosin (Rapid H&E) and Leishman's stains are usually adequate and the ones most likely to be available in general practice. The staining techniques are summarized in **Tables 3.1** and **3.2**.

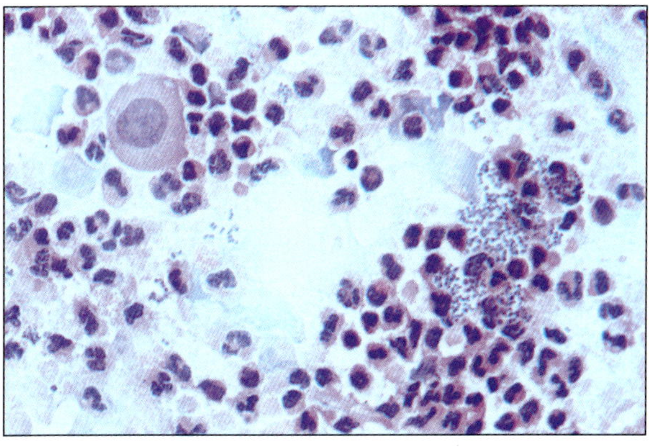

3.23 Cytology of urine from a four-year-old male Irish wolfhound presented with dysuria. The cytology smear (H&E, × 300) revealed numerous polymorphonuclear leucocytes and bacteria, consistent with pyuria. This animal had a staphylococcal prostatitis.

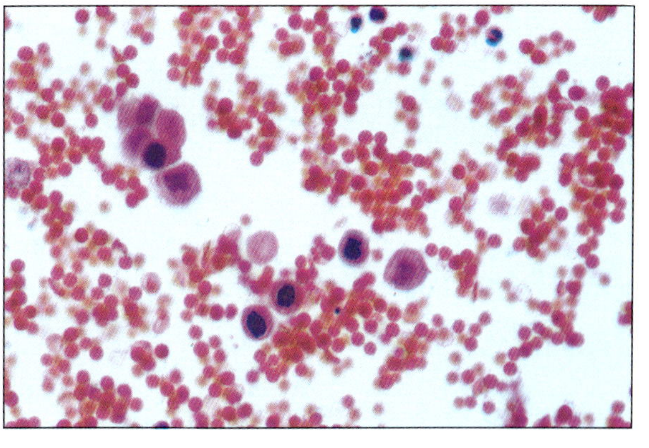

3.24 Cytology (H&E, x 300) of urine from an eight-year-old neutered female Cocker spaniel presented with haematuria and a palpable bladder mass. Numerous red blood cells are present but malignant epithelial cells can also be seen. Histopathological examination of the excised bladder wall mass confirmed a diagnosis of transitional cell carcinoma.

Table 3.1. Rapid H&E stain

1. Fix slide in acetic alcohol (3% acetic acid in 95% alcohol) for one minute.
2. Wash in water.
3. Stain in Harris' haematoxylin for one minute.
4. Wash and 'blue' (wait until the stain turns blue) in running tap water for one minute.
5. Stain in eosin (1% in tap water) for two minutes.
6. Wash in water.
7. Dehydrate in 100% alcohol, rinse in xylene and mount in DPX.

Results: Nuclei –blue;
other cellular components –shades of red and pink.

Table 3.2. Leishman stain

1. Put slide(s) on a rack and cover with 1 ml of Leishman stock (made up of 0.15% Leishman powder in 100% methanol – use within 24 hours); leave for 20 seconds.
2. Add 2 ml of pH 6.8 buffer and tip rack up and down to ensure mixing; leave for seven minutes.
3. Rinse quickly in distilled water.
4. Treat with pH 6.8 buffer for two minutes.
5. Rinse quickly in distilled water.
6. Blot dry. **Do not use alcohol.**
7. Clear and mount.

Results:		
	Nuclei	*purple*
	Acidophils	*pink/red*
	Basophils	*blue*
	Eosinophils	*red/orange*
	Mast cells	*purple (granules).*

Problems

The preparation of good, diagnostic slides and their interpretation comes only with practice and experience. This is unlikely to be acquired in most practices and so the reader is advised to concentrate on preparing an even, air-dried smear on a slide for staining and interpretation at a veterinary pathological diagnostic laboratory. Even then, the results may be unreliable. In most cases, cytology is being used to differentiate malignant from benign conditions, as a guide to treatment and prognosis. Although the finding of malignant cells is diagnostic of malignancy, the converse is, unfortunately, not true. The absence of malignant cells on cytology does not exclude a diagnosis of malignancy; such cells are not always found. In the author's experience, cytology is less reliable than the biopsy techniques described below in the differentiation of malignant and non-malignant urological disorders.

Biopsy techniques

Indications

- To differentiate inflammatory and neoplastic lesions of the urinary tract (e.g. urethritis versus urethral carcinoma).
- To determine the nature of the disease present, more accurately to prescribe treatment and/or obtain a prognosis (e.g. malignancies, glomerular renal diseases).

Techniques

Although biopsy material can be obtained by surgical exposure of the organ concerned, less-invasive methods include needle biopsies and biopsies taken endoscopically (see 'Endoscopy' below) or using a urethral catheter.

The kidney and prostate can be biopsied using a Tru-cut (Travenol) or Bard Biopty-cut (Bard Urological Division) biopsy needle, whereas the catheter biopsy technique is suitable for lower urinary tract urothelial lesions and the para-urethral prostate.

3.25 Renal cortical biopsies can be taken using a biopsy needle (top right). Accurate placement of the needle is necessary in order to obtain a meaningful biopsy while minimizing renal trauma (see **lower right**). Thus, although a biopsy can be taken from a sedated animal using local analgesia, the author prefers to perform the technique under general anaesthesia, if possible. The development of veterinary ultrasonography has made renal biopsy a less hazardous technique and ultrasound-guided biopsies are preferred. The skin over the kidney (see **3.3**) is prepared for aseptic surgery and sterile ultrasound gel applied (e.g. Ultra/phonic Conductivity Gel, Pharmaceutical Innovations Inc.) (surgical drapes have been omitted to facilitate orientation). The biopsy needle is inserted through a stab incision in the skin into the renal cortex under ultrasonic guidance and the biopsy taken, in this case using an 18Fr Biopty-cut needle and automatic biopsy 'gun' (Biopty Instruments, Bard Urological Division). If a Tru-cut biopsy needle is used, it is important to familiarize oneself and one's assistant with the functioning of the biopsy needle before inserting it. This may seem obvious but most veterinary surgeons perform needle biopsies infrequently and once the needle has been inserted, the effects of manipulations cannot be seen. The novice is advised to have two needles available; one to take the biopsy and the other in case he/she forgets what to do once the first needle has been inserted! The biopsy needle is introduced via a small stab skin incision and inserted into the kidney cortex, taking care to avoid the medulla or corticomedullary junction (see **lower right**). In cats, the kidneys are usually sufficiently palpable and mobile to be held through the skin and abdominal wall. The kidneys of dogs, on the other hand, may be difficult to locate and fix adequately and some authors suggest making a small flank incision through which a finger can be inserted into the abdomen, better to fix the kidney. In both species, the left kidney is easier to biopsy than the right because of its more caudal location: this is the kidney of the author's choice, therefore, in cases of generalized renal disease (e.g. glomerulonephropathies). However, other authors prefer the right kidney as this is less mobile than the left. The author prefers to hold the kidney in one hand (the left if one is right-handed) and to insert the needle with the other. Unless one has access to a biopsy 'gun', this means that an assistant is required to manipulate the needle in order to obtain a biopsy. Once the needle is withdrawn, it should be examined to ensure that the amount of tissue obtained is adequate for laboratory examinations (histology, electron microscopy, and immunohistochemistry), and pieces of tissue should be transferred to suitable containers. **(lower right)** Kidney specimen (from a dog with benign, idiopathic renal haemorrhage) illustrating the correct (solid lines) and incorrect (broken lines) positions of insertion of the biopsy needle.

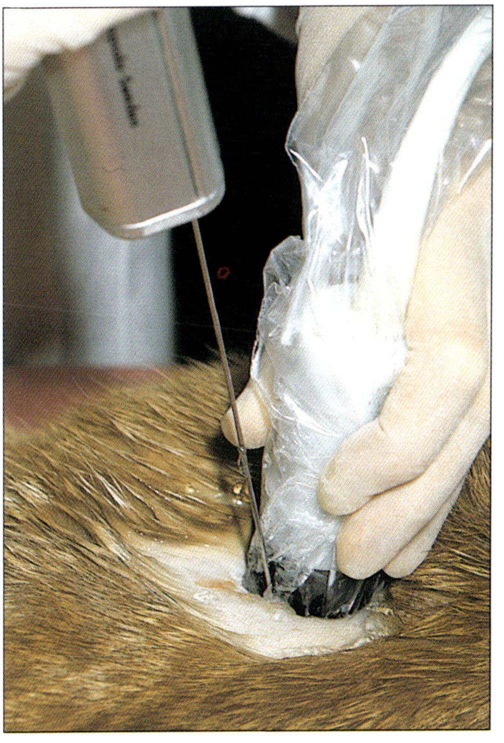

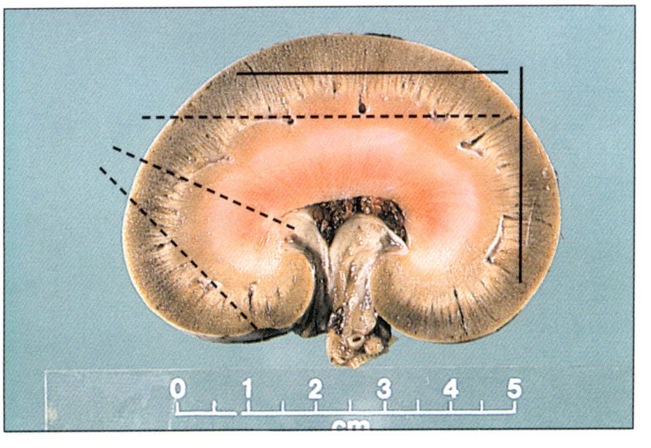

3.26 A needle biopsy of the prostate gland is usually obtained through the perineum, as illustrated (top). The prostate is fixed, in the case of transperineal biopsy using a gloved finger in the rectum. The finger is also used to guide the needle into the area of the gland to be biopsied. Care is taken to avoid the urethra. **(middle)** The rectum is evacuated, either by the administration of an enema or by digital removal of faeces. The anaesthetized dog is placed in left lateral recumbency if one is right-handed; right lateral recumbency if left-handed. The perineum is prepared for aseptic surgery and sterile drapes applied, leaving the anus and perineum exposed (the drapes have been removed from this dog to facilitate orientation). The prostate is fixed with the index finger of the left hand (right-handed people). The biopsy needle or needle for centesis (as shown in this Boxer with a prostatic cyst extending caudally into the perineum) is introduced into the perineum adjacent to the anus and above it, as shown. This reduces the risk of contamination of the needle by faecal organisms as any material leaving the anus will tend to fall downwards, away from the needle. Once the needle is inserted into the prostate, fluids can be withdrawn, or a Tru-cut or Biopty-cut biopsy taken in an identical way to a renal biopsy. The centre of the gland is avoided to prevent iatrogenic prostatic urethral trauma and the biopsy needle is usually inserted into the dorsolateral region of the prostate. **(lower middle)** If the prostate is cranial to the pubic brim, it can be biopsied via a prepubic approach as shown (again, the surgical drapes have been removed to facilitate orientation). The prostate is fixed with the left hand (if one is right-handed) and the right hand used to introduce the biopsy needle, taking care to avoid the urethra in the centre of the gland. The resulting biopsy is also illustrated **(bottom)**. The prostatic enlargement, alopecia and feminisation in this dog were due to excessive, prolonged oestrogen therapy, leading to squamous metaplasia of the prostate gland.

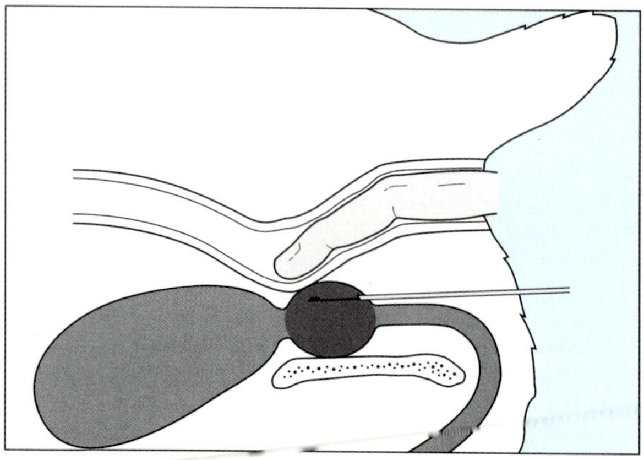

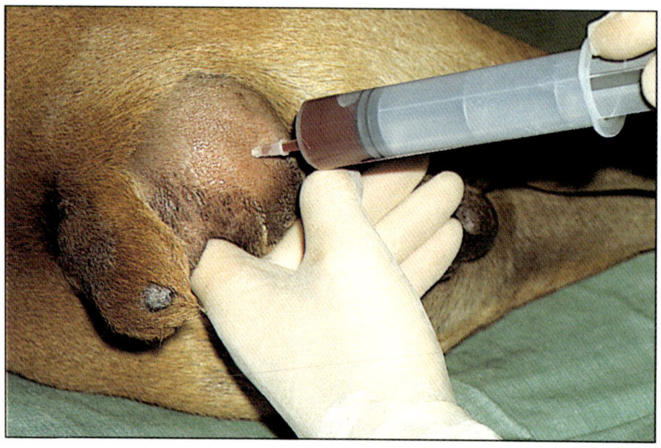

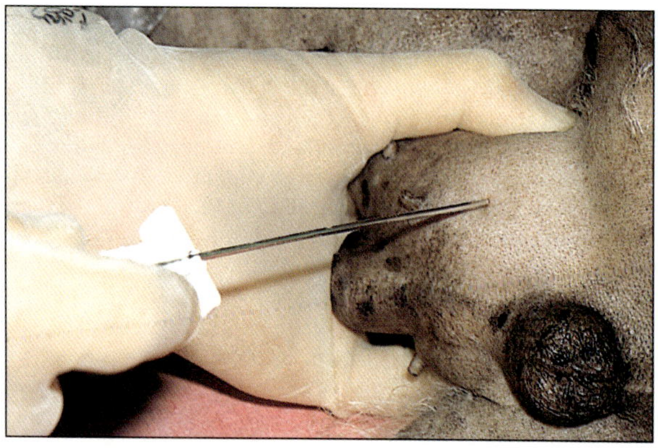

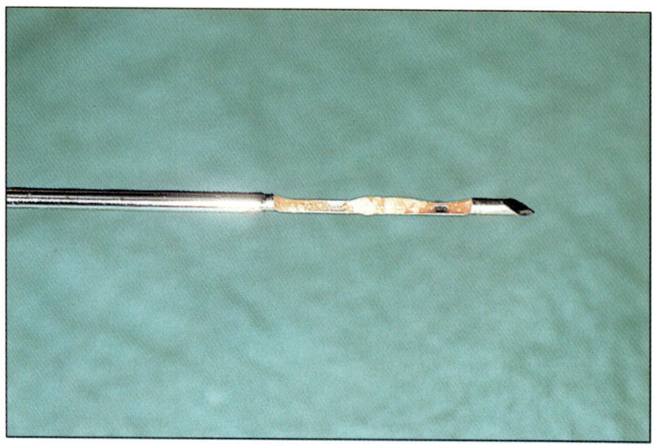

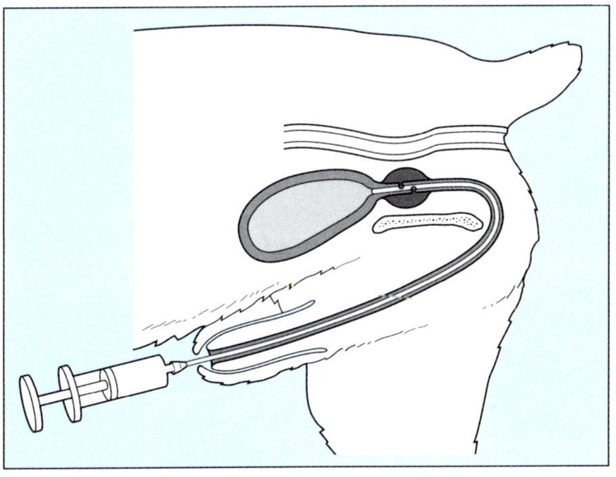

3.27 Diagram illustrating the catheter biopsy technique of Melhoff and Osborne (1977). The catheter tip is introduced to the level of the tissues to be biopsied (in this case, the prostatic urethra), as judged from previous clinical and radiographic investigations. A syringe is attached to the catheter and used to apply suction. Pieces of tissue are sucked into the side holes of the catheter and are dislodged by moving the catheter to and fro. The catheter is then withdrawn and the pieces of tissue flushed out of the catheter (using formol–saline) into a container of formol–saline. Experience suggests that it is easier to obtain biopsies from diseased (e.g. neoplastic or inflammed) tissues than from normal urothelium and its surrounding tissues. The small pieces of tissue which are obtained can be aggregated by centrifugation, fixed, sectioned, stained and examined. The pieces are not always large enough to allow orientation of the sample by a veterinary pathologist but this is often not essential; in most cases, the differentiation of neoplastic from inflammatory tissue is sufficient for diagnostic purposes.

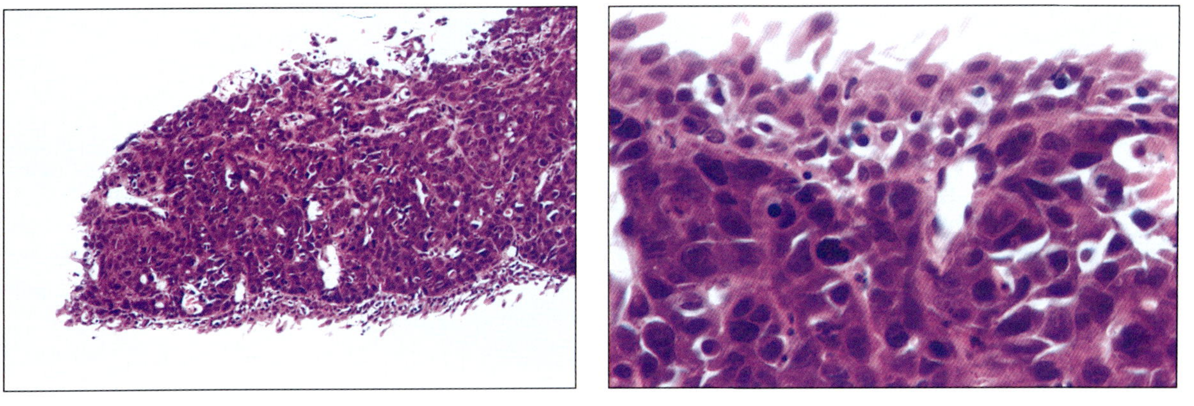

3.28 The histological appearance of the material obtained. H&E stained and illustrated at magnifications of ×100 **(left)** and ×300 **(right)** in this example of a catheter biopsy from a nine-year-old castrated male German shepherd with prostatic urethral carcinoma.

Problems

The main problems with needle biopsy techniques are haemorrhage from or into the organ biopsied and iatrogenic trauma to the organ; the latter may be a particular problem in the kidney. In addition, attempts to biopsy infected (especially abscessed) organs may result in dissemination of infection. The risks of introducing infection with the biopsy needle itself can be minimized by careful attention to sterile technique.

The catheter biopsy technique shares the problems associated with urethral catheterization (see above) but otherwise is free of complications.

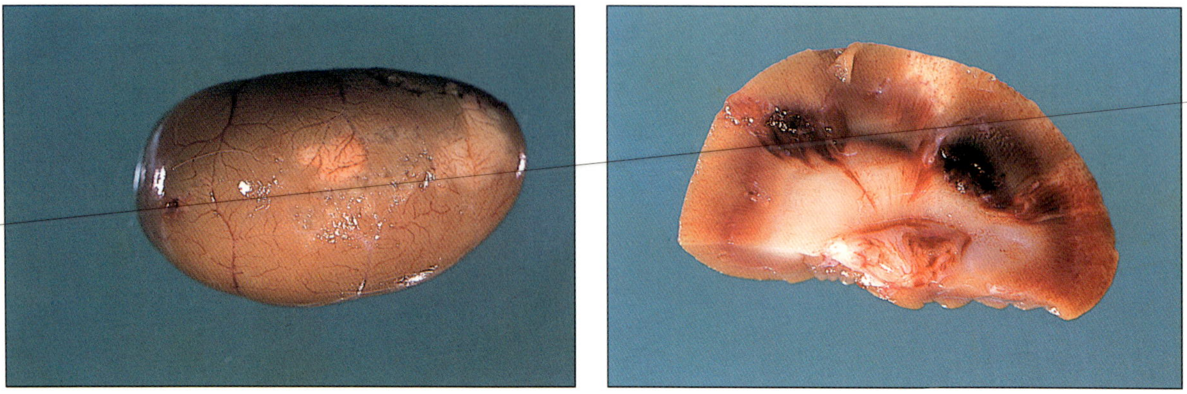

3.29 The post mortem appearance of a feline kidney, one week after a Tru-cut biopsy. Note the pale areas associated with renal infarction **(left)**. A section through the kidney **(right)** demonstrates that the biopsy needle had been introduced too deep, damaging the renal arcuate vessels at the corticomedullary junction and leading to thrombosis and infarction.

Blood and urine analyses

Indications

Haematological and biochemical examinations of blood are indicated in animals with dysuria or haematuria. They are of less value in incontinent animals. Haematology is mainly of use in assessing the degree of anaemia (in animals with severe haematuria), dehydration (for example, the vomiting dysuric patient) and toxaemia/bacteraemia (e.g. acute prostatitis or prostatic abscessation). Biochemistry can be used to evaluate the degree of pre-renal, renal or post-renal azotaemia in dysuric animals but is also valuable in assessing renal function before nephrectomy or nephrotomy is performed. In cases of suspected bladder rupture, comparison of blood and ascitic fluid creatinine levels is a useful diagnostic aid. If uroperitoneum is present, ascitic fluid levels of creatinine will be markedly higher than those in the blood (comparisons of urea levels are less reliable as urea diffuses readily across the peritoneum and thus blood and peritoneal fluid levels tend to equilibrate).

Urine biochemistry may provide further information on the nature and degree of renal damage but is mainly of value (along with urine cytology) in detecting the presence of microscopic haematuria. Urine bacteriology is mandatory in most animals with urological signs; even if urinary tract infections are not the main cause of the clinical signs, they are frequently present as secondary complications and, if possible, should be eliminated before urological surgery is carried out. This is important in animals in which ureteral transplantation is to be performed (see Chapter 4). Dogs with prostatic infections frequently shed organisms into the urine and thus urine bacteriology is valuable in such cases, especially if it is not possible to sample prostatic secretions or abscesses directly.

Techniques

There are a number of commercial laboratories offering a service for the analysis of veterinary samples, although the increasing availability of desk-top analysers means that even those practices without practice laboratories are now perfoming routine laboratory examinations. The analytical techniques required vary between analysers and laboratories and will not be described here. A few basic principles are worth mentioning, however.

It is important to know the range of normal values for the variables being assessed *for that particular laboratory or analyser.* Most commercial laboratories will supply details of their 'normal' values, as may the manufacturers of some analysers. However, in the latter instance, experience with the use of the analyser will lead to a knowledge of the ranges of normality which can be expected. Variations in normality should also be considered. For example, young animals often have a lymphocytosis, lower PCV and haemoglobin levels; fit, working dogs (e.g. Greyhounds, Whippets) normally have PCVs which would be considered high for other dogs.

The ranges of normal values used in the clinical laboratories at the Bristol Veterinary School are given in **Tables 3.3–3.5** as a guide.

Table 3.3. Normal biochemical ranges.

Estimation	*Units*	*Dog*	*Cat*
Albumin	g/l	36–44	25–40
Globulin	g/l	20–35	21–51
A:G ratio		0.7–2.0	0.4–1.7
ALT	U/l	20–60	15–45
Ammonia	μmol/l	0–50	0–50
Amylase	U/l	800–2000	800–2000
AST	U/l	20–35	0–20
Bile acids	μmol/l	0–50	0–50
Calcium	mmol/l	2.15–2.5	2.12–2.44
Chloride	mmol/l	102–112	
Cholesterol	mmol/l	3.5–7.0	4.0–10.0
CPK	U/l	75–230	50–150
Creatinine	μmol/l	70–110	110–160
Glucose	mmol/l	3.5–5.0	3.5–5.0
Inorganic phosphorus	mmol/l	0.75–1.25	0.95–1.55
LDH	U/l	35–450	130–470
Lipase	U/l	0–300	0–300
Magnesium	mmol/l	0.8–1.1	0.8–1.1
Potassium	mmol/l	3.5–4.5	4.0–5.0
SAP	U/l	0–110	15--60
Sodium	mmol/l	135–150	149–157
Total bilirubin	μmol/l	0–10	0–10
Total proteins	g/l	63–71	77–91
Urea	mmol/l	2.0–7.0	6.5–10.5

Table 3.4. Normal haematological values.

Estimation	*Units*	*Dog*	*Cat*
PCV	%	40–50	30–40
RBCs	$\times 10^6$/mm^3	5.1–6.8	5.5–8.5
Haemoglobin	g/dl	12.5–16.5	9.5–14.0
MCHC	%	31–35	30–35
MCV	μ^3	68–75	42–55
WBCs	$\times 10^3$/mm^3	8.5–14.0	8.0–21.0
Differential WBC counts:			
Bands	%	<3.0	0.9
Neutrophils	%	74.0	60.4
Lymphocytes	%	20.0	28.2
Monocytes	%	4.0	1.7
Eosinophils	%	2.0	8.8
Basophils	%	0	0

Table 3.5. Normal urinalysis values.

Estimation	*Dog*	*Cat*
pH	5.0–7.0	5.0–7.0
Specific gravity	1.015–1.045	1.015–1.060
Protein	negative	negative
Blood	negative	negative
Haemoglobin	negative	negative
Glucose	negative	negative
Ketones	negative	negative
Bilirubin	negative/trace	negative/trace
Urobilinogen	negative	negative
Urine production	24–40 ml/kg/day	22–30 ml/kg/day

Problems

If blood and urine samples are to be posted, they should be prepared and packed in an appropriate way. Most laboratories prefer blood to be clotted and the serum decanted and submitted for analysis rather than whole blood. Apart from the obvious problem that the sample may haemolyse, serum levels of potassium in whole blood tend to increase during transit (as potassium leaks from blood cells). This may lead to misdiagnoses of hyperkalaemia and inappropriate therapy.

If urine is posted to a laboratory for bacteriological culture, there may be overgrowth of organisms of low pathogenicity during transit, masking the significant bacteria. This can be prevented by placing the fresh urine sample in a receptacle containing boric acid powder (e.g. Boricon Sterile Tube, Medical Wire and Equipment Company Ltd) in the proportion of 20 ml of urine to 200 mg of boric acid powder. There is increasing evidence that urine bacteriology should be quantitative as well as qualitative and that low counts of bacteria are of no clinical significance. Opinions vary on what is meant by 'low counts' but, in general, if a sample is obtained by aseptic catheterization, counts of <1000 and <100 organisms per ml are taken to be due to contamination in dogs and cats, respectively. If the sample is taken by cystocentesis, this figure is <100 organisms per ml in both species.

If samples are posted to a commercial laboratory, it is a legal obligation that the Post Office guidelines are followed for their package and labelling. Apart from the illegality of inadequate packing and labelling and health hazards to handlers, urine and blood samples squeezed from sodden envelopes are of little diagnostic value!

Urodynamics

Indications

- Suspected abnormal functioning of the lower urinary tract such as urethral sphincter mechanism incompetence, detrusor instability, reflex dyssynergia and neurogenic abnormalities.

Techniques

Techniques included within urodynamics are:
- Urethral pressure profilometry ('resting' or 'stressed').
- Cystometry.
- Electromyography.

In small animal practice, most work has been done on resting urethral pressure profilometry and indications for other urodynamic techniques are uncommon. However, all of these techniques are subject to a wide variety of artefacts and variations in the results obtained (see Holt and Gregory, 1993 for a review). Apart from the fact that they are not available in most veterinary practices (and unlikely to be so in the forseeable future), they have proved to be of less diagnostic value than was first hoped. A brief description only, therefore, will be given of urethral pressure profilometry. The reader who wishes to learn more about urodynamics will find additional information in 'References and Further Reading' at the end of this book.

.30

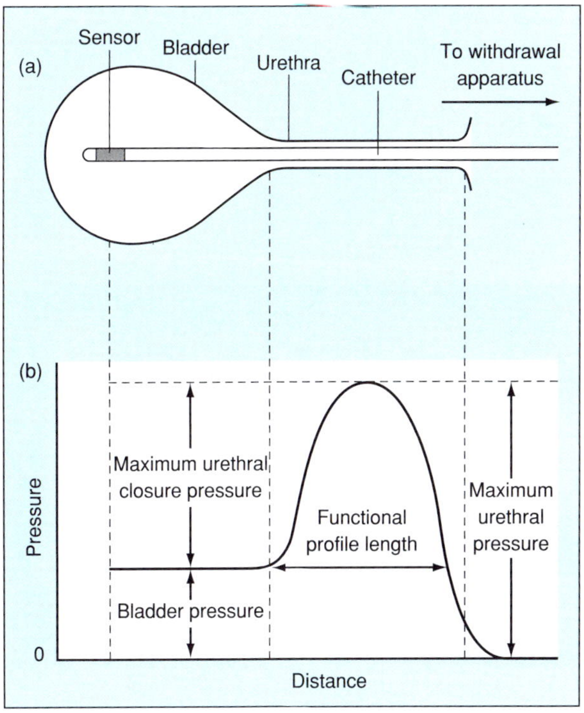

3.30 During urethral pressure profilometry, a catheter, with a pressure-measuring device at or near the tip, is inserted into the bladder and then withdrawn along the urethra. The pressure can be measured by the resistance to outflow of fluid from catheter side holes (perfusion profilometry), pressure changes within balloons or by using microtip pressure transducers. The latter are preferable but are expensive. As the catheter passes along the urethra, a graph of pressure against distance is produced on a recorder: this is the resting urethral pressure profile. A number of variables can be measured from the graph. They have been defined by the International Continence Society and are shown in **3.30**.

3.31 Subtracted urethral pressure profile recordings from a continent bitch (top) and an incontinent bitch (bottom). A 'subtracted' profile makes allowances for variations in intravesical pressure (e.g. those due to respiration, as shown by regular small peaks). Subtracted profilometry involves the simultaneous measurement of intra-urethral and intravesical pressures. The intravesical pressure is continuously subtracted from the intra-urethral pressure to give a more accurate representation of urodynamic events, the subtracted urethral pressure profile. This is summarized in the top graph, but the lower graph shows only the subtracted profile. The profile from the continent animal conforms to **3.30** but urethral resistance in the incontinent bitch is less than intravesical pressure throughout the profile. It would be helpful if all profiles were as diagnostic of good or poor urethral function as these two examples, but unfortunately this is not the case.

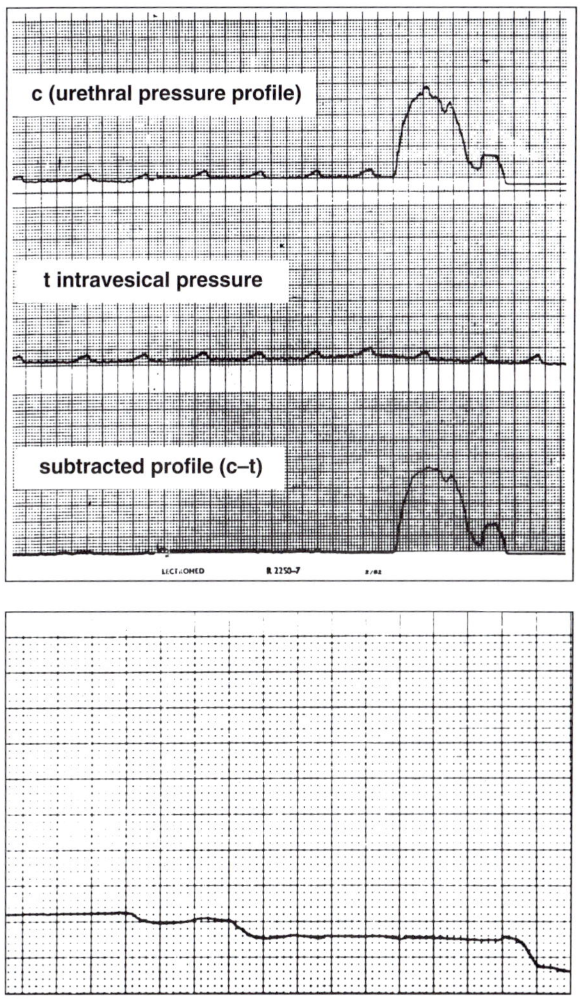

Problems

In order to minimize variations, it is imperative that a standard technique is used. This should include the position of the animal, orientation of the catheter within the urethra, method of chemical restraint, size of catheter, catheter material, catheter withdrawal rate and degree of bladder filling.

From studies of some of these variables, the following standards have been suggested:

- The animal should be positioned in right lateral recumbency.
- The catheter should be orientated so that the side hole (if a perfusion technique is used) or microtip transducer is facing dorsally within the urethra.
- The catheter should be as narrow and soft as possible; in practice, this usually means a 3–4Fr polyurethane catheter in cats and a 6–8Fr silicone rubber catheter in dogs. Softer catheters are available but are more difficult to insert and, if microtip catheters are used, more liable to damage.
- A standard method of chemical restraint should be used in all cases. However, a perfect anaesthetic or relaxant (i.e. one that has no effect on the urodynamic variables being measured) has yet to be discovered.
- The catheter should be withdrawn at a speed of 1 mm/s or less.
- The bladder should be filled with sterile saline or emptied of urine to achieve a resting intravesical pressure of 5 cm H_2O.

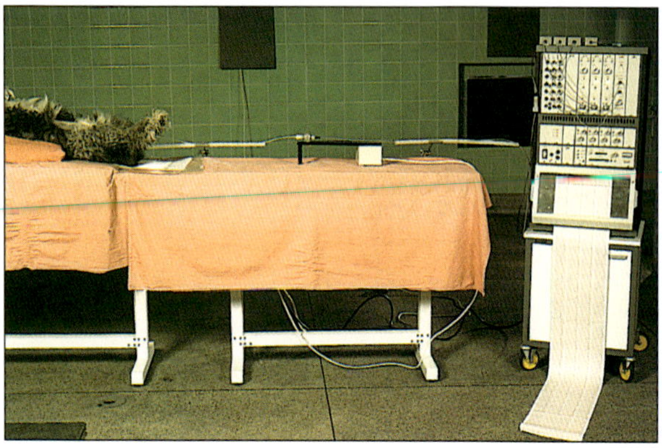

3.32 The use of a belt-driven catheter withdrawal device during profilometry in this bitch necessitates the use of channels to support the catheter and its lead. This device does not prevent the weights of the catheter and catheter lead from pulling the catheter from the urethra, resulting in urethral pressure profile artefacts. In addition, it fails to prevent catheter rotation during withdrawal (a source of artefacts) as it does not secure the catheter. The bitch is in dorsal recumbency which is an inappropriate position for urethral pressure profilometry; right lateral recumbency results in a more diagnostic profile.

Once the method has been standardized, it is important to determine the range of normality using that method as this will vary from centre to centre. Meaningful conclusions can be drawn only when normal values are known. Even then, the situation is far from black and white!

Belt-driven catheter withdrawal devices are unsuitable as they do not prevent the weight of the catheter or its lead from pulling the catheter from the urethra. It is preferable to use a rod-driven device which clips directly on to the catheter.

The use of a single sensor on the catheter makes the assumption that intravesical pressure remains constant as the sensor passes along the urethra. This problem can be overcome by the use of two sensors – 'simultaneous' urethral pressure profilometry.

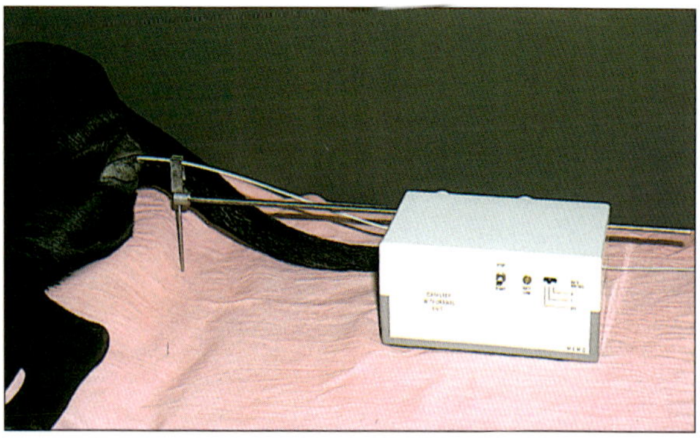

3.33 The problems of inadvertent pulling of the catheter from the urethra and catheter rotation are overcome by the use of a rod-driven device which clips directly on to the catheter.

3.34 Double sensor catheter used to measure (simultaneously) intravesical and urethral pressures. The microtip transducer at the tip of this silicone rubber catheter remains in the bladder throughout profilometry whereas the second sensor starts in the bladder but then passes along the urethra during withdrawal. An electronic subtraction unit in the recorder continuously subtracts the intravesical pressure from the intravesical pressure, resulting in a more accurate 'subtracted' pressure profile (see **3.31a**). In most animals in which urethral pressure profilometry is indicated (i.e. large incontinent breeds of female dog with suspected urethral sphincter mechanism incompetence), the tip and second sensors should be separated by 8 cm to allow the tip sensor to remain in the bladder throughout profilometry.

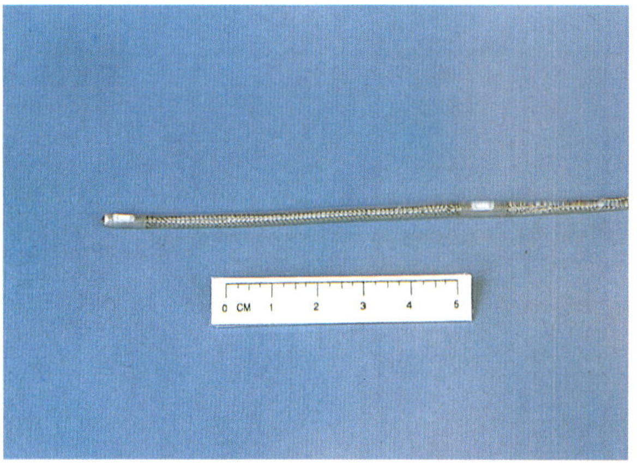

Endoscopy

Indications

Although laparoscopy can be applied to small animals, in urological cases the most commonly used endoscopic technique is urethrocystoscopy. The main indications, therefore, are suspected lesions of the bladder or urethra. In humans, surgical procedures (e.g. transurethral prostatic resection) can be performed endoscopically. Unfortunately, the smaller size of the canine urethra means that surgical endoscopic procedures are limited as the diameters of resectoscopes are usually too great to permit introduction into the urethras of small animals.

The main advantage of urethrocystoscopy is the ability to visualize, and thus take an accurate biopsy from, urethral or bladder lesions. If lithotrypsy equipment is available, endoscopic fragmentation of vesical calculi can be performed. The cystoscope can also be used to guide catheters into the ureters, thus allowing sampling of urine from individual kidneys (e.g. in suspected cases of idiopathic renal haemorrhage) as a less traumatic alternative to cystotomy.

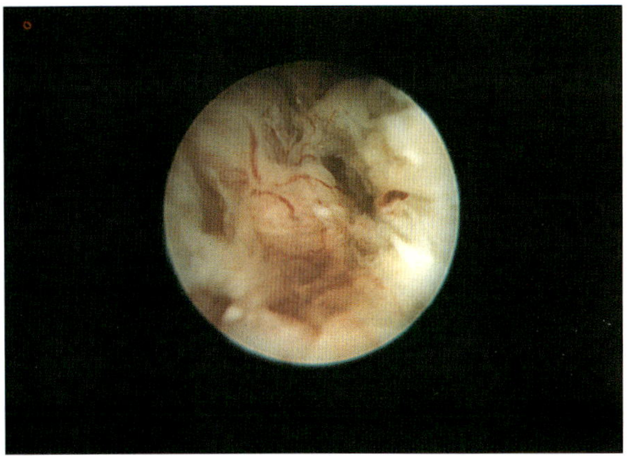

3.35 Urethroscopic appearance of a urethral carcinoma in a bitch. This bitch was dysuric and the urethra can be seen to be almost completely occluded by abnormal, white, vascular tissue. The lesion was readily detectable on retrograde positive contrast vagino-urethrography and the diagnosis was confirmed by means of a catheter biopsy.

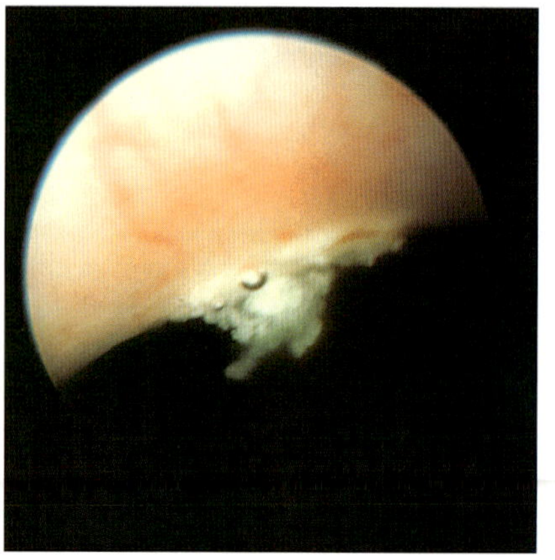

3.36 Urethrocystoscopy allows more accurate collection of biopsy material if the lesion is more discrete, as in this case of localized, diphtheritic cystitis. In this German Shepherd bitch, double contrast cystography had revealed a proliferative lesion near the bladder neck ('skylined' in this illustration). It would have been difficult to obtain an accurate biopsy using the catheter biopsy technique in this case.

Techniques

A variety of equipment is available and most is designed for use in humans rather than animals. It is also rather expensive. Urethrocystoscopy will not be described in this atlas. Rather, the reader is referred to the more extensive descriptions of the apparatus available and its use in the section on urethrocystoscopy in the endoscopy atlas by Brearley, Cooper and Sullivan (1991).

Problems

Urethrocystoscopy is associated with the same potential problems as introduction of other instruments into the lower urinary tract (see 'Catheterization') and is contraindicated in the presence of acute bacterial infections which it may exacerbate.

4 Urological Surgical Techniques

In this chapter, a variety of urological surgical techniques are presented. In addition, the indications for each technique, the pre-operative and peri-operative considerations and possible surgical/post-surgical complications (and their avoidance) are described and illustrated.

Suture material sizes in this chapter and the next are given in BPC gauges (e.g. '5/0 polyglactin'). For those who prefer metric gauges, **Table 4.1** gives a conversion table.

Table 4.1. Conversion table of BPC and metric gauges.

*BPC gauge**	*Metric number*
5/0	1
4/0	1.5
3/0	2
2/0	3
0	3.5
1	4
2	5

* N.B. BPC gauges refer to synthetic absorbable materials. Chromic catgut of the same gauge is actually thicker; that is, chromic catgut gauge 2/0 is equivalent to synthetic absorbable gauge 0 and so on.

Nephrectomy

Indications

- Severe, unilateral lesions such as renal and/or ureteral neoplasia, hydronephrosis, severe chronic pyelonephritis, idiopathic renal haemorrhage, severe renal and/or ureteral trauma.

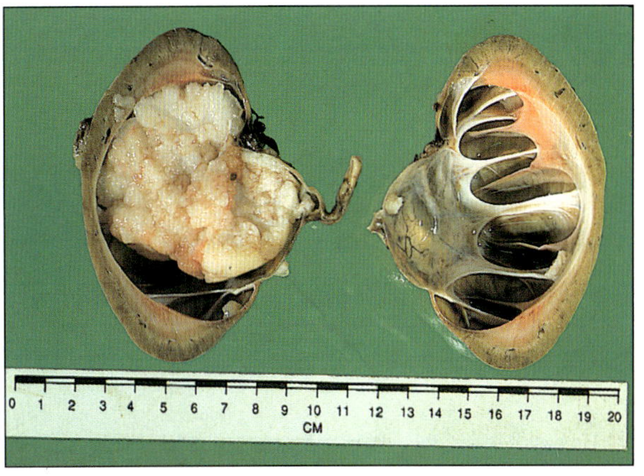

4.1 The excised kidney (sectioned sagittally), shown ultrasonographically in 3.1, from a Golden retriever bitch. This proved to be an embryonal nephroma. The section of tumour from the right half of the kidney has been removed to demonstrate the secondary hydronephrosis which was present.

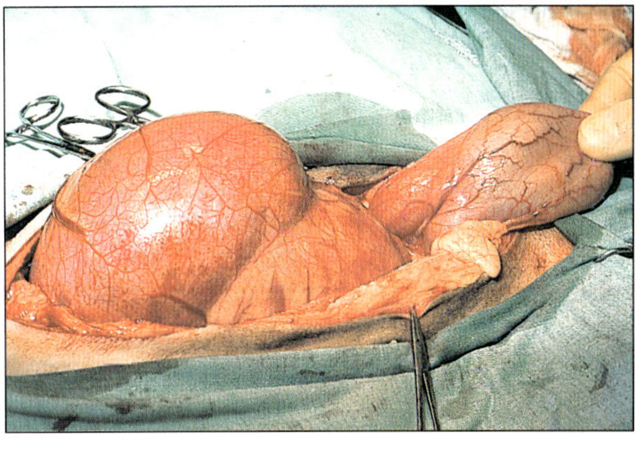

4.2 Gross hydronephrosis and hydro-ureter secondary to ureteral ectopia in a juvenile male Golden retriever. The radiographs and excised kidney of this dog are illustrated in **2.4**, **2.16** and **2.17**.

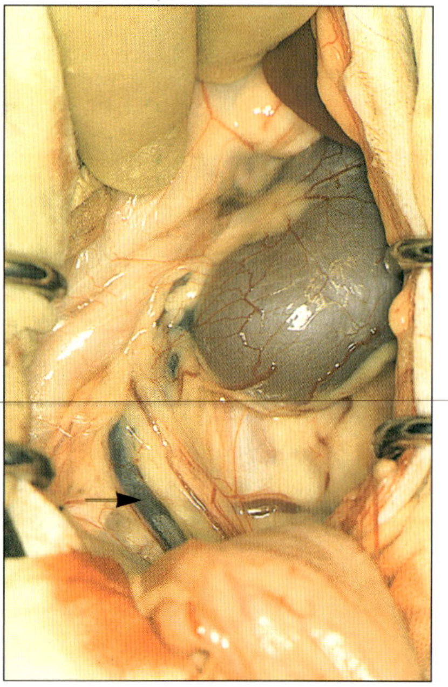

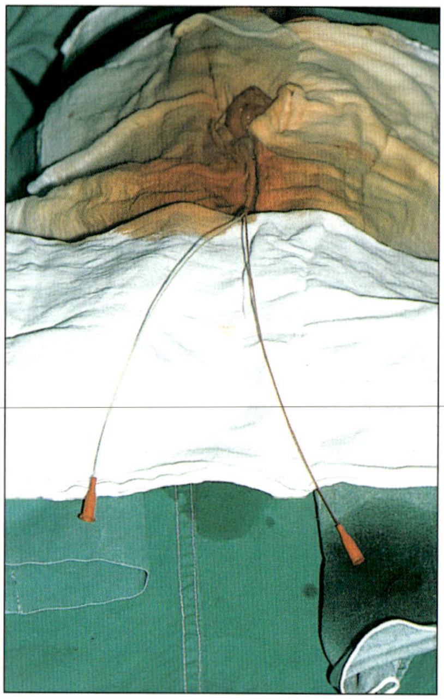

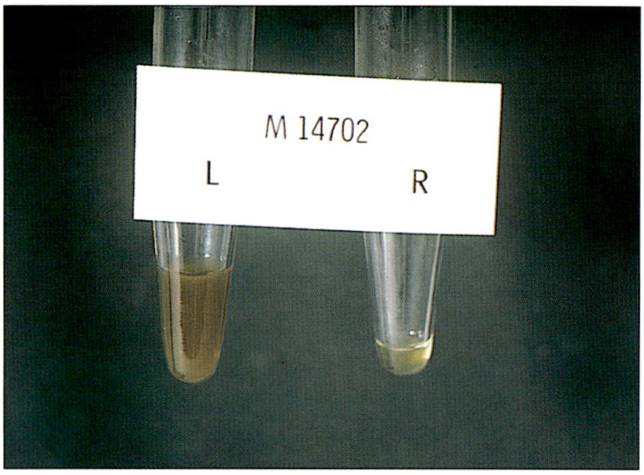

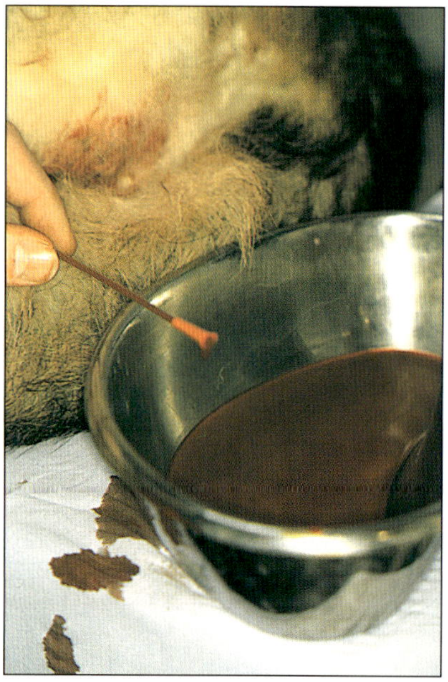

4.3 In cases of renal haemorrhage (top left), the ureter (arrowed) may be filled with blood and resemble a blood vessel but this is unusual. More often, the diagnosis is made by ureteral catheterization, either via a ventral cystotomy **(top right)** or cystoscopically. Urine samples are collected from each ureter **(lower left)**. If bleeding is unilateral, nephrectomy is usually performed to prevent further blood loss (some animals become anaemic) and, sometimes, to obtain a diagnosis; idiopathic renal haemorrhage can be confirmed as a diagnosis only by eliminating other possible conditions through pathological examination of the excised kidney. For example, the German shepherd dog illustrated in **(lower right)** has severe haematuria and secondary anaemia but the renal haemangiosarcoma responsible was so small as to be undetectable by any means other than pathological examination of the excised kidney.

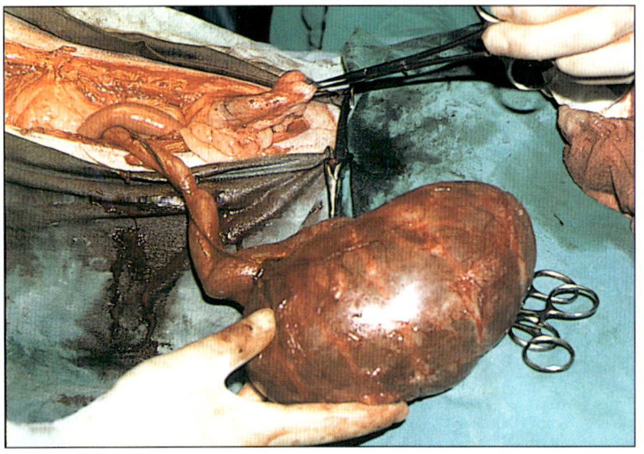

4.4 Iatrogenic ureteral trauma, resulting in hydro-ureter and hydronephrosis and necessitating uretero-nephrectomy. This injury resulted from iatrogenic transection of the ureter during ovariohysterectomy. The severed distal ureter had become adherent to the linea alba incision and thus obstructed.

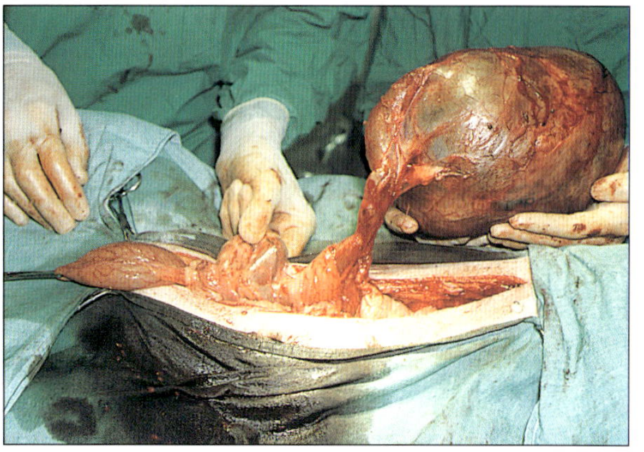

4.5 A similar situation may result from a distal ureteral tumour, as in this Rough collie bitch with a ureteral fibro-epithelial polyp.

Pre- and peri-operative considerations

It must be ensured that a second, functional kidney is present. In cases of partial renal trauma, partial nephrectomy of the affected renal pole should be considered. This is accomplished by incising the peritoneum and capsule over the traumatized pole, bluntly or sharply excising the affected tissues, ligating local bleeding points and oversewing the peritoneum/ capsule back over the remaining healthy tissues. The animal may be anaemic (renal neoplasia, trauma, idiopathic haemorrhage) or polycythaemic (renal carcinoma); appropriate blood or fluid transfusions should be given.

In renal neoplasia cases the animal should be examined for evidence of metastases, both before and during surgery. Discussions with the owners concerning the prognosis and treatment options should take place before surgery is performed. If severe widespread malignancy is suspected but requires laparotomy for diagnosis, the owners should be prepared for the possibility of euthanasia *while the animal is still anaesthetized*. This is much less stressful for all concerned than discussions and euthanasia of the animal after its recovery from anaesthesia. It should be noted that renal tumours in cats are usually lymphosarcomas.

There is some debate over which structures should be ligated first during nephrectomy: the blood vessels or the ureter? The author prefers to ligate the vessels first because ligation of the ureter before the vessels results in renal swelling as urine continues to be produced but not excreted.

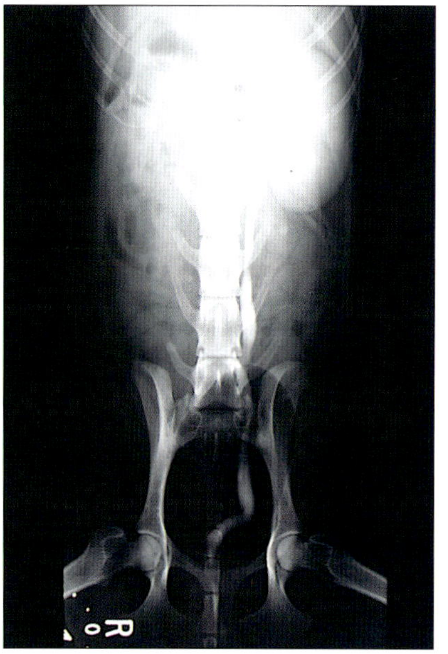

4.6 Ventrodorsal abdominal radiograph of an incontinent female Shetland sheepdog, ten minutes after intravenous injection of contrast medium. Nephrectomy would be an inappropriate form of treatment for the ureteral ectopia in this dog as it has only one functional kidney.

Possible surgical/post-surgical complications

Haemorrhage may occur, peri- or postoperatively; double ligation of renal vessels (one transfixing) is suggested. An intravenous cannula should always be placed before surgery and kept patent in case of haemorrhage requiring administration of blood or plasma expanders.

Urine contamination of the peritoneal cavity can result if vesico-ureteral reflux occurs; ureteral ligation is mandatory.

It has been suggested that an arteriovenous fistula may develop after surgery if the renal artery and vein are ligated together. The author believes this to be a theoretical rather than a practical problem using the technique described and, in some animals, the size of the kidney and its vessels makes separation of the artery and vein hazardous.

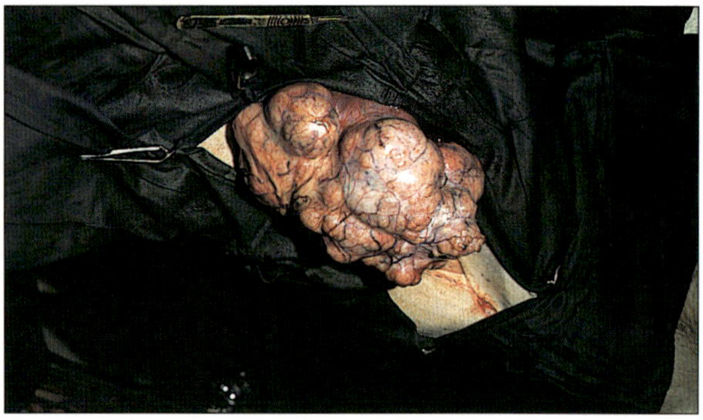

4.7 A large renal carcinoma in a German shepherd dog. The technique for ligation of blood vessels described below is designed to prevent surgical or post-surgical haemorrhage but, in cases like this, it may be difficult to expose the vessels adequately for double ligation. In these circumstances, one may have to rely on single ligation of the renal vessels, if possible, using a crushing ligature technique. In addition, large vessels in the overlying peritoneum should be ligated individually as the peritoneum is stripped from the kidney.

Technique

4.8

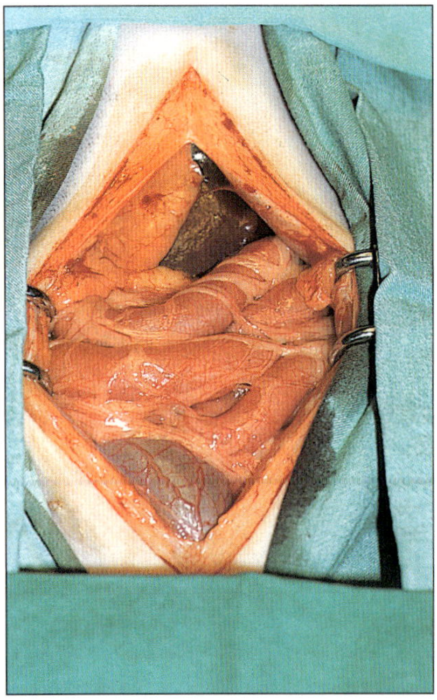

4.8 The kidneys can be approached from flank or ventral abdominal incisions. The author prefers a ventral mid-line abdominal approach, extending from the xiphisternum to just caudal to the umbilicus (for nephrectomy alone) or to the pubis (for ureteronephrectomy). The advantage of the mid-line approach over a flank approach is that it allows access to a greater area of the abdomen. This is important in cases of renal neoplasia (to examine for the presence or absence of metastases) and/or if the ureter is also diseased and requires removal. In addition, most surgeons are more familiar with this approach than the use of flank incisions. Once the abdomen is opened, the kidneys must be located.

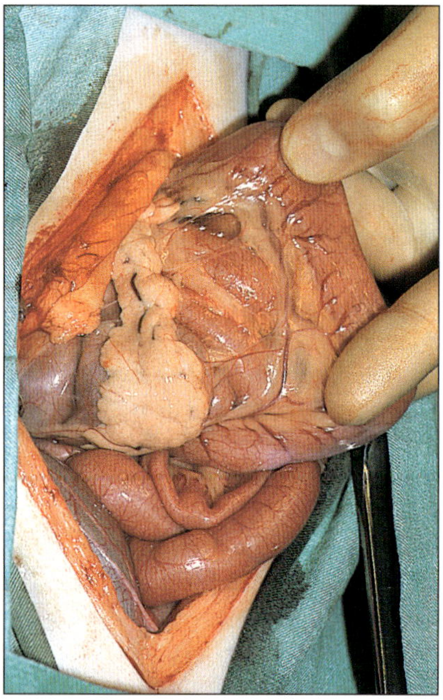

4.9 The right kidney is found by locating and elevating the duodenum, as illustrated.

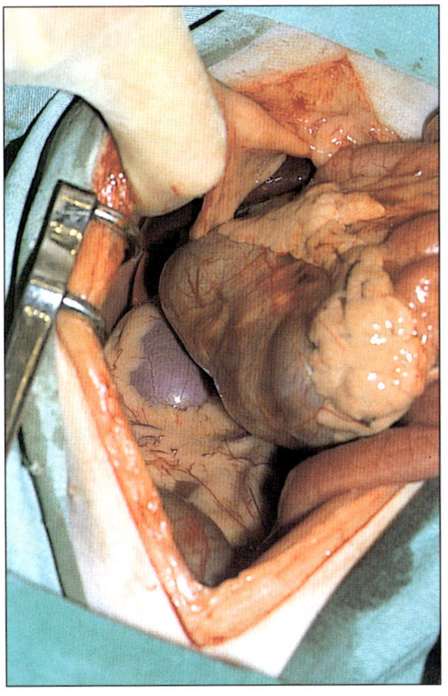

4.10 If the duodenum is now reflected medially, the right kidney is exposed and the mesoduodenum is used to prevent the intestines from returning to the right side of the cranial abdomen.

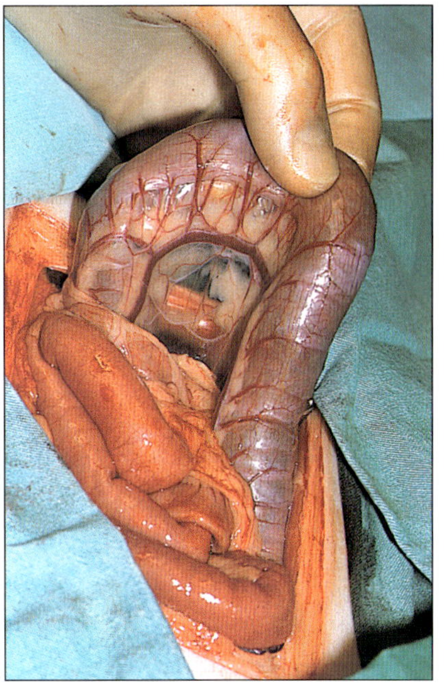

4.11 The left kidney is located in a similar fashion except that the descending colon is found and elevated.

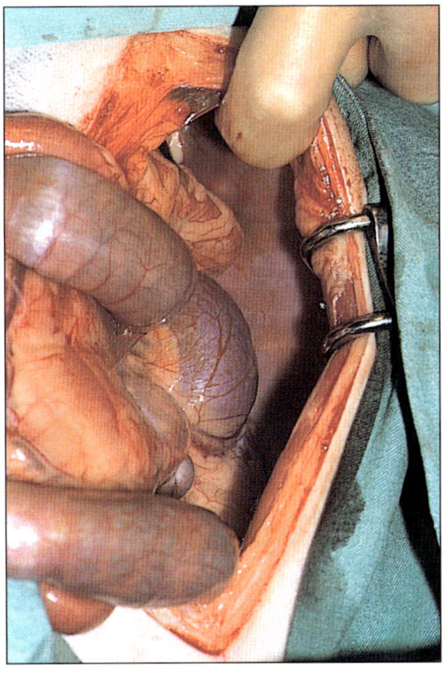

4.12 The descending colon is reflected medially, the mesocolon retaining the intestines and allowing access to the left kidney. The kidneys are attached to the dorsal abdominal wall by the overlying peritoneum and cannot immediately be raised to the level of the abdominal incision. Access to the kidneys can be improved if an assistant depresses the ipsilateral side of the abdominal incision, thus reducing the distance between incision and kidney.

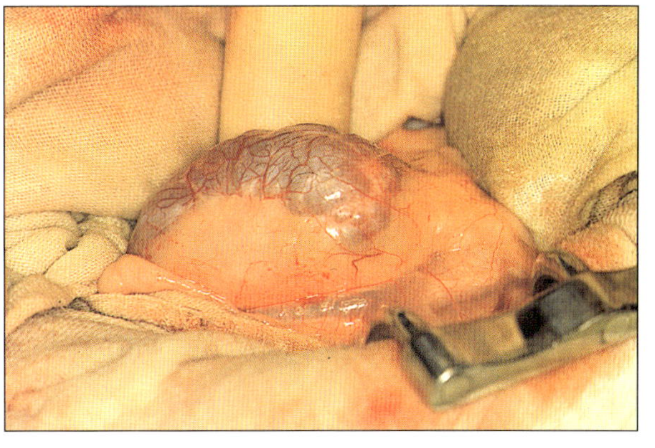

4.13 The kidney is gently elevated and the surrounding viscera packed off with moistened swabs. This particular animal has severe chronic pyelonephritis associated with ureteral ectopia. Prolonged tension in the kidney should be avoided because the transference of traction to the renal vessels may result in tension on the major abdominal vessels, particularly the vena cava, reducing venous return of blood to the heart. Any tension placed on the renal hilus during surgery should, therefore, be intermittent and not prolonged.

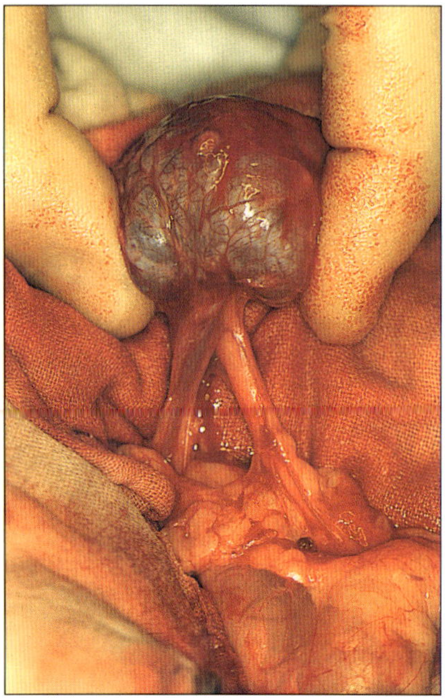

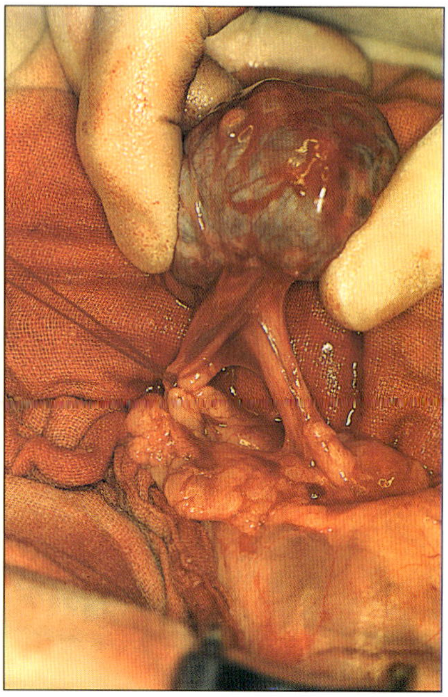

4.14 The peritoneum overlying the kidney and the hilar fat are freed from the kidney, allowing the renal vessels (cranial – to the left in the illustration) and ureter (caudal – to the right in the illustration) to be isolated. Blunt, finger dissection is the safest way to free these tissues. The peritoneum may be firmly attached to the kidney by the disease process, making separation difficult and resulting in haemorrhage from multiple points on the kidney surface. Such haemorrhage is usually minor and ceases when the renal vessels are ligated. More severe haemorrhage is controlled by direct application of pressure (it is not usually possible to clamp and ligate vessels as the bleeding points are often on the surface of the kidney). Large peritoneal vessels are ligated. Obviously, great care should be taken when dissecting around the hilus to avoid damage to the major renal vessels.

4.15 Once the kidney, its vessels and proximal ureter are freed from their attachments, the renal vessels are ligated. It has been suggested that the renal artery and vein should be ligated separately to avoid the possibility of postoperative arteriovenous fistulation. In the author's opinion, this is not necessary: such fistulation appears to be more of a theoretical rather than a practical consideration and, in cases of gross renal enlargement and disease, it would be hazardous to attempt to separate the renal vessels. The author's preferred technique is to use two ligatures. The first is a simple ligature placed proximally around both the artery and vein, as illustrated.

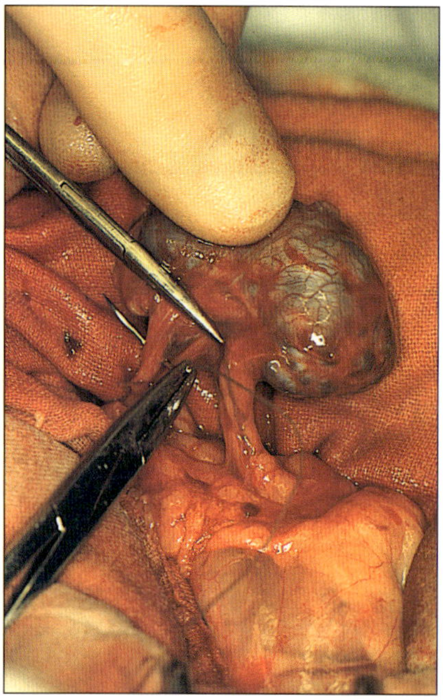

4.16 Once the first ligature has been tied, a transfixing ligature is placed distal to it. The second ligature is transfixed by taking it between the renal artery and vein. If this is not possible, the ligature can be taken through one of these vessels as haemorrhage is prevented by means of the first, simple ligature and by clamping of the vessels adjacent to the renal hilus.

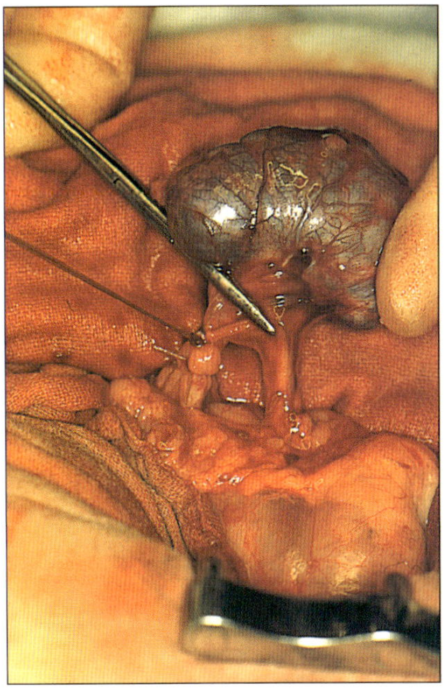

4.17 The transfixing ligature is now tied as shown. The material used for ligation is a matter of personal preference; the author prefers to use synthetic absorbable material. It should be noted that such double ligation of the renal vessels is not always possible, particulary if the kidney is grossly enlarged and/or diseased (see **4.5** and **4.7**). In such cases, the enlarged kidney and the presence of local adhesions may make access to, and identification of, renal vessels difficult and sometimes only single ligation is possible.

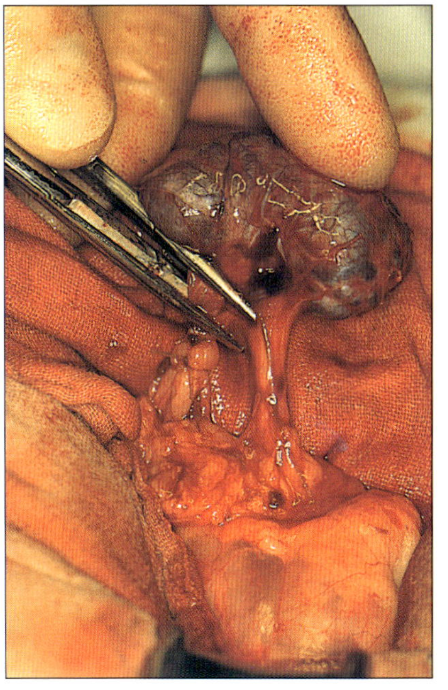

4.18 The vessels are now sectioned between the distal transfixing ligature and the clamps.

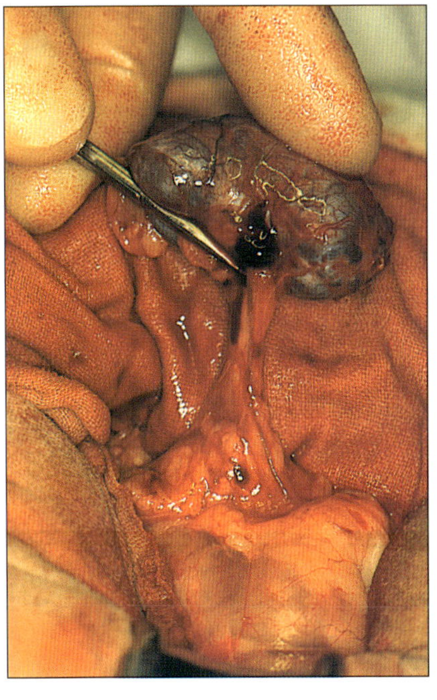

4.19 Only the ureter now remains attached to the kidney. If the ureter is not diseased (as in this case), it can be clamped at the hilus and a simple ligature applied approximately 2 cm distally. The kidney can now be removed by sectioning the ureter between the clamps and ligature. Some authors suggest that the ureter should be excised down to its insertion into the bladder as otherwise it may act as a reservoir for stagnant urine (especially if vesico-ureteral reflux is present), predisposing to recurring urinary tract infections. However, normal ureteral peristalsis in an undiseased ureter results in ureteral emptying and the author has experienced no difficulties in animals in which healthy ureters have not been excised during nephrectomy.

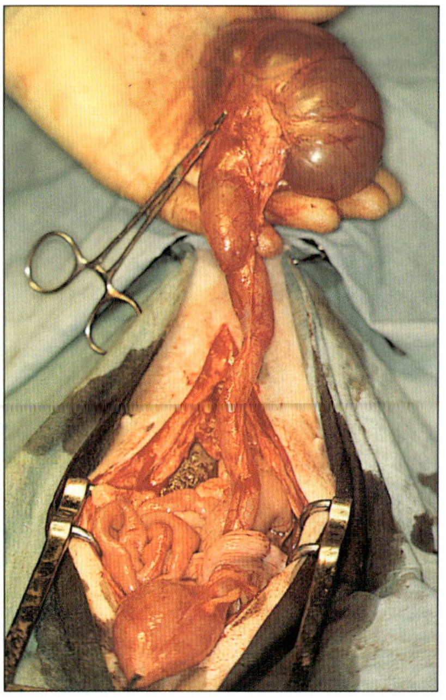

4.20 If the ureter is diseased, it should be removed along with the kidney. In this example, both hydronephrosis and hydro-ureter are present. If the ureter is not removed, it may act as a reservoir for urinary tract infections (ureteral peristalsis is usually poor in animals with such gross ureteral disease). If gentle traction is applied to the ureter, it can be pulled from its retroperitoneal position. Note, however, that the distal ureter passes beneath the uterine horn and its broad ligament (or vas deferens in the male). There is no need to perform traumatic dissection on the uterus or broad ligament; the distal ureter can be freed as illustrated in **4.21–4.27**.

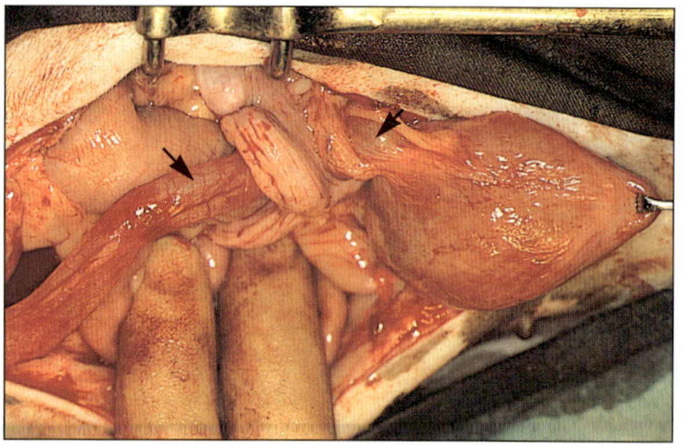

4.21 The distal ureter is identified (arrowed) as it passes beneath the uterus and broad ligament and inserts into the dorsal wall of the bladder.

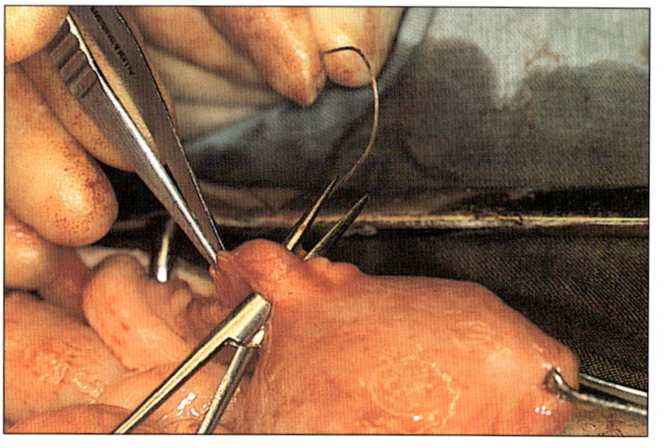

4.22 The tip of a pair of artery forceps is passed through the peritoneum and beneath the ureter as it enters the dorsal wall of the bladder.

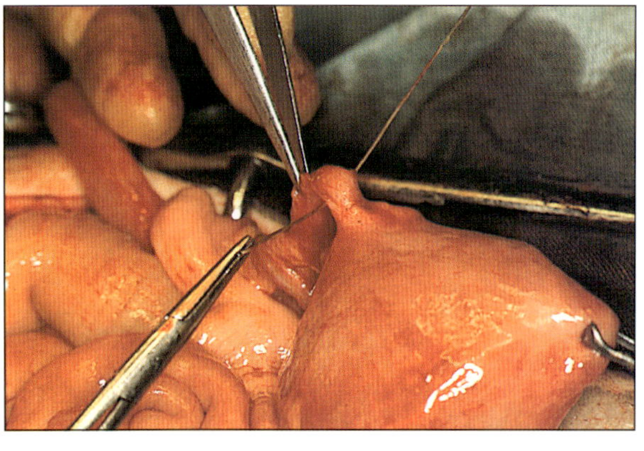

4.23 The forceps are used to place ligature material beneath the ureter, as the forceps are withdrawn.

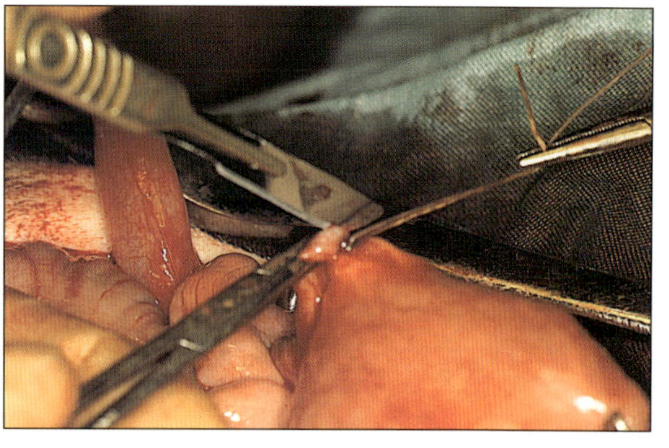

4.24 The ureter (and its associated vessels) are ligated adjacent to the bladder wall, clamped approximately 1 cm cranially and sectioned between the clamps and ligature.

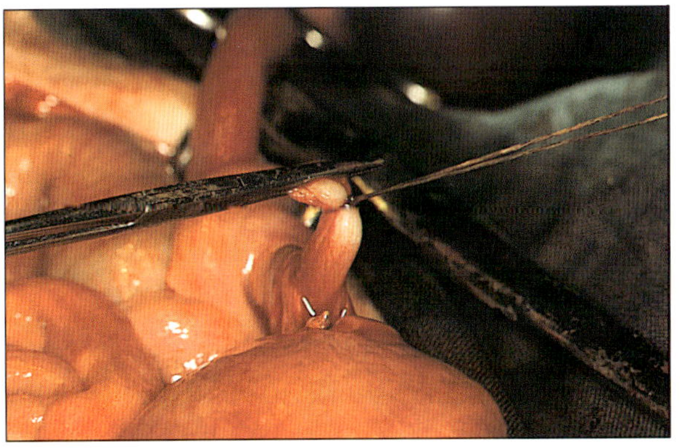

4.25 The freed, distal ureter is now ligated as shown to prevent urine leakage following removal of the clamps.

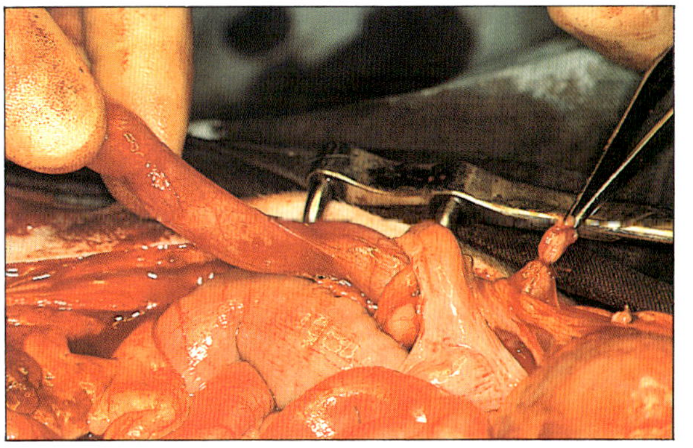

4.26 The clamps are removed, the ureter cranial to the uterus is grasped and gentle cranial traction applied.

4.27 The distal ureter can be pulled retroperitoneally below the uterus and broad ligament (or vas deferens in the male) until it is completely freed. The kidney and ureter can now be removed from the abdomen. The stumps of the renal vessels are checked for the absence of bleeding before the abdomen is closed routinely.

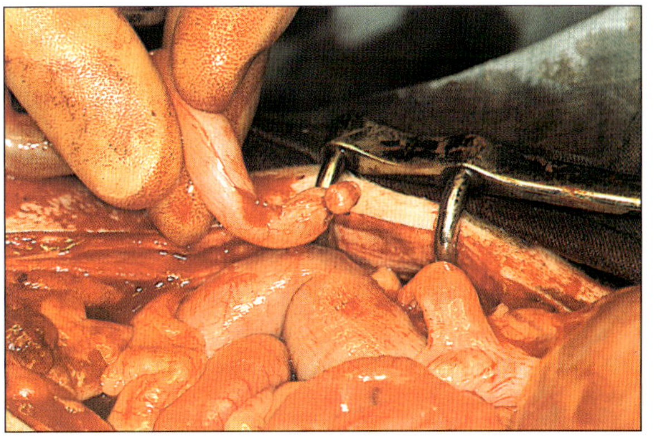

Nephrotomy

Indications

- Nephrolithiasis.

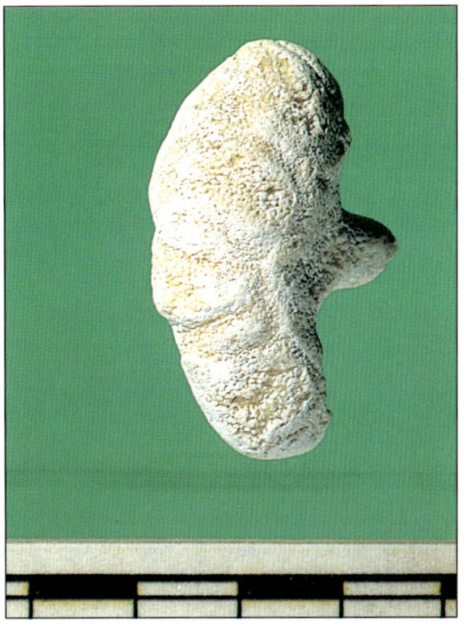

4.28 Renal calculus (struvite) removed from a Labrador bitch. The calculus conforms to the shape of the renal pelvis with a 'beak' corresponding to the proximal ureteral orifice.

Pre- and peri-operative considerations

Nephrotomy is traumatic to a kidney, the function of which may already be impaired, and should not be carried out unless absolutely necessary. An attempt should be made to dissolve the calculus *in situ* first by the use of appropriate dietary measures, antibiotics and urinary pH changes. The success or failure of attempts at dissolution is determined by follow-up radiography and/or ultrasonography.

Care must be taken to ensure that the animal's presenting signs are due to nephrolithiasis and not something else; renal calculi are often asymptomatic and may be seen on plain abdominal radiographs of animals which appear to be clinically normal. However, the calculi may also be indicators of severe renal disease; blood and urine laboratory analyses should be performed to assess renal function pre-operatively or, if surgery is not to be performed, such analyses should be repeated from time to time to ensure that renal function is not deteriorating as a result of the presence of calculi which cannot be dissolved *in situ*.

Even if renal function appears to be satisfactory, an intravenous cannula should always be placed pre-operatively for fluid administration as nephrotomy inevitably results in a temporary impairment of function in the operated kidney.

For this reason, if nephrolithiasis is bilateral, it is inadvisable to perform bilateral nephrotomy on the same occasion; nephrotomies on the animal's individual kidneys should be separated by a period of 4–6 weeks to allow the first kidney to recover before surgery is performed on the second kidney.

It is worth repeating that nephrotomy should be a last resort. In the author's experience, this operation is rarely required nowadays as most renal calculi can be dissolved *in situ* by appropriate dietary and antimicrobial measures.

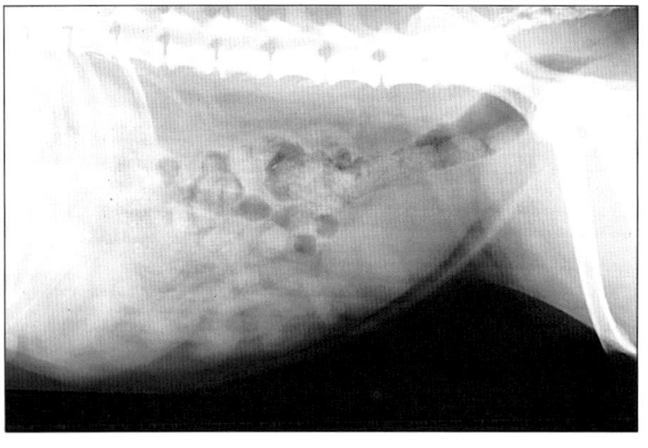

4.29 Lateral abdominal radiograph of the same animal illustrated in 2.1, four months later. This Cavalier King Charles spaniel was presented with severe, acute abdominal pain. Abdominal radiography revealed renal and vesical calculi (**2.1**), which were assumed to be the cause of the signs. However, blood laboratory analyses revealed that the pain was associated with acute pancreatitis, for which the animal was treated with prophylactic antibiotics (ampicillin) and a bland diet (chicken and rice). The radiograph illustrated above reveals that all calculi have disappeared. This animal had triple phosphate crystals and bacteria in its urine; presumably the calculi were of the same material and dissolved in response to elimination of urinary tract infection and a high biological value, low-protein diet. This case underlines two points: the renal calculus or calculi may not be responsible for the presenting signs and nephrotomy may not be required to eliminate nephroliths.

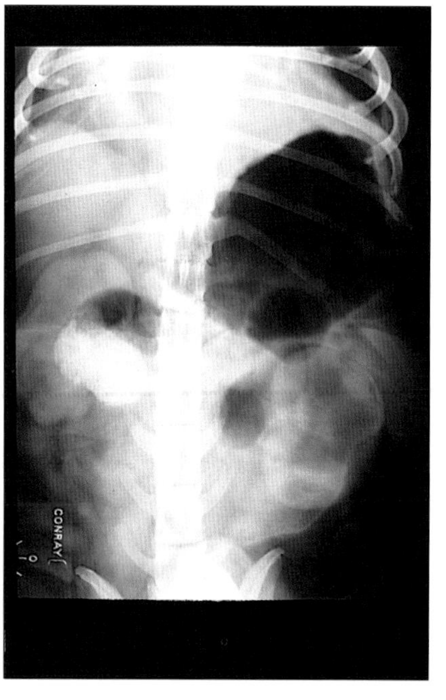

4.30 Ventrodorsal nephrogram during IVU of an 11-year-old debilitated Pug with chronic haematuria. A large renal calculus was present in the right renal pelvis. However, note also the irregular outline of both kidneys and the poor renal opacification by contrast medium. This animal had severe, chronic bilateral pyelonephritis, and nephrotomy to remove the calculus was sufficient to induce acute, fatal renal failure. The case illustrates the potential hazards of nephrectomy and the need for good laboratory work-up before surgery is considered. This type of case would probably be managed best medically.

Possible surgical/post-surgical complications

Haemorrhage occurs from the renal parenchymal blood vessels; attention should be paid to suturing. Non-suturing nephrotomy techniques have been described but are not advised by this author. Although they are intended to reduce the likelihood of iatrogenic postoperative renal vascular damage, there is the risk of haemorrhage or urine leakage from the unclosed nephrotomy. At the time of writing, there is insufficient data on the use of non-suturing techniques in significant numbers of clinical cases (as opposed to healthy experimental animals) to evaluate their safety. The author remains to be convinced and, if serious complications occurred due to blood loss or urine leakage from a nephrotomy wound which was not sutured, it would be difficult to defend a case of negligence brought to court by the owners.

Renal infarction may develop postoperatively. This is iatrogenic and usually results from poor suturing technique (hence the use by some authors of non-suturing methods). Care should be taken to avoid placing mattress sutures, in particular, too deep and/or tying them too tight (see below).

Technique

The technique is illustrated by means of line diagrams only, as no suitable cases were available for photography. As described above, nephrotomy is a traumatic procedure and is rarely indicated nowadays because it is usually possible to dissolve renal calculi *in situ* using calculolytic diets and appropriate antimicrobial therapy to eliminate urinary tract infections. Indeed, at the time of writing, it is over five years since the author last had to perform a nephrotomy, all cases of nephrolithiasis being treated successfully by calculus dissolution. As no suitable cases were available for photography, the technique is illustrated by line drawings.

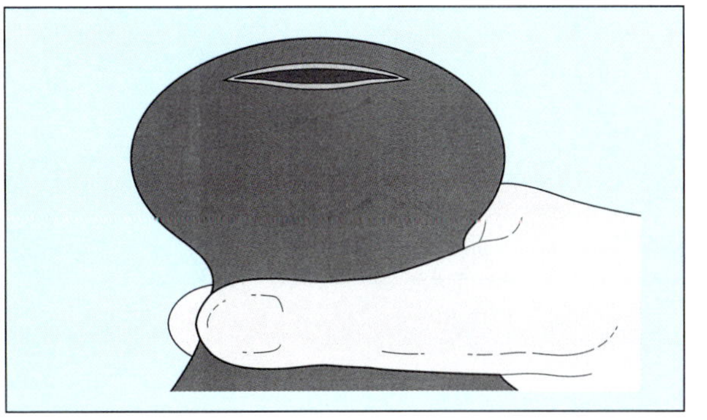

4.31 The kidney is approached and located as illustrated in 4.8–4.12. In the author's opinion, nephrotomy (like nephrectomy) requires the help of a surgical assistant. The assistant grasps the hilus of the kidney between the thumb and index finger of one (gloved) hand and uses the other hand to depress the ipsilateral side of the abdominal incision to improve access to the kidney by the surgeon. As well as supporting the kidney for surgery, the assistant can feel the pulse in the renal artery through the perihilar peritoneum and fat and can thus occlude the renal vessels during surgery (for haemostasis). Similarly, pressure on the hilus will occlude the ureter, preventing fragments of the calculus from passing into the ureter during surgical manipulations. The alternatives to the use of an assistant's finger and thumb involve dissecting through the perihilar tissues, isolating the renal vessels and occluding them temporarily with atraumatic vascular clamps or loops. In the author's view, the use of an assistant's digits is quicker, easier and less traumatic, and there is no need to move the kidney during surgery if it is desirable to resume renal blood flow; the assistant merely relaxes his/her grip slightly. An incision is made through the peritoneum, renal capsule and renal parenchyma into the renal pelvis. The location of the renal pelvis can be appreciated when the scalpel blade contacts the calculus. The size of the incision is related to the size of the calculus but it usually extends approximately over the middle third of the greater curvature of the kidney. The calculus is removed using forceps and submitted for analysis. Any remaining fragments of calculus are removed with forceps and by flushing the renal pelvis with sterile saline. If the surgery thus far has taken more than 10 minutes, the assistant should allow blood to flow through the kidney for a minute or so. Haemorrhage from the nephrotomy can be reduced by gently holding the incision closed during this period.

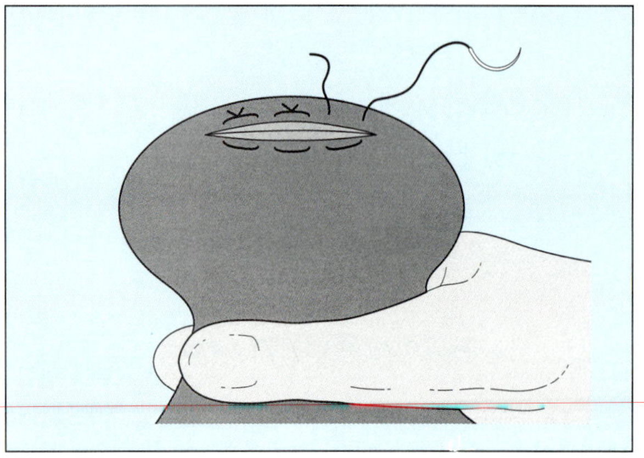

4.32 The nephrotomy incision is closed. The author prefers to appose the renal parenchyma using horizontal mattress sutures of synthetic absorbable material. The sutures should be placed through the peritoneum, renal capsule and renal cortex but should not be placed too deep or too tight, to avoid damage to the arcuate vessels at the cortico-medullary junction. They should be placed to a depth of approximately half that of the renal cortex.

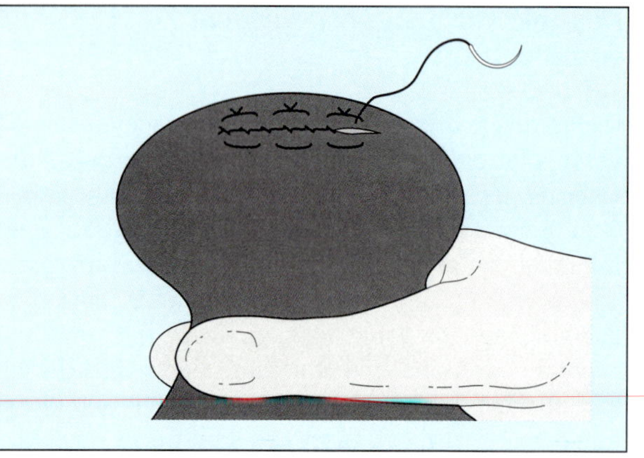

4.33 After apposition of the renal parenchyma, the renal capsule and peritoneum are closed in a single layer using a simple continuous suture, again of synthetic absorbable material. The abdomen is closed routinely. Note:some authors compromise between the technique described here and non-suturing methods by closing only the renal capsule and peritoneum.

Ureteral repair

Indications

- Ureteral trauma.

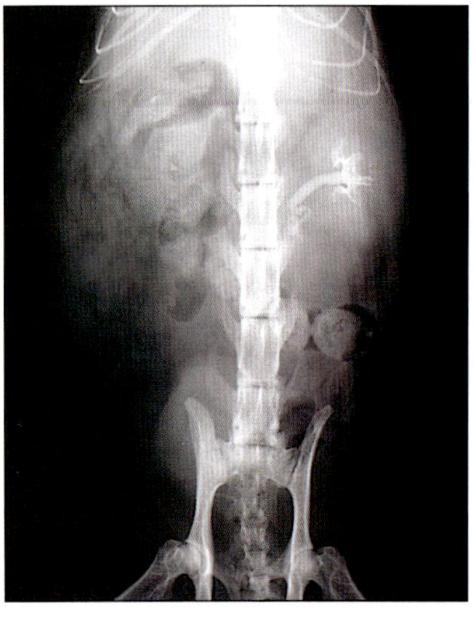

4.34 Proximal ureteral rupture in a cat after a road traffic accident, demonstrated by intravenous urography. Note the increase in soft tissue density surrounding the left kidney due to retroperitoneal leakage of urine (see also **2.18**).

Pre- and peri-operative considerations

Uraemia, acidosis, hyperkalaemia are likely to be present but, because urine leaks predominantly into retroperitoneal tissues, these changes occur more slowly than would be the case if bladder rupture had occurred. It may be difficult to find the ureter and/or tear because of the swelling and urine cellulitis in surrounding tissues. Pre-operative IVU is essential. During surgery, one should be prepared for ventral cystotomy and ureteral catheterization (using a 3Fr or 4Fr catheter). If cystoscopy is available, it may be possible to pass a ureteral catheter non-invasively, pre-operatively under endoscopic guidance in dogs. The small size of cats makes this procedure more difficult. Ureteral catheterization allows palpation of the ureter (because of the presence of the catheter) and, if necessary, retrograde flushing of the ureter with sterile saline to identify the site(s) of small leaks during surgery. The catheter can be left *in situ* postoperatively as a stent (see below).

Finally, ureteral surgery is delicate and requires fine surgical instruments; a major pre-operative consideration should be whether the case is best referred to a veterinary urologist with more experience and/or better instrumentation.

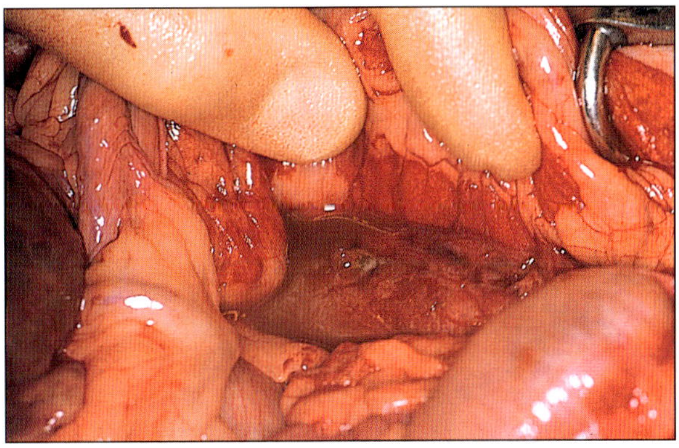

4.35 The laparotomy appearance of a ruptured ureter in the Golden Retriever bitch illustrated in 2.18. Urine can be seen leaking from the retroperitoneal tissues, the swelling of which (due to infiltration of urine and cellulitis) prevents visualization of the ureter. Retrograde catheterization of the (ectopic) ureter was used in this case to facilitate identification of the ureter and the tear during dissections through the swollen peri-ureteral tissues.

Possible surgical/post-surgical complications

Ureteral stricture may develop after ureteral trauma and repair. It is important to debride all devitalized tissues before repair. The ureter should be repaired or anastomosed using fine (5/0) synthetic absorbable sutures in a simple interrupted pattern. An in-dwelling ureteral catheter can be placed during surgery and left as a stent for three to five days. The catheter should be long enough to pass from proximal to the site of repair, down the ureter, through the bladder and urethra and is sutured to the prepuce or vulva (as illustrated in **3.4**). The animal should be fitted with an Elizabethan collar or body brace to prevent it from removing the catheter. Fluid diuresis is useful both during surgery and postoperatively to flush debris and small blood clots from the ureter and to stimulate ureteral patency.

Technique

The technique is illustrated by the repair of an iatrogenic ureterovaginal fistula in a female dog.

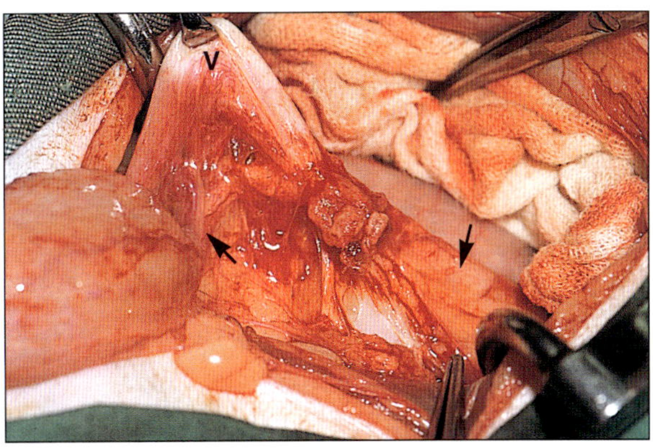

4.36 Laparotomy findings in a juvenile Cocker spaniel bitch with an iatrogenic ureterovaginal fistula (following ovariohysterectomy). The bladder has been reflected caudally (to the left) and its dorsal wall exposed. The vagina (v) has been elevated and the site of fistulation exposed. Cranial to the granuloma on the anterior vagina, the ureter is identified (arrowed) surrounded by peritoneum and fat. In this animal, the insertion of the caudal ureter into the bladder can also be seen (also arrowed) – this was not detectable on pre-operative contrast radiography. An intra-operative decision was made to resect the cranial vaginal granuloma and traumatized section of ureter and to perform ureteral anastomosis. If insufficient caudal ureter remains in these cases and/or gross hydro-ureter (+/– hydronephrosis) exists, re-implantation of the ureter into the bladder (using an extravesical technique – see **4.60–4.76**) or ureteronephrectomy (see **4.8–4.27**) is required.

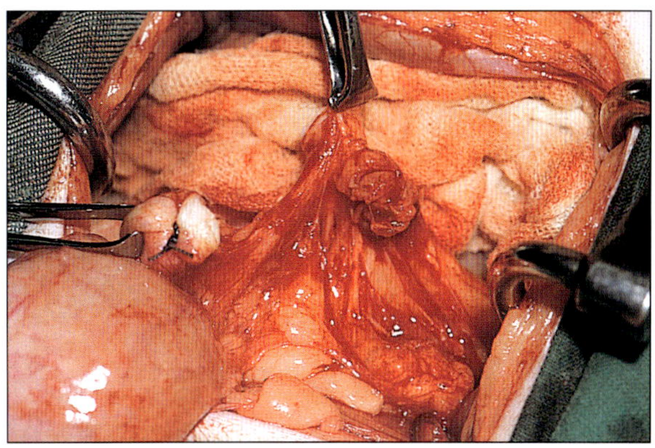

4.37 The cranial vagina is ligated and sectioned caudal to the granuloma, as shown.

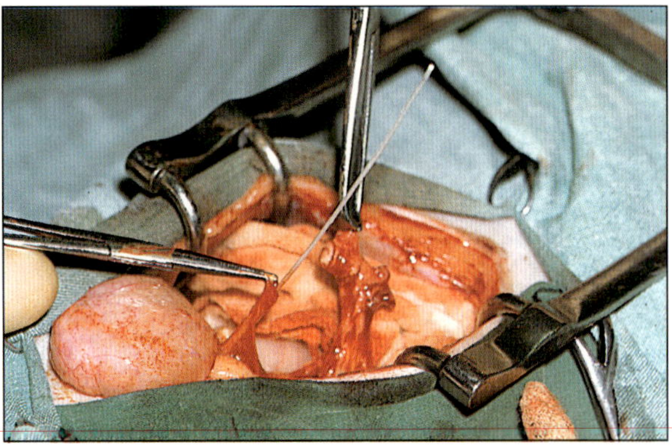

4.38 The granuloma containing the ureterovaginal fistula is excised, leaving caudal and cranial sections of ureter which require anastomosis. The ends of the ureter can be cut obliquely or/and spatulated (see **4.66 and 4.67**) to reduce the risk of postoperative stenosis at the site of anastomosis, but this was not considered to be necessary in this case. Any bleeding ureteral vessels should be clamped and ligated level with the ends of the ureter. The hub of a 3Fr urinary catheter has been cut off and the catheter passed, hub end first, through the caudal ureter (identified by the artery clamps on the ureteral vessel), bladder and urethra to exit at the vulva.

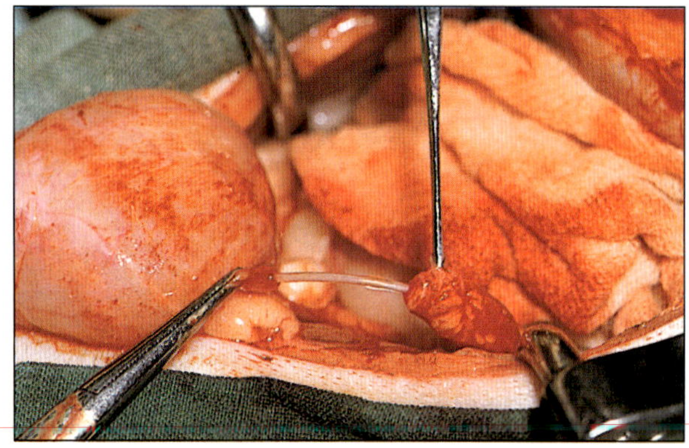

4.39 The catheter tip is now introduced into the cranial section of ureter (being held by fine rat-toothed forceps) and passed cranially to a level just distal to the ureteropelvic junction.

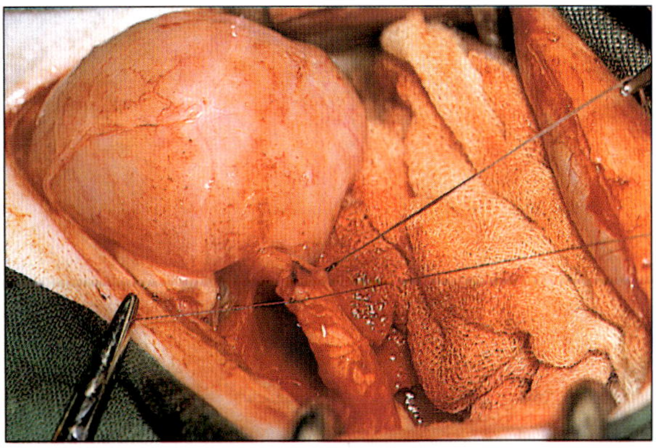

4.40 The ureter is now anastomosed, taking care to avoid rotation of the ureteral sections around their longitudinal axis. Simple interrupted sutures have been placed 180° apart to facilitate orientation and handling. Fine synthetic absorbable sutures (e.g. 5/0 polyglactin – Vicryl, Ethicon) should be used in a simple interrupted pattern. Ureteral surgery is less traumatic and suture placement improved if fine ocular instruments are used.

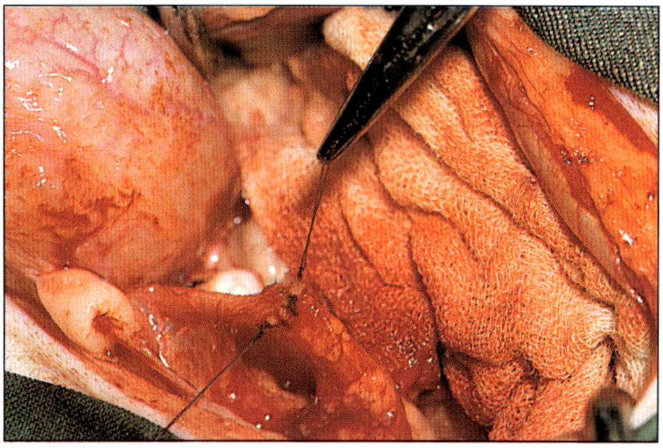

4.41 Anastomosis is completed and the ureter observed for leakage during peristalsis. Alternatively, if ureteral peristalsis is poor, a few millilitres of sterile saline can be injected slowly up the catheter to test for leaks. Any leakage sites should be sealed by further suturing, as required. Following routine abdominal closure, the catheter is sutured to the paravulval perineal skin (or preputial skin in male animals), as illustrated in **3.4,** and left *in situ* for three to five days. In some animals, despite being sutured in place, the in-dwelling ureteral catheter will come out within 72 hours, presumably as a result of ureteral peristalsis and urine flow pressures.

Ureteral transplantation

Indications

- Ectopic ureter (see **2.15** and **2.35**).
- Ureterovaginal fistula.
- Irreparable distal ureteral trauma.
- Distal ureteral or trigonal neoplasia.

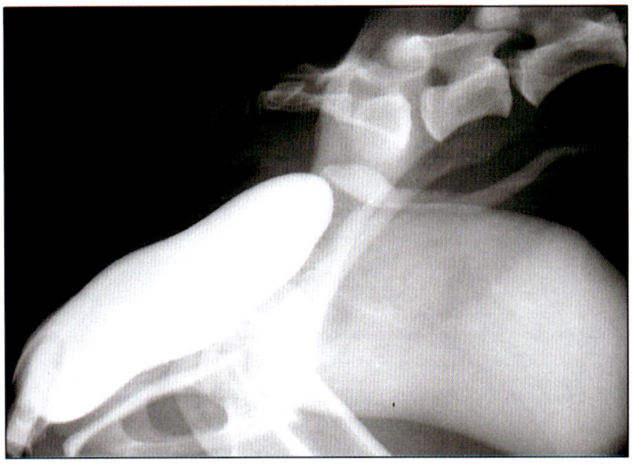

4.42 Iatrogenic ureterovaginal fistula after ovariohysterectomy in a bitch. The fistula has been demonstrated by retrograde positive contrast vaginography during which contrast medium passes from the cranial vagina into a distal, dilated ureter. Another case is illustrated in **4.36–4.41**.

Pre- and peri-operative considerations

There are species differences in ureteral ectopia. Ectopic ureters in dogs usually enter the bladder at the normal site and travel intramurally, but instead of entering the bladder lumen at the trigone, they continue intramurally beyond the bladder neck to open ectopically, usually into the urethra or vagina. In the cat, ectopic ureters usually bypass the bladder completely to terminate in the urethra or vagina. This means that in cats (and in animals in which the distal ureter has to be excised – e.g. trauma, neoplasia, ureterovaginal fistulation) the ureter must be tunnelled through the bladder wall during transplantation. In most dogs, particularly bitches, transplantation makes use of the fact that the ureter is in its normal position within the bladder wall but travels too far intramurally. In some male dogs, the presence of the prostate, particularly if this extends cranially around the bladder neck, may make access to the trigone difficult and necessitate the use of a tunnelling technique.

The presence of two kidneys should have been determined by the pre-operative contrast radiography which was used to diagnose the condition (see Chapter 2). If only one kidney is present (e.g. **4.6**), an indwelling ureteral catheter (see 'Ureteral Repair' above) should be used for a few days postoperatively to ensure adequate patency of the distal ureter in the event of bladder wall oedema. If marked bladder wall oedema develops during surgery in animals with bilateral ectopia, it is safer to transplant one ureter only at this stage, leaving the second until 4–6 weeks later. Oedema may obstruct the distal transplanted ureter(s) and, if this is bilateral, may result in acute post-renal renal failure and death. This is particularly true in the case of juvenile animals, which are much more prone to oedema of the bladder wall during surgery than older animals. In uncomplicated cases of ureteral ectopia, therefore, it is best to delay transplantation until the animal is five months old. This age is something of a compromise; surgery on younger animals may be hazardous whereas delaying further may allow complications such as hydronephrosis or pyelonephritis to develop or worsen.

It is imperative that any urinary tract infection is eliminated before surgery is performed. If not, severe complications may result (see below).

If severe hydro-ureter and hydronephrosis are present, ureteronephrectomy is indicated, rather than ureteral transplantation (e.g. **2.4**, **2.16 and 2.17**).

Renal function in the majority of animals with ureteral ectopia is usually not impaired. However, in bilateral cases in which there is radiographic evidence of bilateral renal disease, pre-operative renal function tests are mandatory to determine if surgery is likely to result in overt renal failure (see **Table 3.3**).

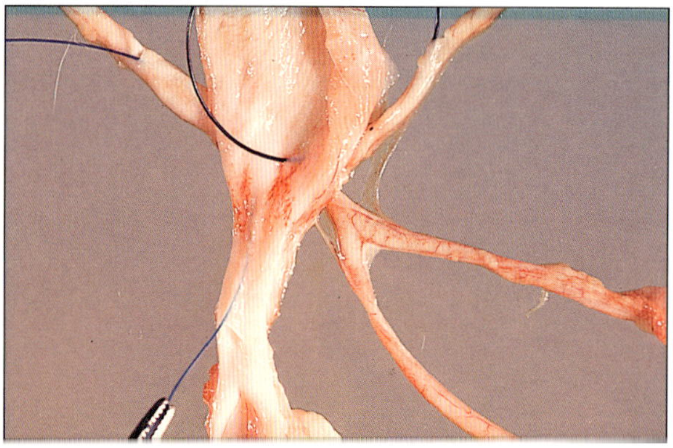

4.43 ***Post mortem*** **specimen illustrating the usual site of ureteral ectopia, in a Golden retriever bitch puppy.** Blue nylon has been inserted into the ureters. Note that the abnormal ureter enters the bladder wall at the same level as the normal ureter but then travels intramurally beyond the bladder neck to open ectopically into the urethra, the commonest site of termination of ectopic ureters in the dog. This means that ectopia cannot be diagnosed by exploratory laparotomy (unless a cystotomy is performed and absence of a trigonal ureteral termination detected – even then, the situation may be confused by the presence of distal ureteral branches). More diagnostic information is obtained with less trauma to the patient by performing good contrast radiography than by an exploratory laparotomy. The intramural route of the ectopic ureter also means that this part of the ureter can be stomatized into the bladder (see below).

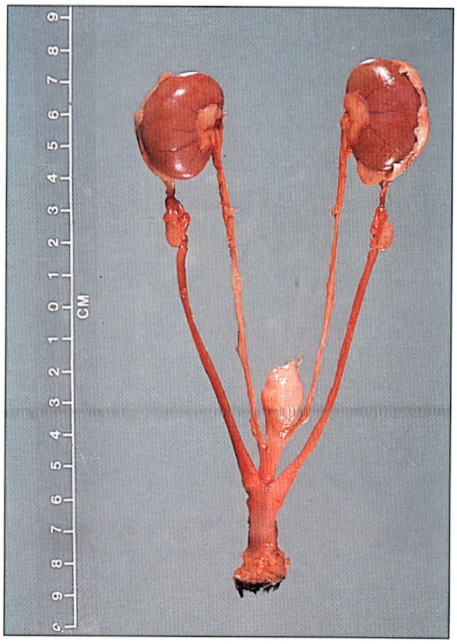

4.44 The situation is different in most cats, as can be seen from this ***post mortem*** **specimen.** The cat had bilateral ureteral ectopia, with both ureters bypassing the bladder and opening ectopically into the proximal and distal parts of a hypoplastic urethra. The animal also had a hypoplastic bladder and absence of a vagina, the latter due to congenital failure of the Müllerian ducts to unite. The extramural route of the ureter in cats and a minority of dogs means that the ureter has to be tunnelled through the bladder wall during transplantation (see below).

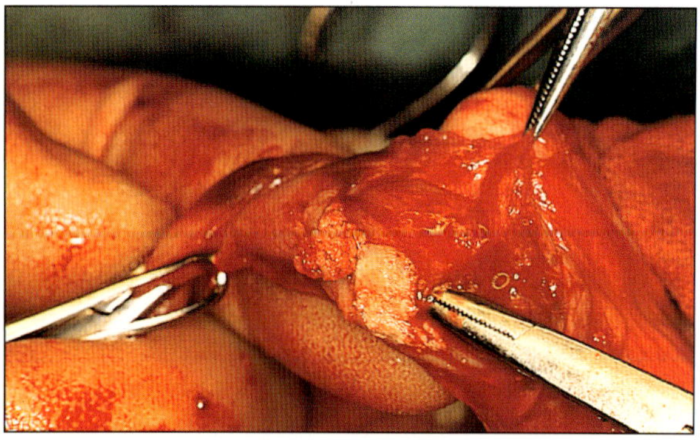

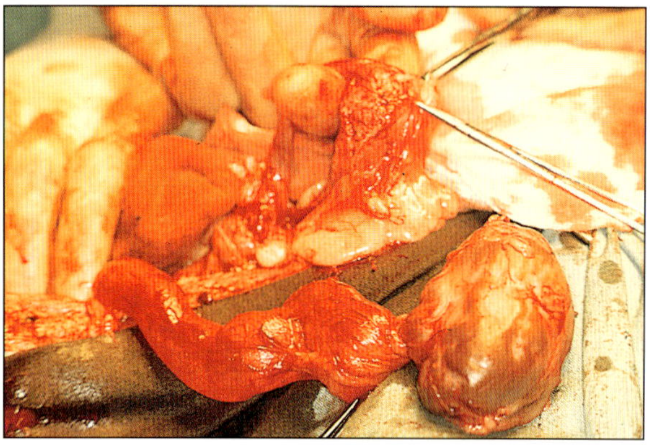

4.45 The potential effects of urinary tract infection on ureteral transplantation. The ectopic ureter of this Golden retriever bitch was transplanted before the results of urine cultures were known. These revealed the presence of *Proteus* infection and, despite prolonged antibiotic therapy based on bacteriological sensitivities, the infection persisted (*Proteus* can be a notoriously difficult organism to eliminate and rapidly develops resistance to an antibiotic). The infection resulted in severe cystitis, with mineralization of areas of bladder urothelium. One such area was the ureteral stoma **(top)**, which became obstructed, resulting in hydro-ureter and hydronephrosis **(bottom)**. Ureteronephrectomy was performed but, despite months of antibiotic therapy based on cultures and sensitivities, the *Proteus* colonized the remaining kidney. This in turn led to unresponsive acute renal failure, necessitating euthanasia eight months after the original operation to transplant the ureter. The experiences with this case are the reasons why the author now postpones surgery until any urinary tract infection has been treated and the success of treatment confirmed by negative cultures on follow-up urine bacteriology.

Possible surgical/post-surgical complications

The impairment of ureteral emptying associated with bladder wall oedema, particularly in young animals, has been described above. A further, rare postoperative problem associated with bladder wall oedema or intramural haematoma is dysuria. If transplantation has been performed at the level of the trigone (and thus close to the bladder neck) bladder wall swelling can sometimes obstruct the internal urethral orifice. This is more of a problem after the stomatization technique. An in-dwelling catheter should be used until the swelling has settled down (usually within five to seven days). In this situation, the author prefers a catheter inserted *per urethram* to a prepubic catheter as the latter may result in further bladder wall oedema and/or haemorrhage and worsen the situation.

The transplanted ureter can become obstructed by blood clots resulting from the surgery. This is a rare (and usually temporary) complication and can be avoided by the use of adequate parenteral fluids during surgery and immediately postoperatively so that any small clots are flushed from the ureter.

Hydro-ureter and hydronephrosis can develop, persist or worsen after ureteral transplantation. However, although at the time of writing there is insufficient data on large numbers of animals, the impression of the author and other veterinary urologists is that pre-existing hydro-ureter and hydronephrosis (unless severe) will often be reduced in severity by successful transplantation.

In bilateral cases, IVU should be repeated 4–6 weeks after transplantation of the first ureter to determine the presence (if any) and degree of hydro-ureter and hydronephrosis in the transplanted ureter/kidney before surgery is performed on the second ureter. If severe disease is present in the transplanted ureter and kidney, renal function tests should be carried out, especially if complications are present in the remaining ureter and kidney. If severe hydronephrosis has developed or worsened in the first kidney/ureter, retransplantation or even ureteronephrectomy may be required at the same time as the second ureter is transplanted.

It is possible that the stoma of a transplanted ureter may stenose, leading to hydro-ureter and hydronephrosis. This is rare and can be avoided by attention to suturing when making the stoma during surgery (see below) and ensuring that all urine from the associated kidney passes through it by adequate ureteral ligation distal to the stoma (in the case of the stomatization technique).

A minority of animals fail to become continent after successful ureteral transplantation. Persistence of urinary incontinence has been associated with undiagnosed bilateral ureteral ectopia, concomitant urethral sphincter mechanism incompetence, failure of a hypoplastic bladder to expand to accommodate the increased inflow of urine (this is rare) and distal ureteral branches (these are extremely rare). Distal ureteral branches may also occur following ureteral stomatization if recanalization of the ligated intramural portion of ureter takes place.

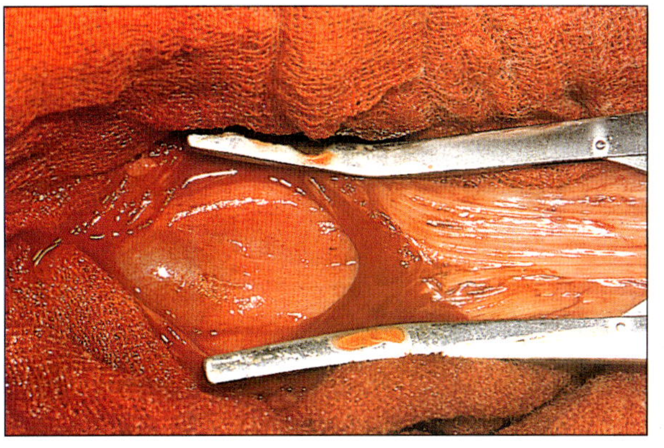

4.46 Distal ureteral branches have been reported as a cause of persistence of urinary incontinence after ureteral transplantation using tunnelling techniques. In these cases, the distal ureter opens ectopically but also communicates with the bladder lumen. Thus, following transplantation using a tunnelling technique, urine may pass from the bladder into the ureteral remnant and exit distally from the termination of the ectopic ureter, bypassing part of the urethral sphincter mechanism and leading to persistence of the incontinence. Although such branches may be congenital, they may also be acquired if a ureterocoel ruptures into the bladder. A case of bilateral ureteral ectopia is illustrated. A ventral, caudal cystotomy has been performed revealing a dilated intramural ureter (uppermost). Note the appearance of the second (lowermost) ectopic ureterocoel which is separated from the bladder by only a thin layer of tissue. This ruptured as soon as the overlying tissue was grasped with fine rat-toothed forceps. Rupture of a ureteroceol into the bladder lumen may result in so-called distal ureteral branches. The potential problem of distal ureteral branches is overcome if a stomatization technique is used (see below); all that is required is ligation of the intramural ureter distal to the opening into the bladder.

4.47 The appearance of a stomatized ureter (arrowed) two months after transplantation in a Yorkshire terrier bitch. Although the stoma has remained patent, the ureter distal to the stoma has recanalized, allowing urine from the ureter and bladder to exit via the ectopic part of the ureter and resulting in recurrence of the incontinence. This was successfully treated by re-ligation of the ureter distal to the stoma.

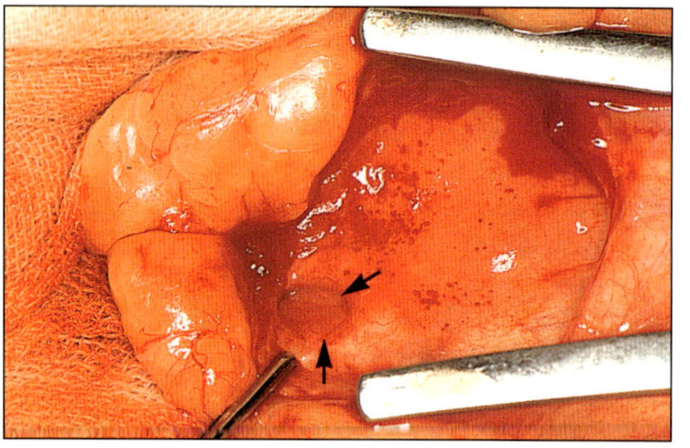

Techniques

Two techniques are described. The first is a stomatization technique, suitable for transplantation of ectopic ureters which enter the bladder normally but travel intramurally to open ectopically (see **4.43**). The second technique is suitable for transplantation of ureters which completely bypass the bladder (see **4.44**) or when access to an intramural ectopic ureter is difficult (e.g. in a male dog with an enlarged prostate).

Stomatization technique

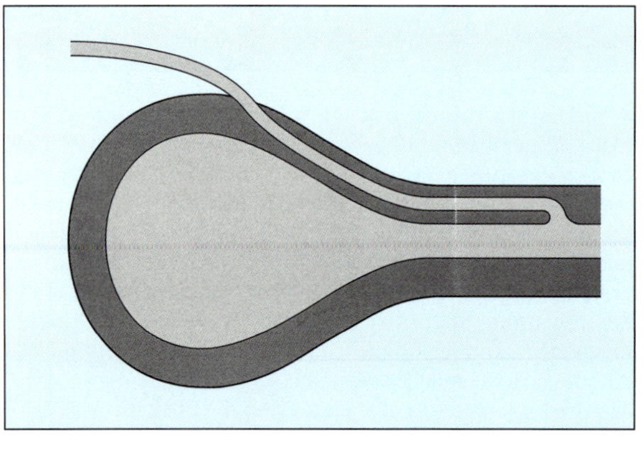

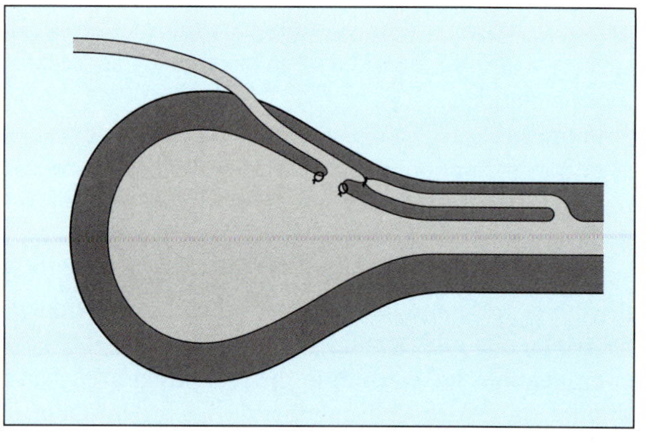

4.48 Diagrams summarizing the stomatization technique used to treat an intramural ectopic ureter (left). The ureter is stomatized into the bladder at the level of the trigone and ligated just distal to the stoma (**right**). The technique is described in detail below.

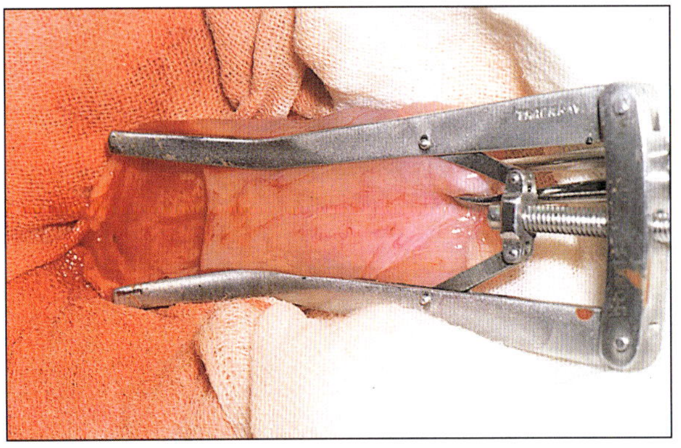

4.49 The intramural part of the ectopic ureter is approached via a ventral cystotomy (after emptying the bladder of urine by centesis or catheterization), just cranial to the bladder neck. Alms self-retaining retractors are useful for keeping the edges of the bladder incision apart. Alternatively, retention sutures can be used.

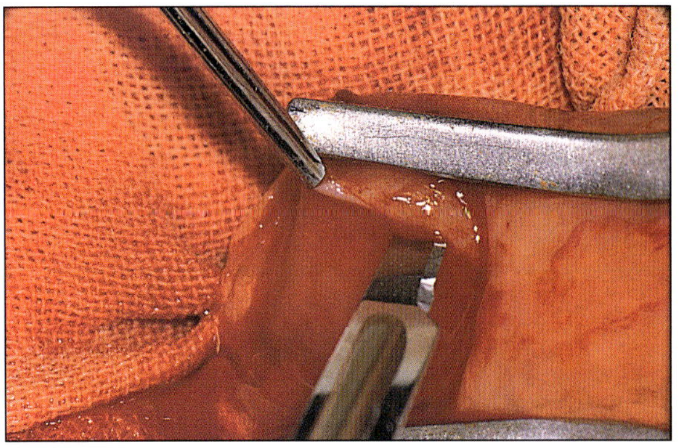

4.50 The urothelium of the dorsal bladder wall is incised over the intramural ureter at the level of the trigone. If the ureter is dilated (e.g. **4.46**), the site of incision is easy to identify but difficulty may be encountered in locating an intramural ureter of normal size. Applying pressure to the bladder neck may result in retention of urine in the ureter and facilitate identification, as may passage of a small (3Fr or 4Fr) urinary catheter up the ectopic ureter from its termination, if possible.

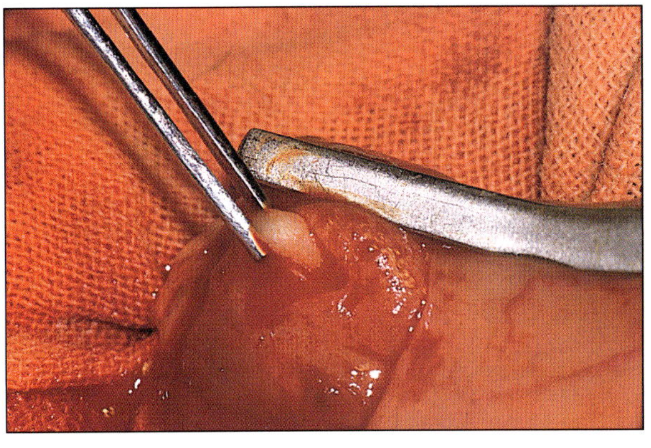

4.51 The ureter is then located within the bladder wall. It is usually much paler in colour than the bladder wall tissues and feels firmer when grasped with forceps.

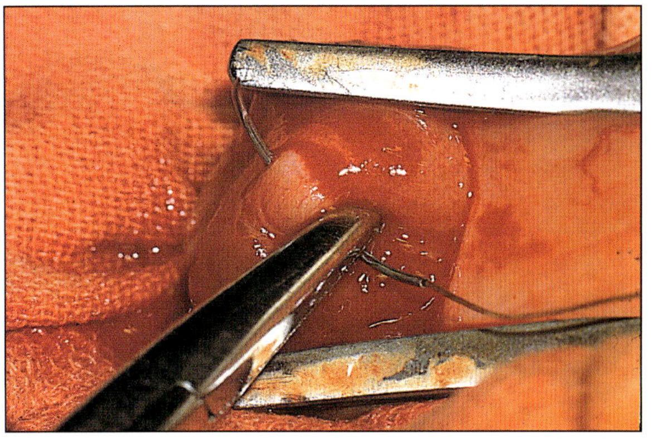

4.52 A ligature is passed around the ureter. Although synthetic absorbable ligature materials are suitable, the author prefers to use no. 0 chromic catgut in the hope that the resultant fibrous reaction may help to prevent recanalization of the ureter.

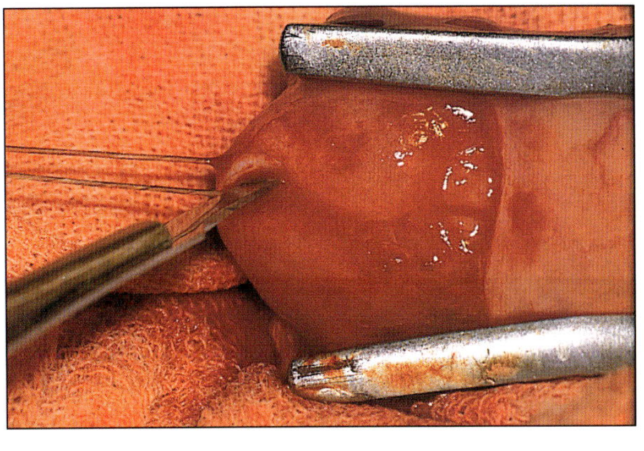

4.53 Gentle traction is applied to the ligature in a caudal direction. This supports the ureter while it is incised.

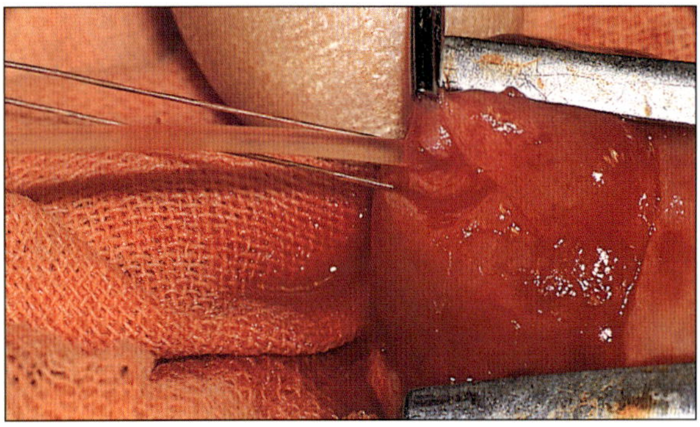

4.54 A 3Fr or 4Fr catheter can be passed cranially into the ureter through the incision to facilitate identification of the ureteral stoma and to divert urine from the surgical site. Note the ooze of blood from small suburothelial vessels; although not serious, this makes visualization difficult and necessitates frequent swabbing.

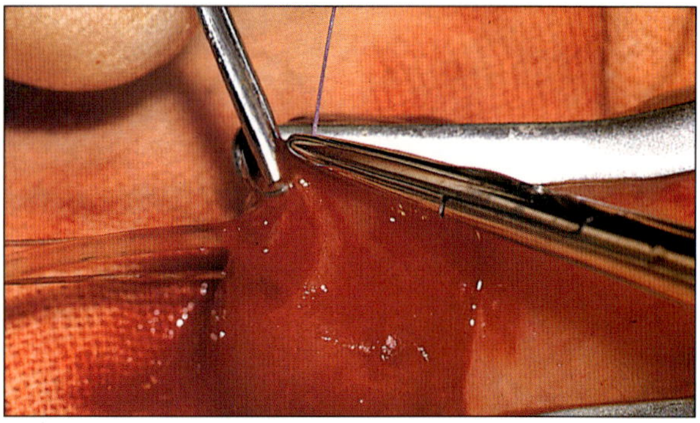

4.55 The edges of the stoma in the ureteral wall are anastomosed to the edges of the bladder urothelial incision using simple interrupted sutures of fine, synthetic absorbable suture material. The author prefers to use 5/0 polyglactin (Vicryl, Ethicon). Suturing is greatly facilitated and the degree of surgical trauma reduced by the use of fine ocular instruments.

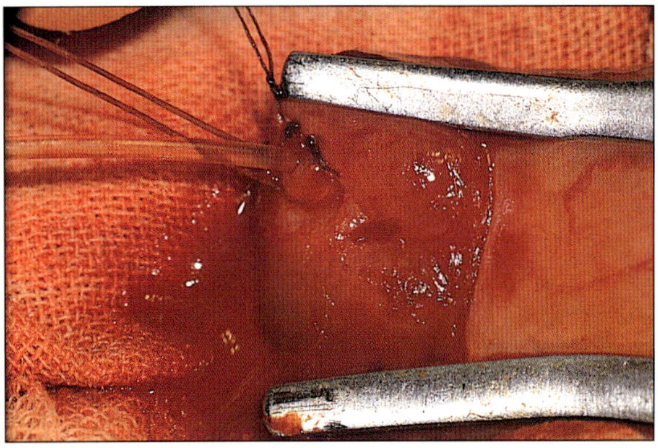

4.56 Suturing is continued along one edge of the stoma.

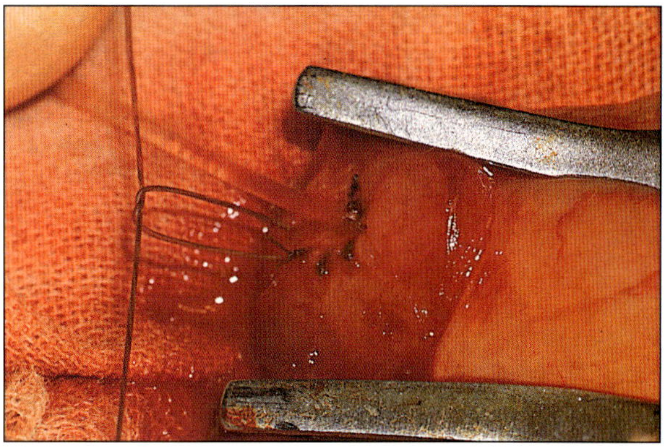

4.57 Once stomatization of the ureter into the bladder lumen has been completed by anastomosis of the ureteral and bladder urothelial incisions, the catgut ligature is tied just caudal to the stoma.

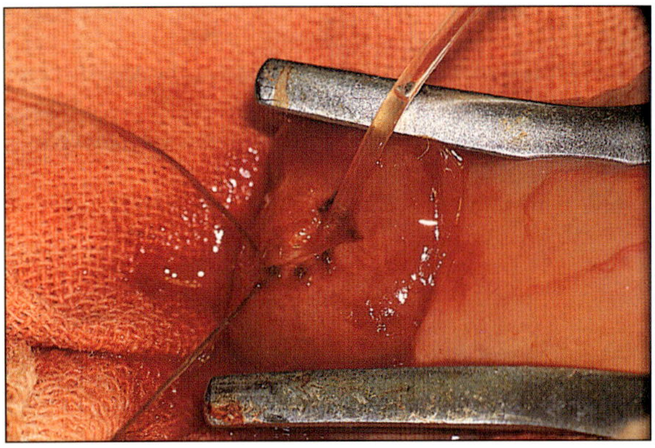

4.58 The catheter is removed from the proximal ureter and used to confirm that the ureter distal to the stoma has been occluded by the ligature.

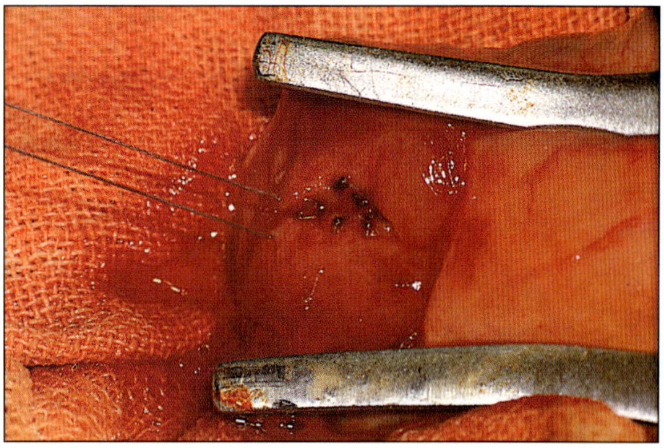

4.59 The knot of the ligature is buried within the bladder wall by suturing the bladder urothelium over it with a further suture of 5/0 polyglactin. The ventral bladder incision is then closed routinely (see 'Cystotomy', etc., below).

Tunnelling technique

4.60 Diagrams summarizing the tunnelling technique used to transplant a ureter which completely bypasses the bladder (left). The ureter is ligated, transected and tunnelled through the bladder wall (**right**). Its terminal opening is then stomatized into the bladder. The surgery is described below.

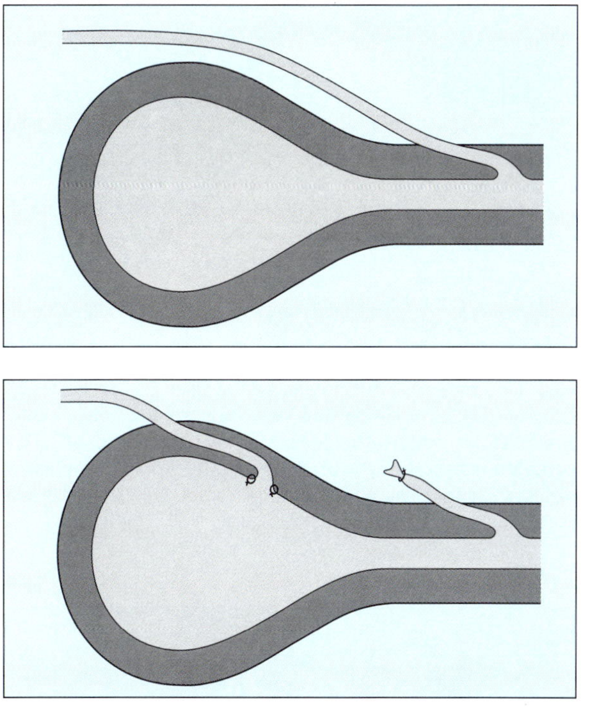

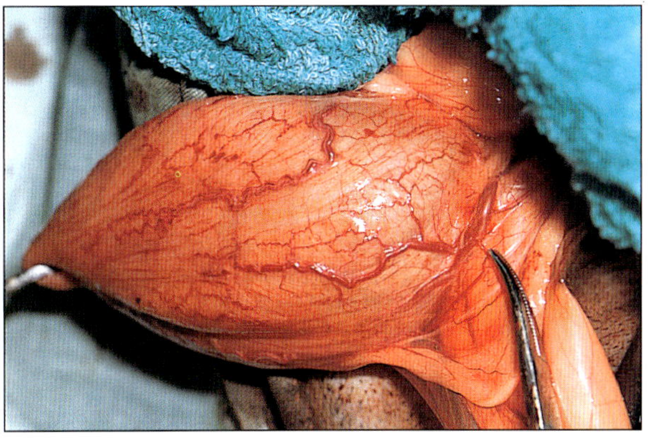

4.61 If the ureter does not travel within the bladder wall or the intramural ureter is inaccessible due to the presence of a large prostate in male dogs, a tunnelling technique has to be used. The ureter can be tunnelled through the bladder wall via an intravesical or extravesical approach. An extravesical approach in a male Labrador with ureteral ectopia is illustrated. The bladder is approached via a caudal mid-line or paramedian abdominal incision. The bladder is exteriorized and reflected caudally to expose its dorsal surface. The entrance of the ureter into the bladder wall (if intramural) can be identified by a plexus of vessels on the dorsal bladder wall, as indicated by the artery forceps. Note that 'cranial', 'caudal', 'dorsal' and 'ventral' relate to directions on the bladder when it is in its normal anatomical position, ignoring the fact that the bladder has been reflected caudally so that its dorsal surface is exposed.

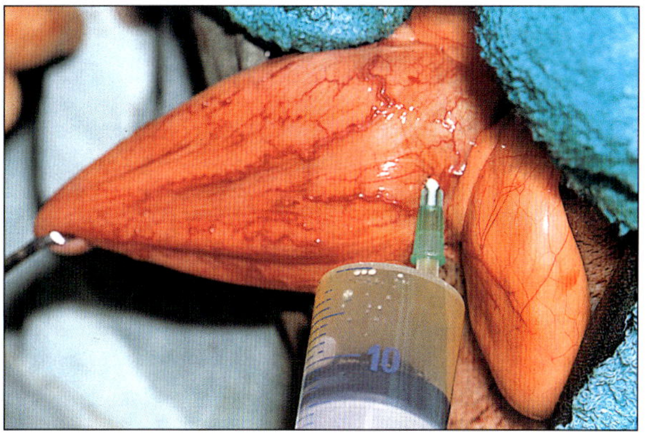

4.62 The bladder is emptied of urine by catheterization or, as in this case, by cystocentesis.

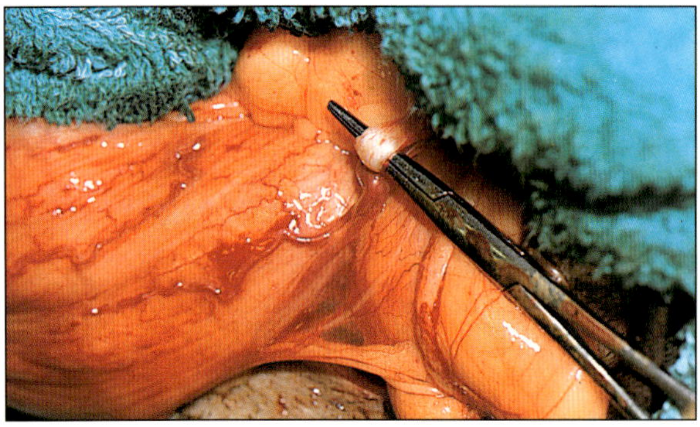

4.63 Two to three centimetres of the ureter is freed from the peri-ureteral fascia and peritoneum at its entry into the bladder (or at the level of the bladder neck if it completely bypasses the bladder) by blunt dissection using artery forceps. The ureteral blood vessels and their fascial attachments to the ureter are preserved.

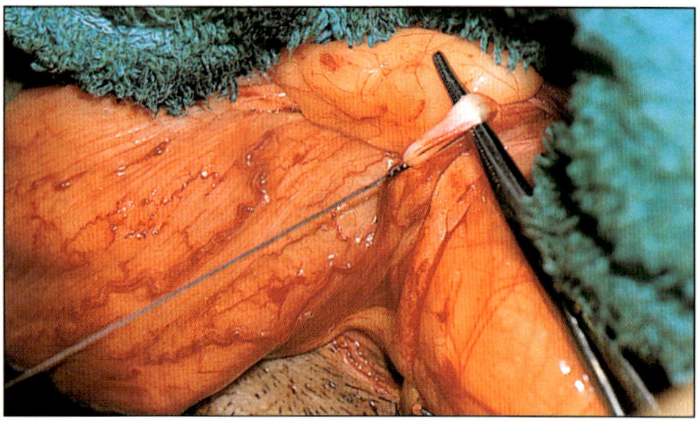

4.64 The ureter is ligated distally using synthetic absorbable material and taking care to avoid damage to the blood vessels in the dorsal wall of the bladder.

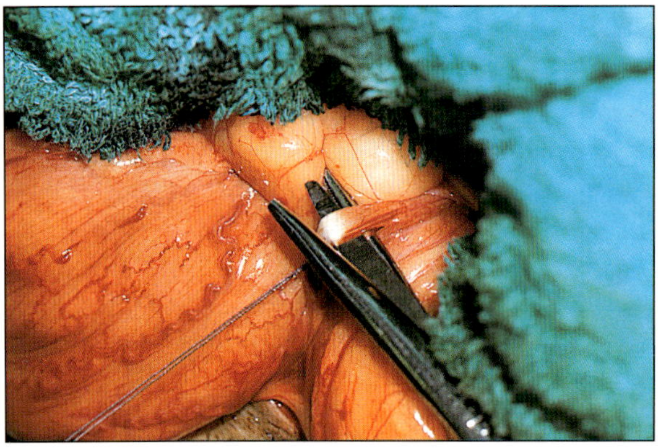

4.65 The ureter is then sectioned just proximal to the ligature and its end placed on a swab to absorb any urine. The use of a catheter to divert urine is not recommended as it makes the remainder of the procedure difficult.

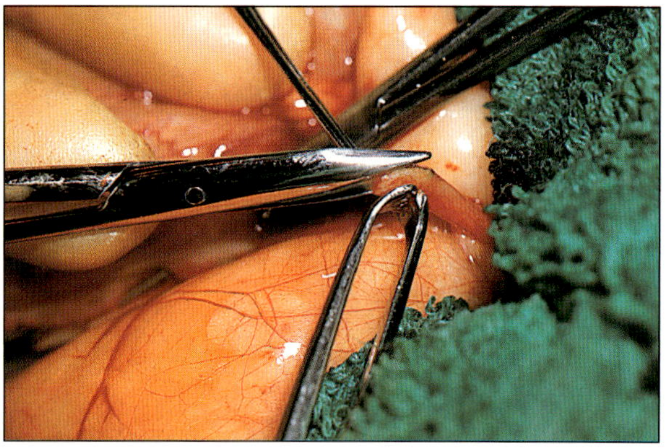

4.66 The ventral wall of the severed end of the ureter is cut with fine scissors for a distance of 1.5–2 times the (normal) diameter of the ureter.

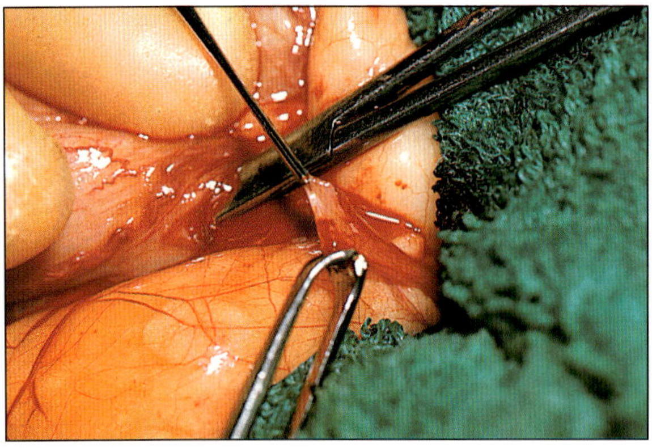

4.67 This allows the end of the ureter to be spatulated, providing a larger opening for stomatizing into the bladder.

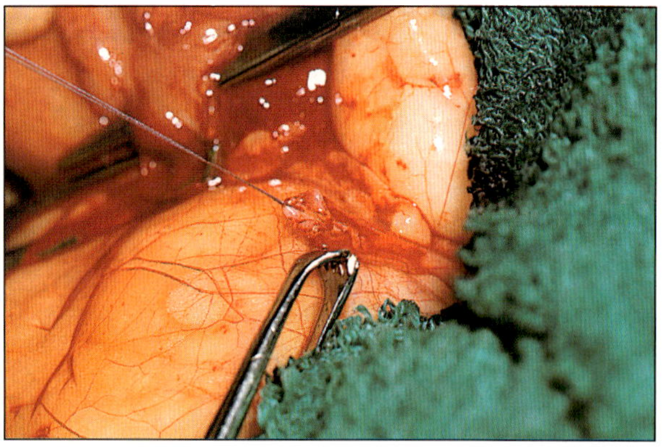

4.68 A fine (5/0) retention suture is placed through the wall of the end of the ureter.

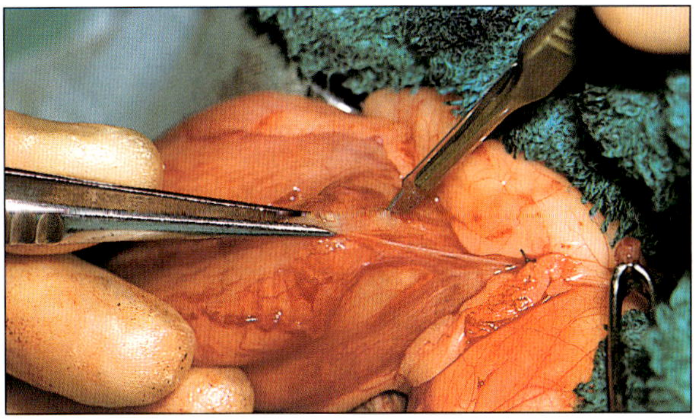

4.69 A stab incision is made into the dorsolateral wall of the bladder, at a level cranial to that at which the ureter originally entered the bladder wall. This is to allow the ureter to be stomatized into the bladder without tension on the suture line.

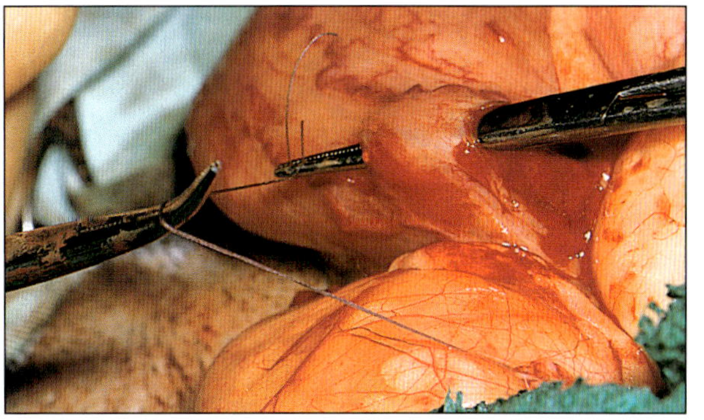

4.70 A tunnel is created in the bladder wall between the urothelium and detrusor muscle using a pair of fine artery forceps, forced through the bladder wall from the stab incision towards the cranial pole of the bladder. The tunnel length should be approximately twice the (normal) diameter of the animal's ureter; this is so that sufficient intramural ureter will be present to collapse under pressure during micturition, thus preventing vesico-ureteral reflux. If the tunnel is too long, however, this may predispose to hydroureter and hydronephrosis. The retention suture is now grasped with the forceps and used to pull the ureter through the tunnel. Note the oozing haemorrhage from suburothelial vessels, necessitating frequent swabbing.

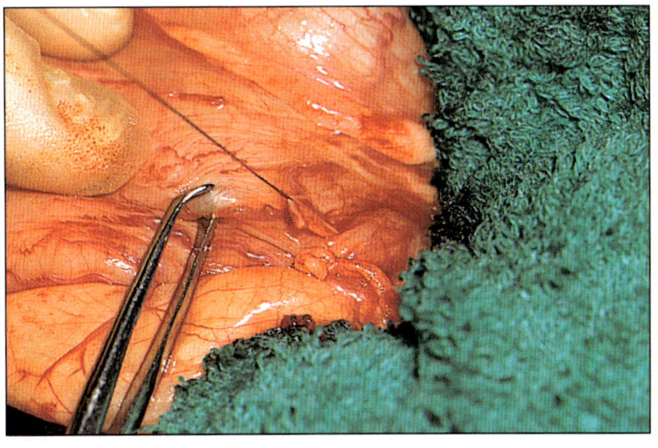

4.71 Care must be taken when pulling the ureter through the tunnel that the ureter is not rotated about its longitudinal axis.

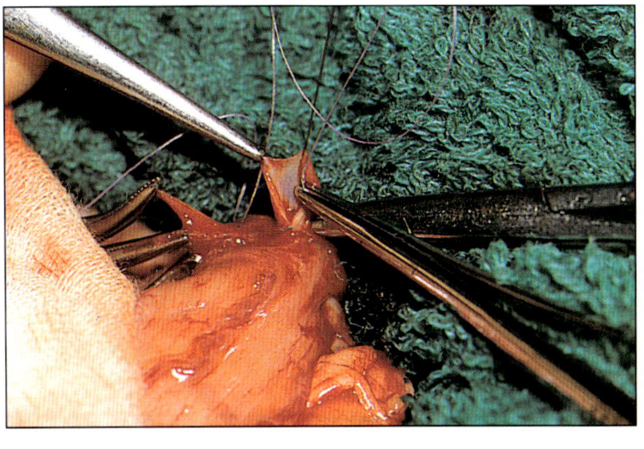

4.72 The spatulated opening in the ureter is now sutured to the opening in the bladder urothelium created by the stab incision shown in 4.69. Fine suture material (5/0 polyglactin – Vicryl, Ethicon) is used to appose ureteral wall and bladder urothelium. The first suture is placed between the proximal end of the cut into the ureter (see **4.66**) – as shown – and the cranial end of the bladder urothelial incision.

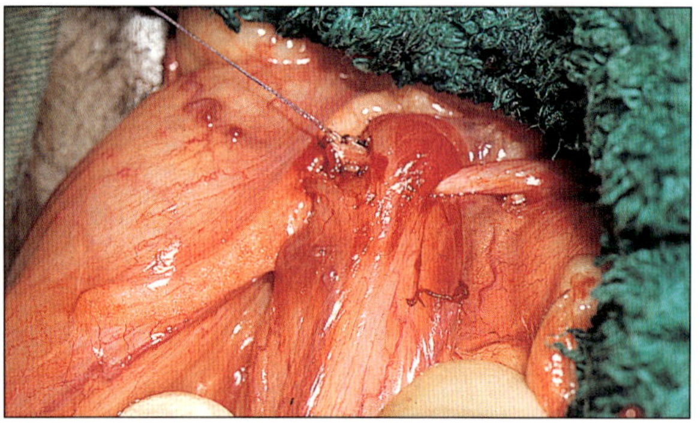

4.73 The sutures are placed so that the knots are outside the bladder lumen.

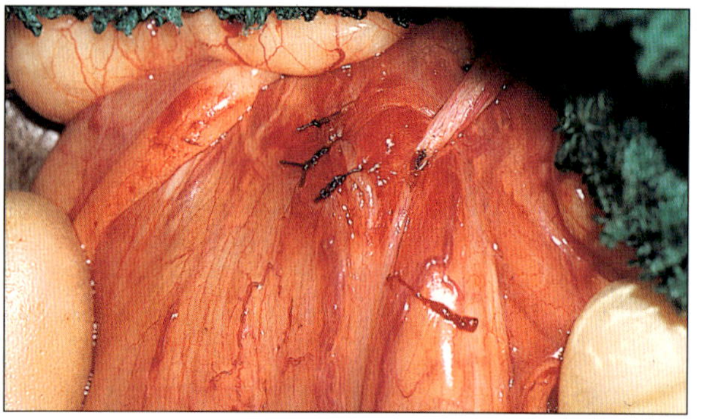

4.74 After the ureter has been stomatized into the bladder, the defect in the overlying detrusor muscle is closed using simple interrupted sutures of 3/0 synthetic absorbable material.

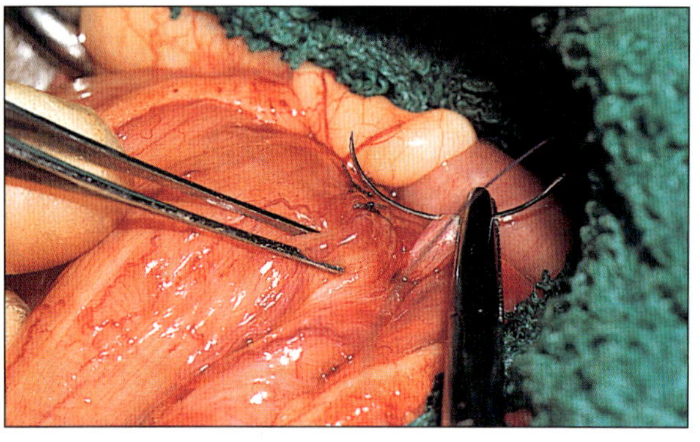

4.75 In order to prevent tension on the stoma suture line, the ureter is anchored to the bladder as it enters the bladder wall. A bite is taken with synthetic absorbable material (3/0 in medium to large dogs, 5/0 in cats and small breeds of dog) through the fascia attached to the ureteral wall.

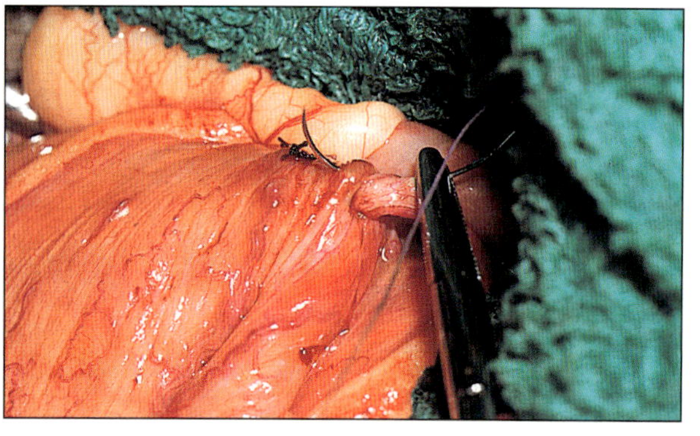

4.76 The suture is then taken through the edge of the detrusor muscle, where the ureter enters the bladder wall, and tied.

Cystotomy/partial cystectomy

Indications

- Cystolithiasis.
- Bladder tumours.
- Bladder ulcers/necrotic urothelium.
- Bladder rupture repair.
- Pervious urachus.
- Infected urachal remnant.
- Ureteral catheterization and transplantation (**4.3b, 4.48–4.76**).
- Removal of blood clots and sloughed urothelium (e.g. post-obstruction).
- Removal of foreign bodies.

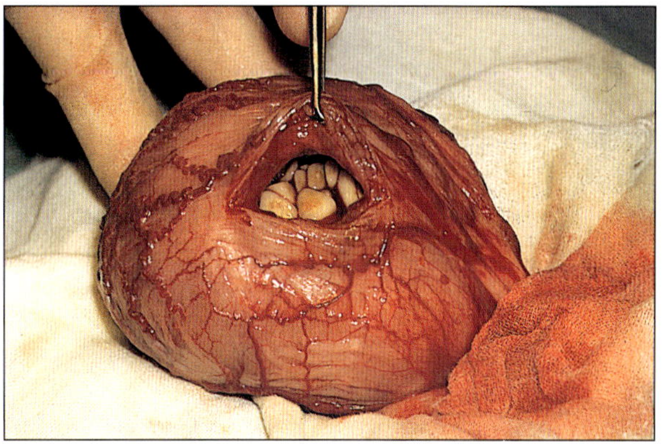

4.77 The commonest indication for bladder surgery is removal of cystoliths.

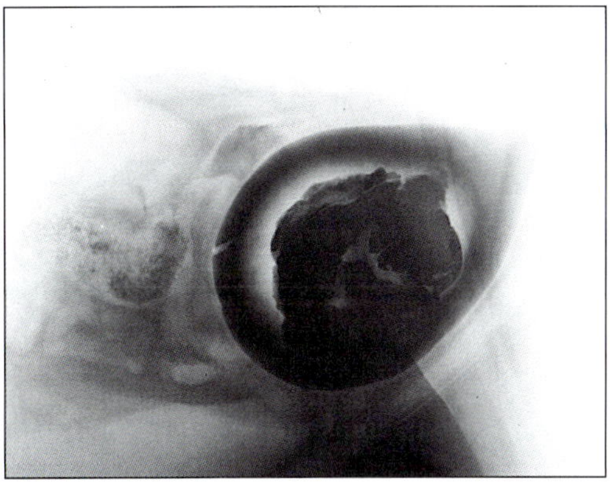

4.78 Although the lateral (left) and ventrodorsal (lower left) double contrast cystograms suggested a large bladder mass with a broad base of attachment in this female Dobermann pinscher, a cystotomy (lower right) revealed that the tumour was attached by a pedicle. This was excised along with a full-thickness margin of bladder wall and histopathology revealed that it was a benign polyp.

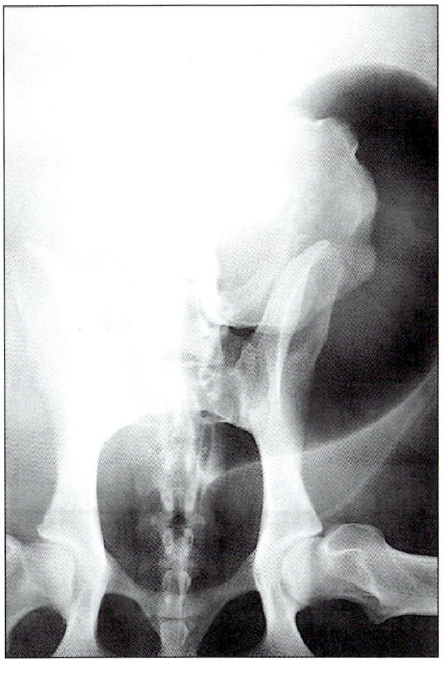

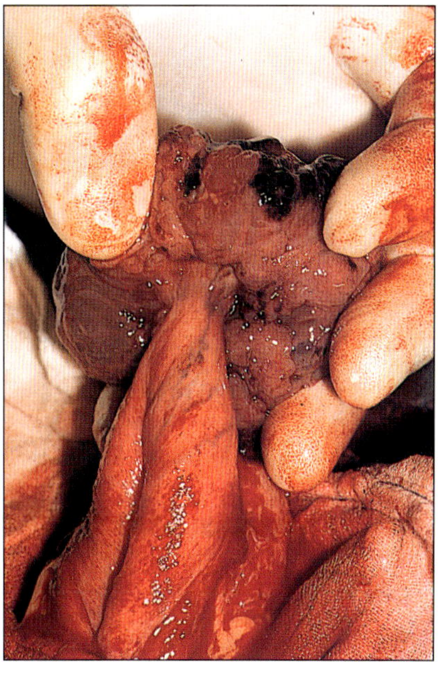

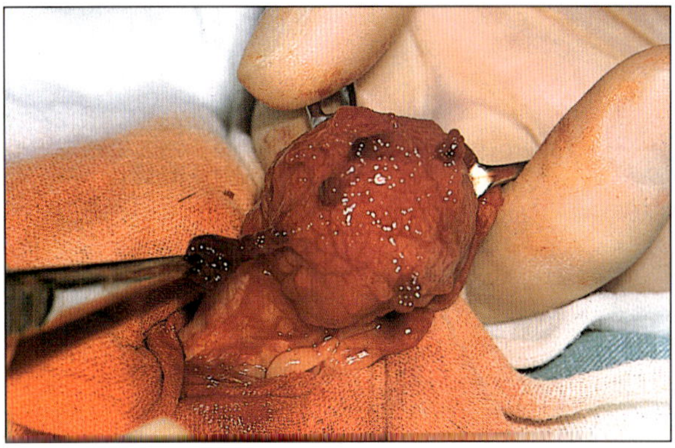

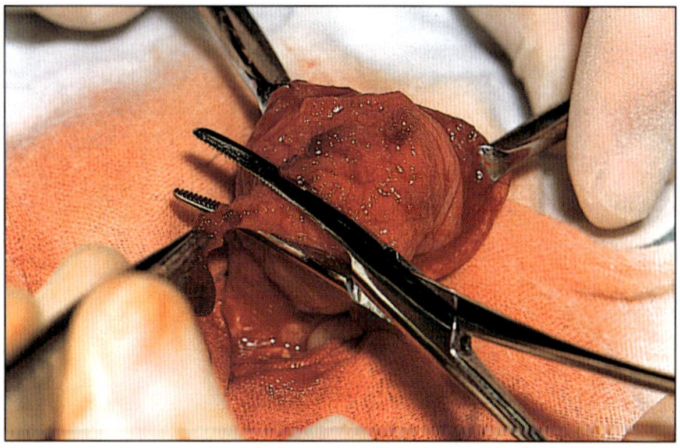

4.79 During cystotomy, benign urothelial polyps (left) can be excised across their base of attachment to the lining urothelium. This can be performed using diathermy excision. If diathermy is not available, each polyp can be clamped across its base on non-neoplastic tissue **(right)** and excised **(lower right)**. After removal of each polyp, the artery forceps are left in place for five minutes to control suburothelial haemorrhage.

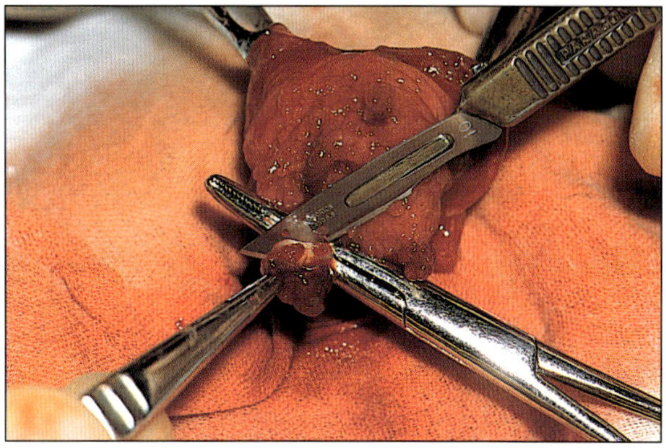

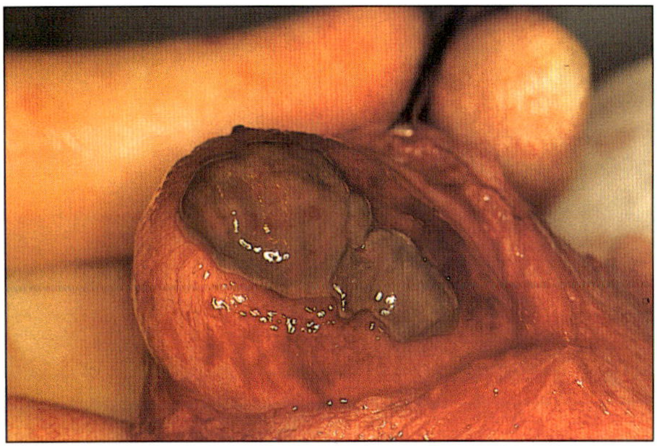

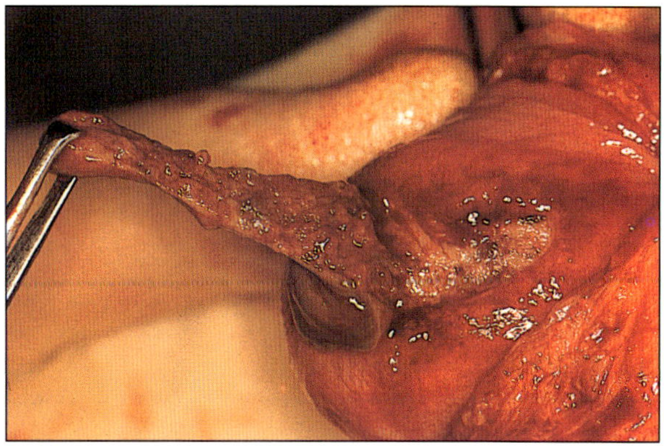

4.80 Occasionally, chronic, localized cystitis fails to respond to antibiotic therapy and it may be necessary to debride ulcerated, necrotic and/or diphtheritic urothelium before healing can take place. Cystotomy in this Great Dane bitch with chronic haematuria revealed the nature of a urothelial lesion **(left)** detected on double contrast cystography. The infected, necrotic urothelium was excised **(right)** and the bitch made an uneventful recovery. It is important that any excised tissues are submitted for histopathological examinations to determine the exact nature of the disease process and obtain a prognosis.

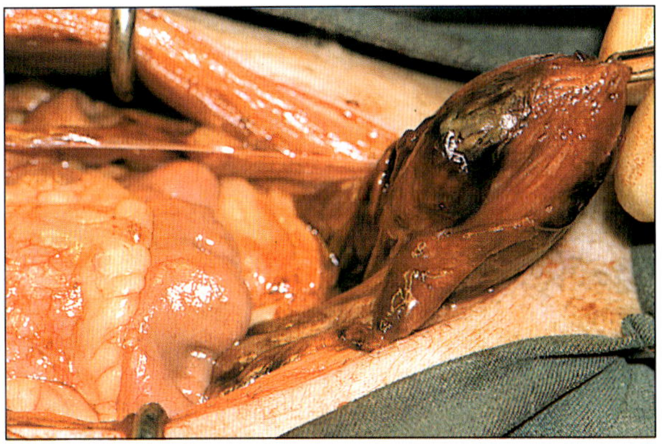

4.81 Rupture of the dorsal wall of the bladder in an Irish setter bitch after a road traffic accident. Note the devitalized tissue, which should be debrided before repair of the defect. Bladder repair in these cases should be deferred until the patient is stabilized (see **3.21**).

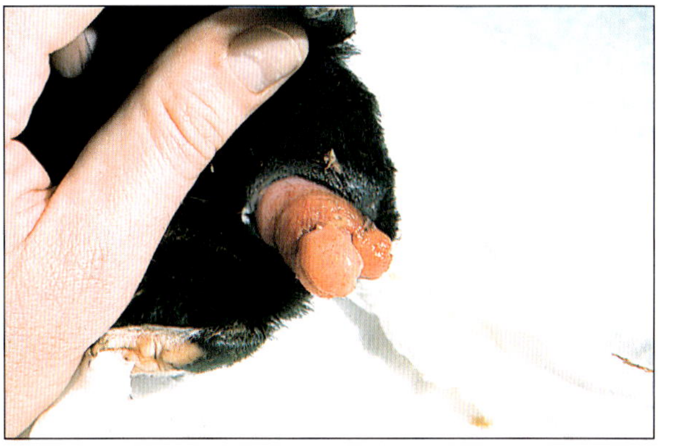

4.82 The bladder may be traumatized and require repair if it is everted. The urethral length of most small animals usually prevents bladder eversion but vagina and bladder eversion in this guinea-pig occurred due to tenesmus. After repair of any trauma, the bladder (and, in this case, vaginal) eversions can be reduced but the cause of the tenesmus must also be treated.

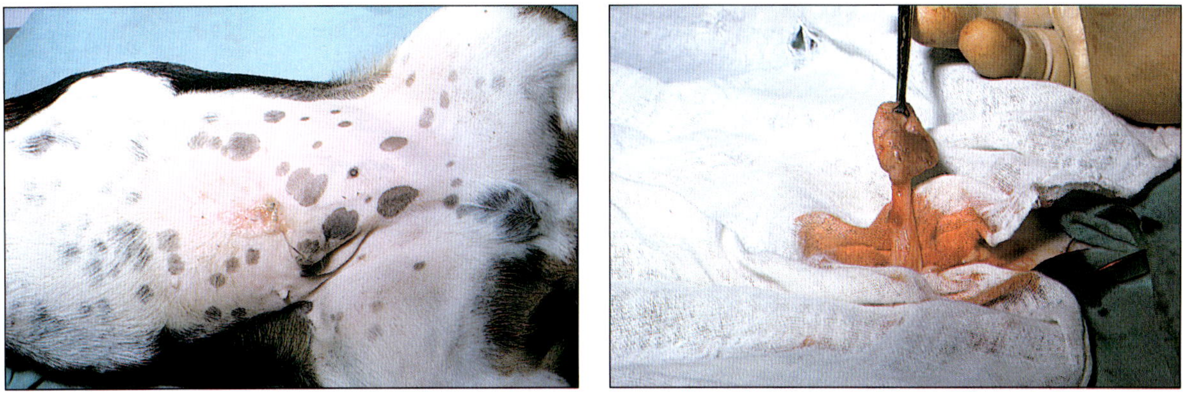

4.83 Pervious urachus in a puppy. This is rare in small animals (compared to horses and farm animals). Affected animals show urinary incontinence through the umbilicus, with urine scalding of the surrrounding skin **(left)**. This is treated by excision of the umbilicus and urachus **(right)**, followed by repair of the resulting cranial bladder wall defect.

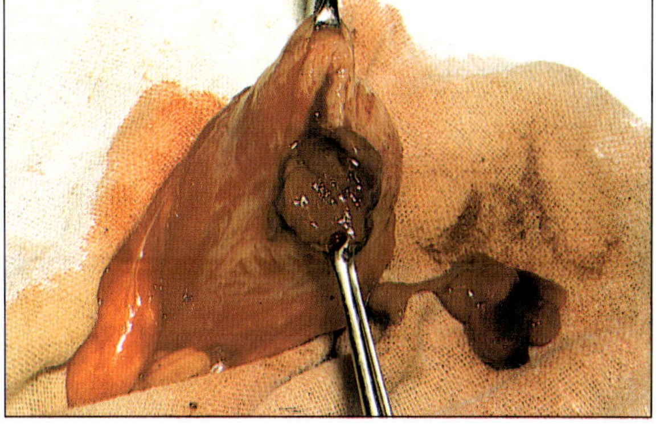

4.84 Sloughed bladder wall urothelium due to dysuria in a cat. This cat was treated five days previously for urethral obstruction. The urethral obstruction (sabulous urolithiasis) was relieved by retrograde flushing and an in-dwelling urinary catheter inserted. After the catheter was removed, the cat became dysuric again and double contrast cystography revealed that this was due to obstruction of the bladder neck by a soft tissue mass. The mass, which was removed via a cystotomy, proved to be sloughed bladder urothelium which had become necrotic as a result of the previous bout of urinary obstruction (see also **1.2**).

Pre- and peri-operative considerations

The bladder should be empty of urine during surgery. This can be achieved by catheterization (see **3.4–3.18**) or cystocentesis (see **3.19**, **3.20** and **4.62**) immediately before or during surgery.

The animal's fluid/electrolyte/acid-base balance should be corrected pre-operatively if bladder rupture (see **3.21**) or dysuria is present. Varying degrees of uraemia, acidosis and hyperkalaemia may be present and can be life-threatening. If these are not corrected pre-operatively, induction of general anaesthesia may be sufficient to kill the animal.

Contrary to previously held beliefs that the bladder should be opened only on its dorsal surface, it can in fact be opened dorsally or ventrally, the site depending upon the indication for cystotomy. For example, a ventral cystotomy is preferable to a dorsal approach for access to the ureteral openings or trigone (e.g. during ureteral catheterization or transplantation – see **4.49**).

Possible surgical/post-surgical complications

Suture material can act as a nidus for the formation of calculi, leading to development or recurrence of urolithiasis. Sutures should therefore not be placed in or through the bladder urothelium unless this is unavoidable (e.g. ureteral transplantation).

Synthetic absorbable sutures are preferred by the author for bladder closure, unless they are likely to come into contact with infected urine. In that case, chromic catgut should be used as there is evidence in the veterinary and human literature that it retains its strength longer than commonly used synthetic absorbable materials such polyglactin (Vicryl, Ethicon) or polydioxanone (PDS, Ethicon)

The potential for wound breakdown can be reduced by the use of a two-layered closure and, if there is a risk of postoperative outflow obstruction and raised intravesical pressure, an in-dwelling urinary catheter can be fitted.

A commonly reported postoperative problem in dogs is early recurrence of cystic calculi following removal of vesicoliths. This is usually due to failure to remove all of the calculi at the time of surgery. Many small stones pass into the pelvic urethra when the dog is placed in dorsal recumbency and these should be removed by retrograde urethral flushing during the operation.

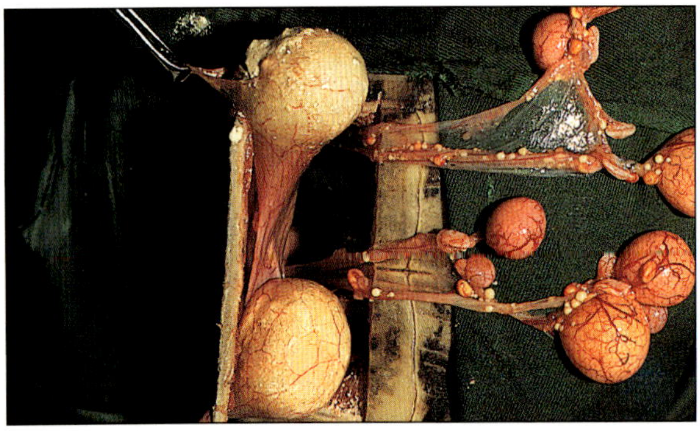

4.85 The bladder wall of most small animals is easily repaired but there are occasional exceptions. A celiotomy on a dystokic tortoise (*Testudo graeca*) is illustrated. There is evidence of egg peritonitis but two shelled ova are present in the urinary bladder (the bladder and oviduct open into a common cloaca in this species: ova retained in the cloaca can pass cranially into the urinary bladder, which opens directly into the cloaca with no urethral tube). The ova were removed from the bladder, the wall of which was extremely friable, as can be seen in the top left of the figure, and was repaired with great difficulty. This animal died 24 hours postoperatively as a result of *Pseudomonas* bacteraemia, originating from the peritonitis.

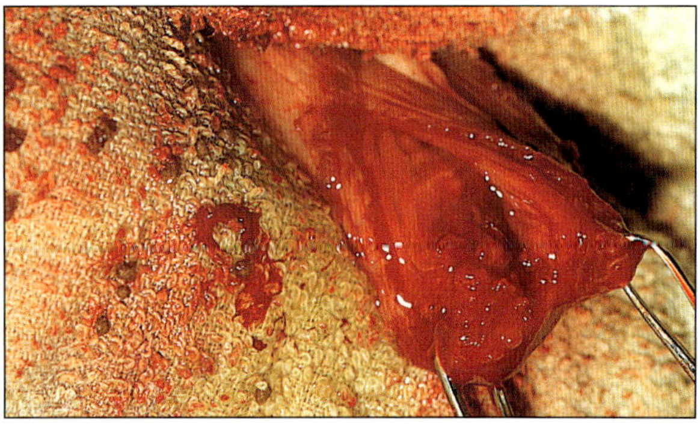

4.86 During cystotomy for removal of calculi, retrograde flushing should be used to remove calculi from the bladder neck and proximal urethra. These are not detectable by palpation. Sterile saline should be used to flush small stones onto a swab placed adjacent to the laparotomy wound, as shown.

Technique

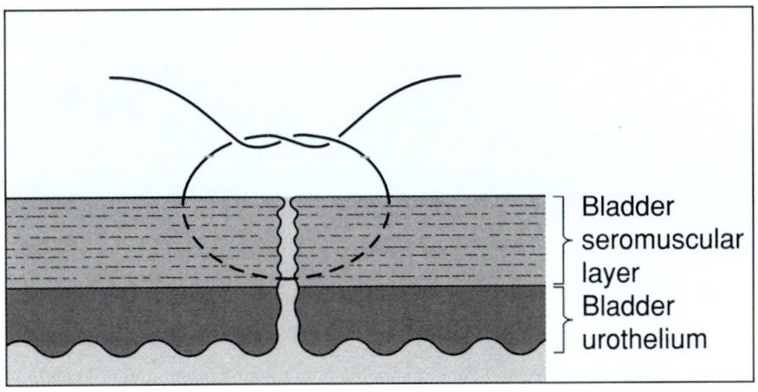

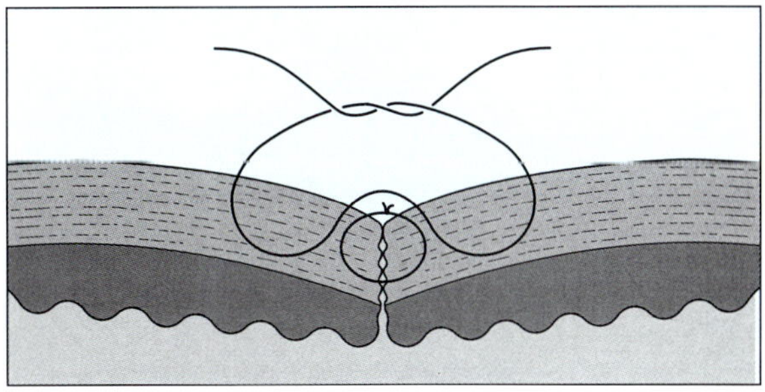

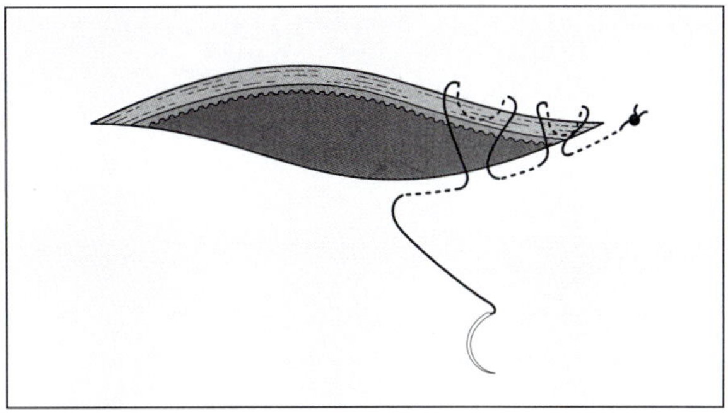

4.87 Diagrams illustrating the author's preferred method of bladder closure. A two-layered closure is used. The first layer is a continuous Czerny suture, shown in a section through the bladder incision in **(left)** to appose the bladder wall edges. The bladder wall is then inverted using Lembert **(right)** or Cushings **(middle)** suture patterns (the Cushings suture pattern is illustrated on an external view of the bladder incision). If the bladder wall is grossly thickened, inversion may not be possible and one may have to rely on appositional closure alone.

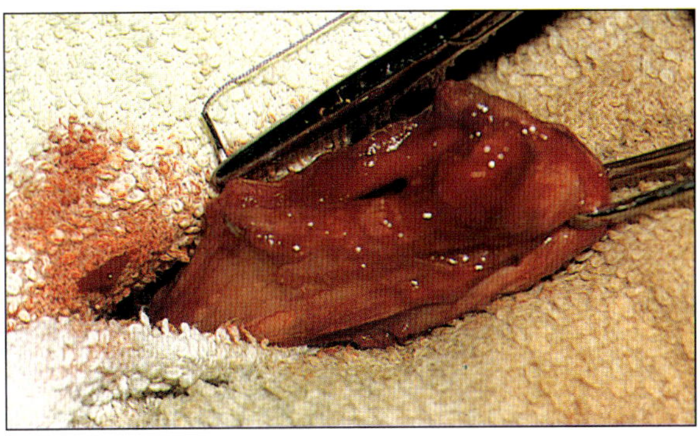

4.88 All sutures begin and end beyond the ends of the bladder wall incision. The author prefers to use synthetic absorbable suture material which should be swaged on to the needle. The Czerny suture is begun by taking a bite through the bladder wall (but not into the lumen) just beyond one end of the incision. After tying the knot, the short end of suture is not cut but is grasped with clamps. This can then be used to support that part of the bladder and to provide something to pull against as the suture is tightened.

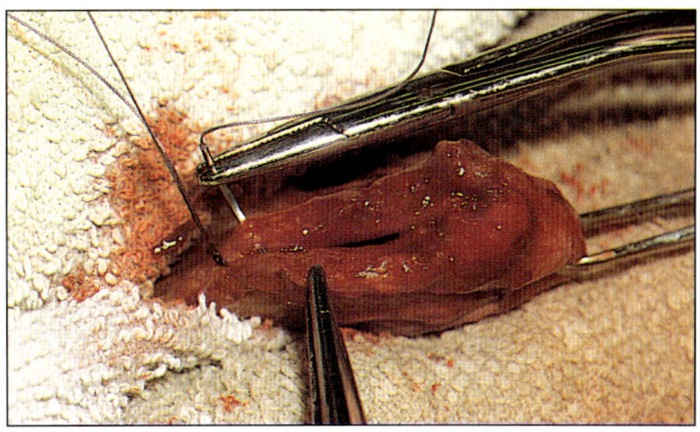

4.89 The Czerny suture is used to appose the edges of the wound without passing through the urothelium (4.87a). In other words, the suture is taken through the bladder serosa and detrusor muscle down to the suburothelium only. The suturing continues from left to right (in this figure) to beyond the right-hand end of the incision and is then tied. The suture is left attached to the right-hand-end knot and an inverting suture placed in a continuous fashion from right to left.

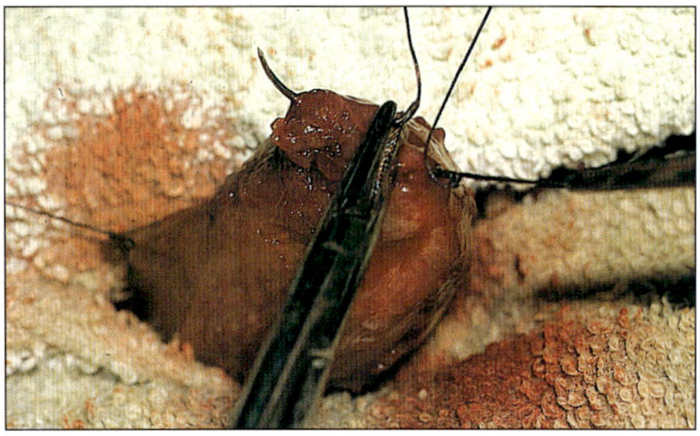

4.90 Here, a continuous Cushings pattern is being used. The suture is taken in and out of the bladder wall adjacent to the far side of the incision and parallel to it without entering the bladder lumen.

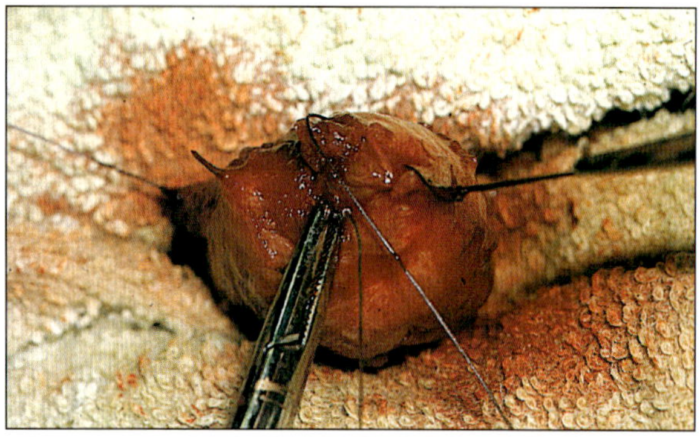

4.91 The suture is then taken into the bladder wall on the near side of the incision at a point just caudal to the level of its exit from the far side. (See **4.87c.**) Again, it is passed through the bladder wall parallel to the incision.

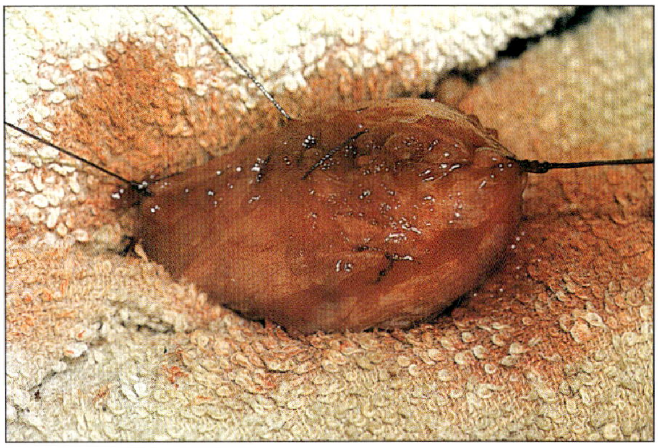

4.92 To illustrate the inversion effect of the Cushings suture, a number of bites of suture have been placed but not tightened. The Czerny sutures are still visible.

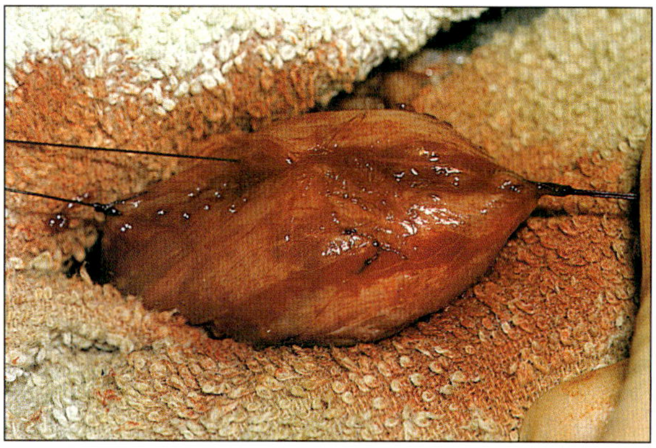

4.93 When the suture is tightened, the bladder wall is inverted, thus burying the layer of Czerny sutures.

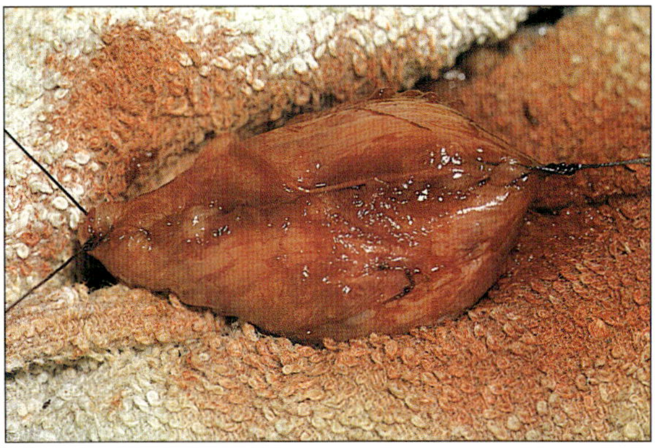

4.94 When the inverting layer has been completed, the suture can be tied either to itself or to the short end of suture material which remains attached to the initial knot of the Czerny suture.

Urethrotomy

Indications

- Removal of urethral calculi, foreign bodies and benign urothelial tumours.

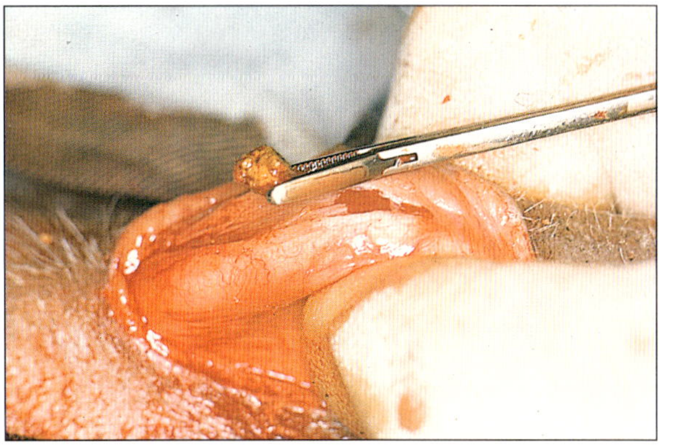

4.95 Removal of urethral calculi. This is the commonest indication for urethrotomy but should be a last resort.

Pre- and peri-operative considerations

The diagnosis of urethral obstruction due to calculi (or foreign body) must be accurate; catheterization alone is unreliable for detecting obstruction of the urethra. Tortuosity of the groove in the caudal os penis can prevent passage of a urinary catheter (and feels like a calculus during attempts at catheterization) but is not a cause of dysuria.

Urethrotomy should be a last resort, and avoided if possible. The complications associated with cystotomy are fewer and less serious than those after urethrotomy. In addition, there are usually additional vesical calculi. It is preferable, therefore, to return the urethral calculi to the bladder using the technique of retrograde hydropropulsion (see below) and then to remove all calculi via a cystotomy. The bladder should first be emptied of urine by centesis. This is part of the treatment of any animal with dysuria associated with outflow obstruction but is also required to facilitate retrograde hydropropulsion and to prevent iatrogenic overdistension of the bladder during retrograde flushing. In addition, the metabolic consequences of dysuria (azotaemia, acidosis and hyperkalaemia) should be corrected by appropriate fluid/electrolyte therapy.

Urethrotomy is not indicated in bitches as urethral calculi can either be returned to the bladder using retrograde hydropropulsion or be removed from the urethra via the external urethral orifice using forceps. In male dogs, if retrograde hydropropulsion fails, then urethrotomy is indicated to relieve the urethral obstruction. Urethrotomy is not indicated in obstructed male cats; if retrograde flushing fails to dislodge the urethral obstruction (see **3.12** and **3.13**), then a perineal urethrostomy may be required (see **4.128–4.136**).

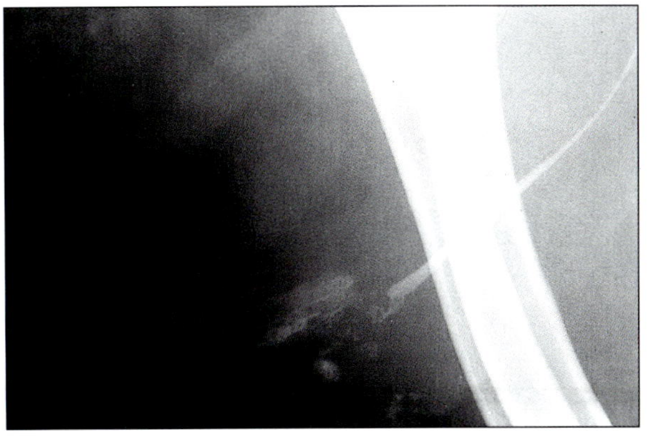

4.96 Repeated urethrotomies for recurring urolithiasis in this German shepherd dog have resulted in urethral stricture. The retrograde positive contrast urethrogram demonstrates the severe disruption of normal urethral anatomy. This case underlines two points: urethrotomy should be avoided if possible and any calculi obtained should be analysed so that suitable prophylactic measures can be instituted and the possibility of recurrence minimized.

Possible surgical/post-surgical complications

Urine passing from the urethrotomy (which is usually left open to heal by secondary intention) may infiltrate the subcutaneous tissues and scrotum, leading to necrosis and sloughing of tissues. This is usually due to poor alignment of the skin and urethrotomy incisions and can be avoided if care is taken to ensure that the urethrotomy incision is directly beneath the skin incision.

Urethral stricture may occur, particularly after poor urethrotomy technique or/and repeated urethrotomies (see **4.96**): this is but one reason for avoiding urethrotomy.

After urethrotomy, it is common for the wound to haemorrhage, particularly following urination or if the dog becomes excited. This is usually self-limiting and stops within 7–10 days but often causes concern to the owner and blood-staining of carpets and furniture, so it is important to warn the owner before urethrotomy of the likelihood of postoperative bleeding. If bleeding is severe and prolonged, the animal may become anaemic (and require a blood transfusion) – but this is very rare. Suturing the urethrotomy wound to control haemorrhage may be necessary but again should be left as a last resort since the reaction to the sutures and blood clots are likely to obstruct the urethra. In addition, if the skin alone is sutured, urothelial pouching may occur.

The urethrotomy may become obstructed by blood clots, causing further dysuria. These can be dislodged and removed using a urethral catheter. The risk of postoperative urethral obstruction after urethrotomy means that it is unwise to perform a urethrotomy and a cystotomy on the same occasion. The increased intravesical pressure may result in bladder wound breakdown. It is safer to delay cystotomy to remove bladder calculi until the urethrotomy incision has just healed

Rarely, a urethrotomy fails to heal (it usually does so within 10 days) and a urethrocutaneous fistula persists. If this happens, the fistula can be repaired by simple closure.

Recurrence of urolithiasis is common if not all calculi have been removed from the lower urinary tract and/or prophylactic measures have not been instituted. Although the urethrotomy is left open to heal by secondary intention, it is rare for additional vesical calculi to be passed via the urethrotomy. It is important, therefore, to ensure that all calculi have been removed, if necessary by performing a cystotomy after the urethrotomy has healed. The author considers it to be unwise (and possibly negligent) to leave calculi in the bladder, even if calculolytic management is instituted, as these may subsequently pass into the urethra, resulting in recurrence of the obstructive dysuria.

It is imperative that any calculi obtained are analysed so that appropriate prophylactic measures can be initiated.

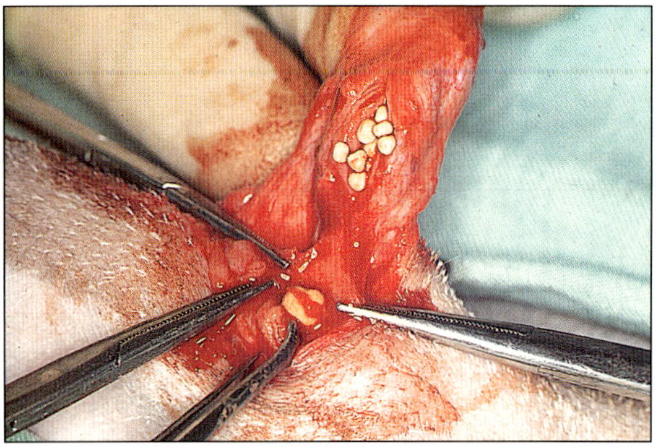

4.97 A urethral diverticulum containing over 30 calculi in a Basset hound. The diverticulum resulted from closure of a urethrotomy skin incision (in an attempt to control postoperative haemorrhage) and subsequent outgrowth of urethral urothelium into the subcutaneous space to form a pouch. As further calculi from the bladder travelled down the urethra, they passed into the pouch which, when full, resulted in compression of the urethra and further dysuria. The pouch and calculi had to be excised.

Techniques

Retrograde hydropropulsion technique (after Piermattei and Osborne, 1977)

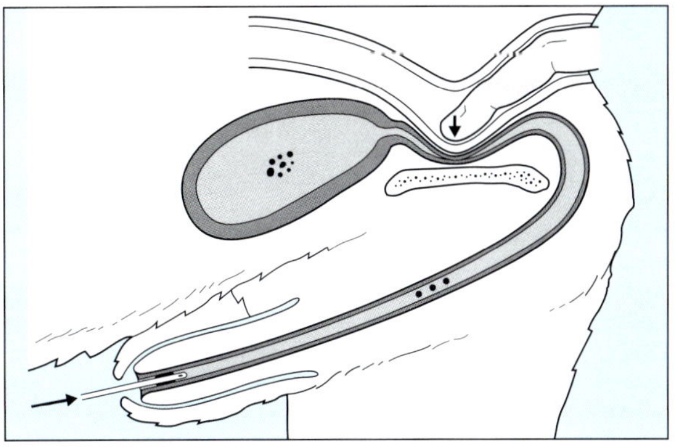

4.98 Diagram illustrating retrograde hydropropulsion of urethral calculi. The bladder is emptied by cystocentesis. A gloved finger is inserted *per rectum* and used to compress the pelvic urethra against the pubis. An 8Fr Foley catheter is inserted into the penile urethra and its cuff inflated with 2–3 ml air (alternatively, a polyurethane catheter can be used and the urethra occluded around it with digital pressure). Sterile saline is injected through the catheter; this results in dilation of the urethra (which can be appreciated beneath the ball of the finger in the rectum), thus freeing the calculi from the surrounding urethral wall. The digital pressure on the pelvic urethra is released (while saline continues to be injected), allowing the calculi to be flushed retrograde into the bladder. Several attempts may have to be made before all urethral calculi are returned to the bladder and the success of the technique should be confirmed radiographically. If all calculi are seen to have been returned to the bladder on a radiograph, the urethra is catheterized (to empty the bladder and to prevent calculi from returning to the urethra) and the animal taken to theatre for cystotomy to remove the vesical uroliths (see **4.87–4.94**).

Urethrotomy technique

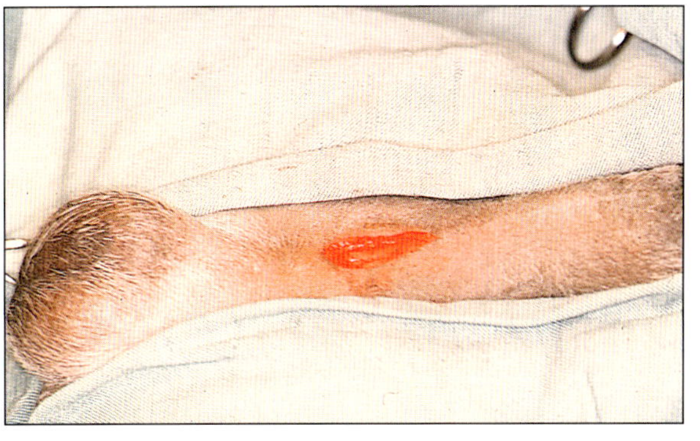

4.99 If retrograde hydropropulsion fails, urethrotomy may be required to remove the calculi. The commonest site for urethrotomy is at the caudal end of the os penis as this is the most likely location of urethral calculi. The incision should not be too close to the scrotum, to reduce the risk of urine tracking subcutaneously into the scrotum, resulting in scrotal necrosis.

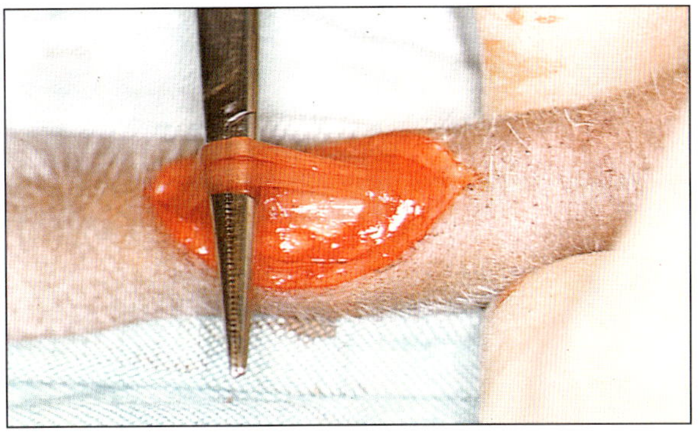

4.100 The retractor penis muscle (which is somewhat vestigial in the dog compared to ruminants) is identified. It can be incised in the mid-line or retracted to one side to allow access to the penis.

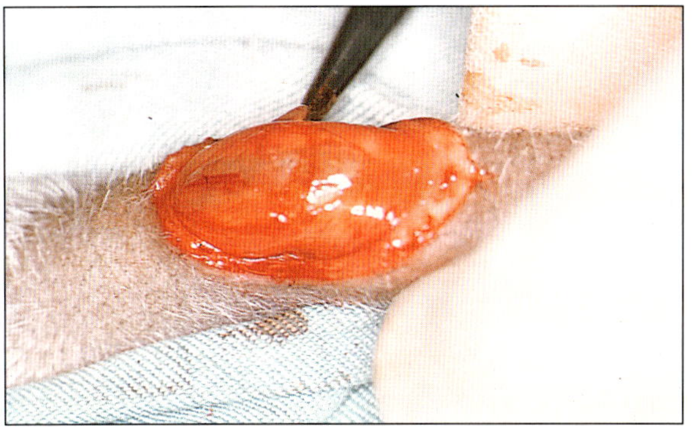

4.101 In this case, the retractor penis muscle is being held aside with forceps and the penis lifted. This allows the ventral groove of the os penis to be seen (or palpated) and used as a guide for a mid-line incision.

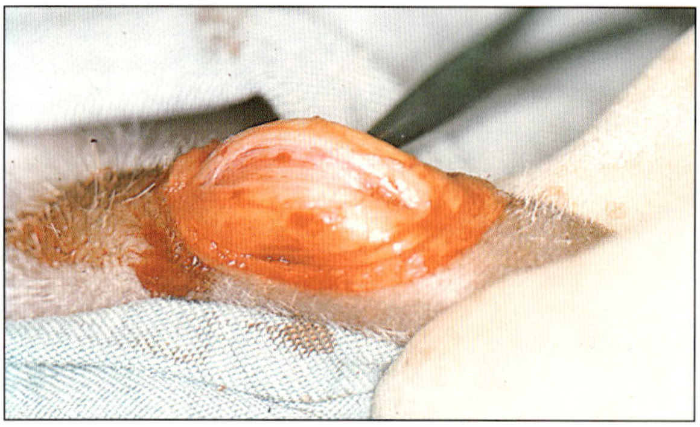

4.102 The penis is incised in the mid-line. Text books often describe an avascular median raphe but this is rarely located during surgery. The incision should pass between the corpora spongiosa and through the ventral urethral urothelium into the urethral lumen, as shown. Once the penis is no longer lifted, haemorrhage usually occurs from the corpora spongiosa. This can be controlled by direct pressure. In the author's experience, local adrenaline has little, if any, effect on the haemorrhage.

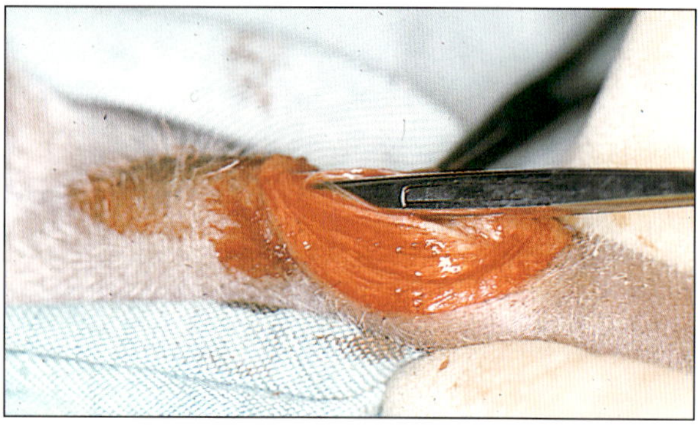

4.103 The calculi are removed from the urethra using alligator forceps (see also **4.95**). Urethral patency is then confirmed by passage of a urinary catheter distally and proximally from the urethrotomy incision. The latter is left open to heal by secondary intention and the owner warned to expect haemorrhage, particularly after the dog urinates. The wound heals usually after 5–7 days.

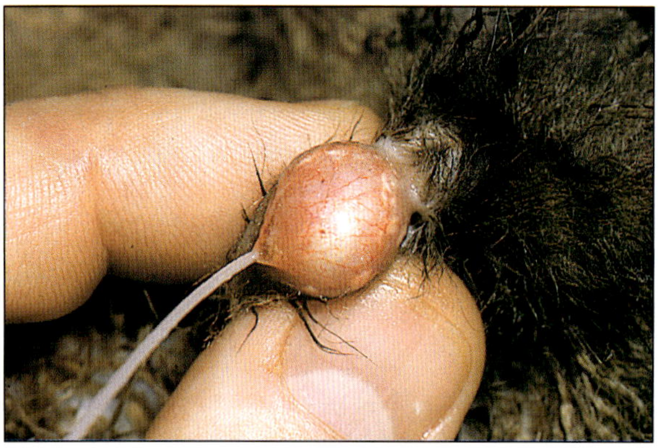

4.104 The urethrotomy technique may have to be adapted to the situation encountered. For example, this male rabbit was presented with acute urethral obstruction associated with a calculus lodged in the terminal urethra.

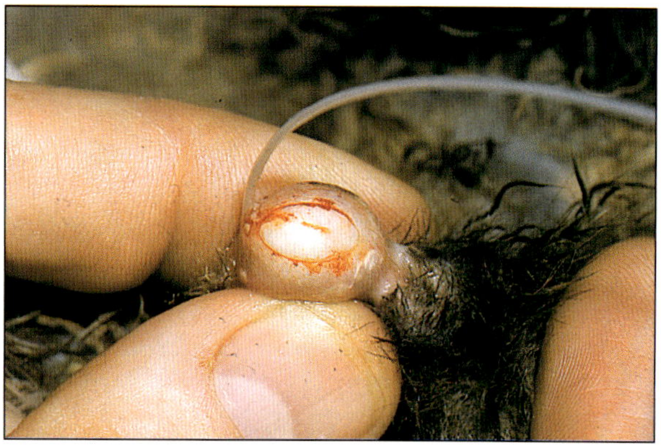

4.105 Under local analgesia (Xylocaine spray, Astra), a urethrotomy was performed directly over the calculus.

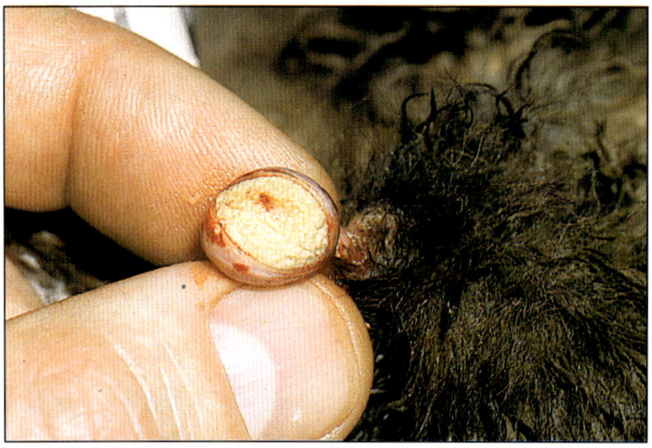

4.106 The calculus (calcium carbonate) was exposed and removed from the urethra, which was left open to granulate. The rabbit had a further calculus in its bladder. This was removed via a cystotomy three weeks after urethrotomy and the animal made an uneventful recovery.

Urethrostomy

Indications

- Unrelievable urethral obstruction – e.g. stricture (see **4.96**), trauma, neoplasia, priapism (in cats).

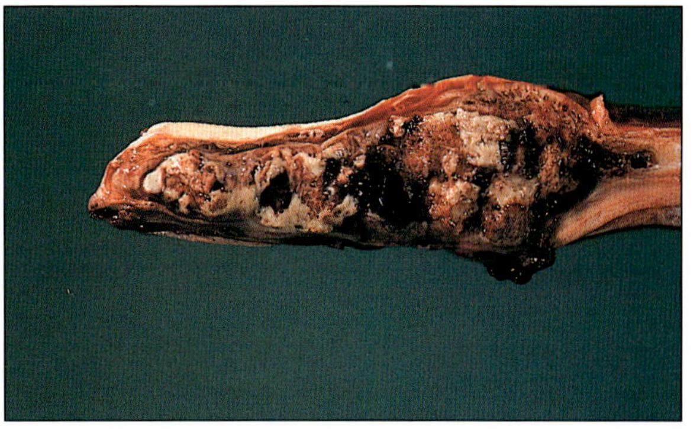

4.107 Penile haemangiosarcoma in a dog. Unfortunately, this animal had widespread metastatic disease but penile neoplasia may be an indication for penile ablation and urethrostomy (see below).

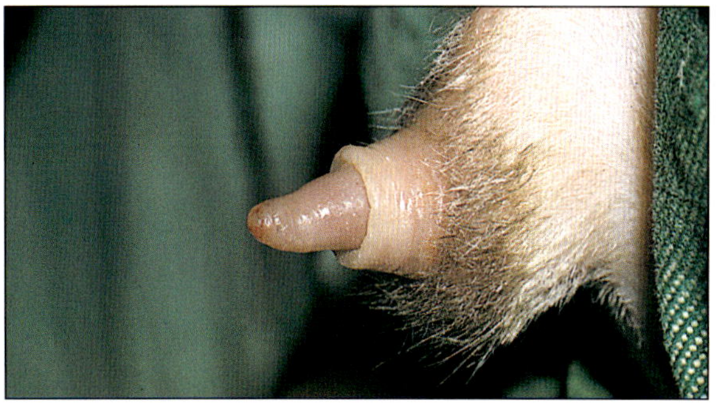

4.108 Feline priapism, an indication for perineal urethrostomy. The persistent erection in these cats results in trauma to and drying of the penile tip. This in turn leads to urethral stricture. The cause of this condition is unknown. Thrombi are often found in the corpora of excised affected penises but it is unclear if these are the cause or effect of the condition.

Pre- and peri-operative considerations

The site of the urethrostomy varies with the level of the obstruction. Obviously, the urethral stoma should be made proximal to the site of obstruction but, in general, should be located as far distally as possible to reduce the likelihood of postoperative complications (see below). The usual sites in the dog are at the levels of the caudal os penis, scrotum (after castration and scrotal ablation) or perineum, but other sites may be indicated (see below).

In cats, perineal urethrostomy is usually performed to prevent urethral obstruction in an animal with recurring urolithiasis which has failed to respond to prophylactic measures. The incidence of feline urethral obstruction has fallen in recent years and so this technique is also less commonly indicated. The technique is best carried out as an elective procedure, once the animal has recovered from the effects of the urethral obstruction. It is sometimes necessary to perform prepubic urethrostomies in cats with irreparable damage to the pelvic urethra, but this is rare.

It may be difficult to locate the urethra in dogs, especially in the ischial region where the overlying ischiocavernosus muscles increase the depth from skin to urethral lumen. The urethral obstruction distal to the stoma site almost invariably means that the urethra cannot be catheterized to facilitate identification.

Possible surgical/post-surgical complications

Postoperative skin scalding with urine may be a problem; barrier creams should be applied locally until the animal adopts a new micturition posture to allow urine to flow from the stoma without running down the surrounding skin. In a minority of animals, this does not occur and skin scalding is a chronic problem

The stoma may stenose, leading to stricture and dysuria. The risks of stenosis can be minimized by:

- Creation of a large stoma at the correct site.
- Attention to suturing (simple interrupted, monofilament non-absorbable sutures; removal of sutures under sedation or general anaesthesia, especially in cats, to avoid tearing of tissues).
- Preservation of preputial mucosa for attachment to the ventral part of the stoma in cats.
- Ligation of the urethra distal to the urethrostomy (unless the distal urethra is excised) to ensure that all urine passes through the stoma, stimulating patency (the stoma is more likely to close if some urine is able to pass distally down the urethra).

Chronic urinary tract infection may occur after urethrostomy. This is more of a problem after perineal urethrostomy in dogs (it is unusual in cats) and is probably associated with the ascent of faecal-borne bacteria such as *Proteus* spp. up the shorter urethra. It can be a real problem throughout the rest of the animal's life and may predispose to urolithiasis; so more distal stoma locations, such as the scrotal site, are preferred.

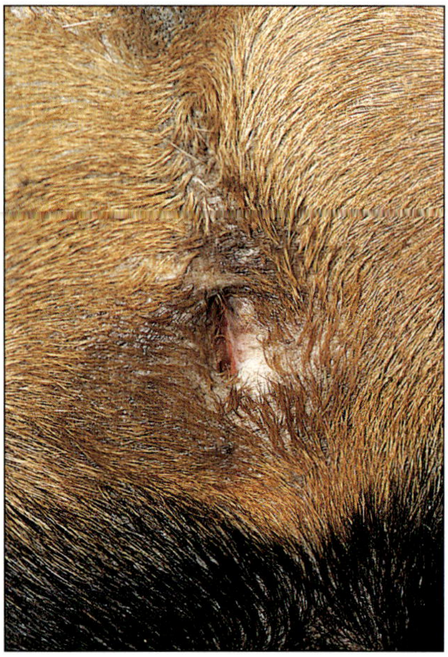

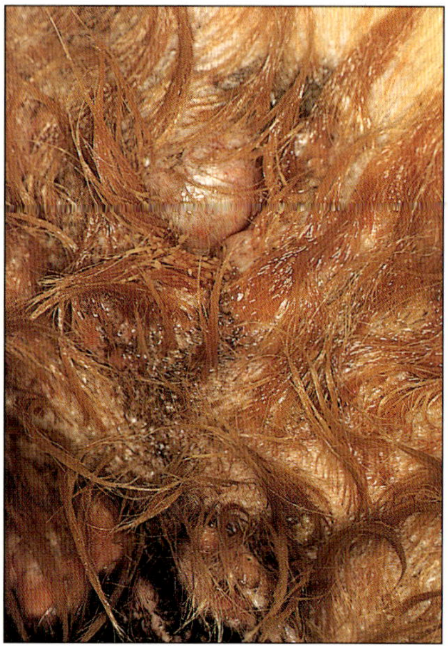

4.109 Urethrostomy may result in urinary tract infection and skin scalding. A perineal urethrostomy stoma in a Dobermann pinscher five years after surgery **(left)**. Apart from minor dampness of the hairs around the stoma after urination, this animal has experienced no ill effects. At the other extreme, the Golden retriever illustrated in **(right)** – also five years after perineal urethrostomy – has serious chronic problems. The skin around the perineal stoma is scalded and the scrotum is ulcerated. Struvite crystals can be seen attached to the hairs around the stoma and are associated with chronic, recurring cystitis and infection by *Proteus* spp.

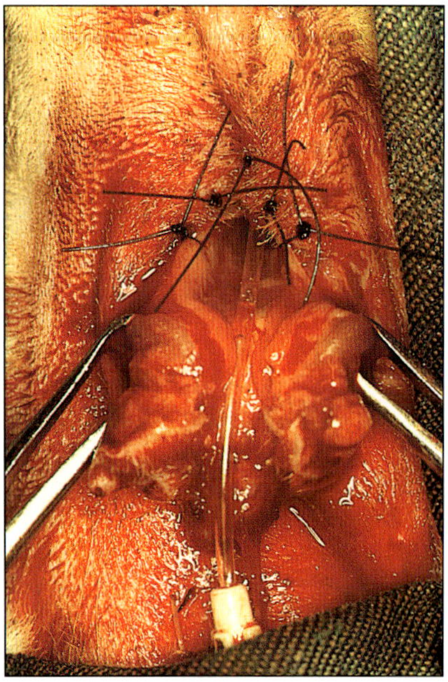

4.110 Stenosis of the stoma may occur. In this cat, the perineal urethrostomy is being repeated to excise the stenosed stoma. The urethra has been opened and the narrowing of the urethra can be seen distal to the patent membranous urethra. The stenosis in this case was associated with stomatizing the urethra at an inappropriate site, resulting in a small stoma on a narrow portion of urethra (the stoma was made into the penile urethra rather than the wider membranous urethra). This was corrected by creating a larger stoma into the membranous urethra, as shown, and excising the stenosed penile urethra and previous stoma.

4.111 The author believes that stricture is less likely after perineal urethrostomy in cats if the ventral part of the stoma is joined to preputial mucosa rather than preputial skin. In addition, the preputial mucosa ventral to the stoma acts as a 'drainage board' and is less likely to be scalded by urine than skin. In this cat (in which perineal urethrostomy is being performed to relieve urethral stenosis after air gun pellet trauma to the penis), the fascia ventral to the stoma has been closed. The preputial mucosa (arrowed) which was left attached to the prepuce will be reflected dorsally and attached to the ventral edge of the urethral urothelium to complete the stoma.

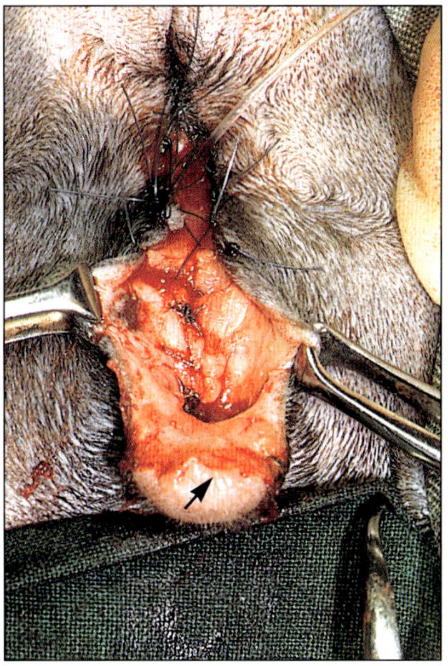

Techniques

Canine urethrostomy techniques

4.112 Urethrostomy should be performed as distally as possible. This male cross-bred is dysuric due to a stricture of the terminal penile urethra associated with previous urolithiasis at that site (which is unusual). This is treated by extending the ventral part of the external urethral orifice caudally. A ventral mid-line incision is made in the urethra from the external urethal orifice to proximal to the stricture using Metzenbaum scissors. A urinary catheter has been placed in the urethra proximal to the stricture. The granulation tissue responsible for the urethral narrowing can be seen in the terminal penile urethra.

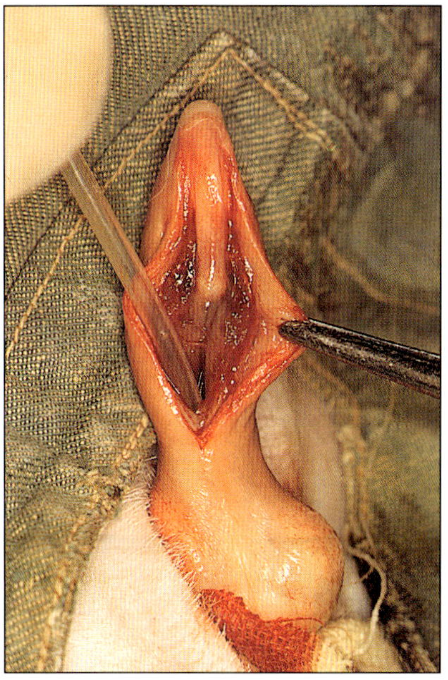

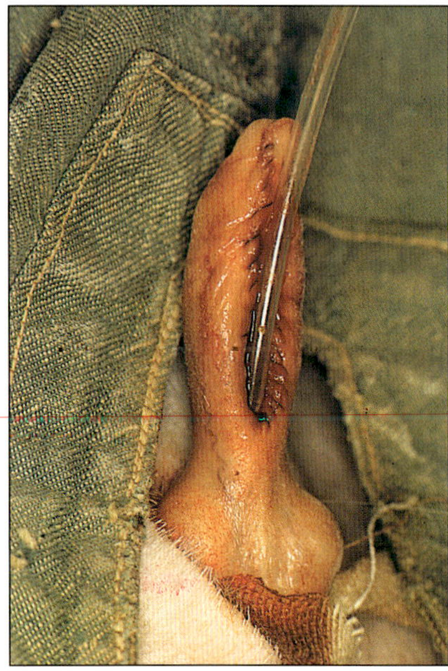

4.113 The penile integument is now sutured to the urethral urothelium, as shown, using a simple continuous pattern of synthetic absorbable material. In this case, 3/0 polyglactin (Vicryl, Ethicon) was used.

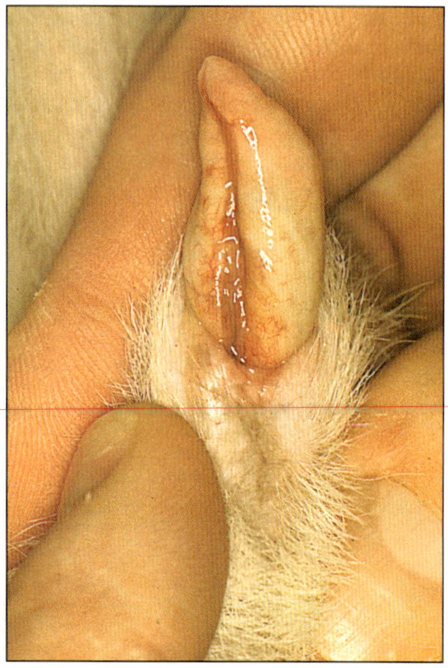

4.114 In effect, this creates a large external urethral orifice (as can be seen in this follow-up photograph one month after surgery) which extends distal to the site of obstruction, thus relieving the dysuria.

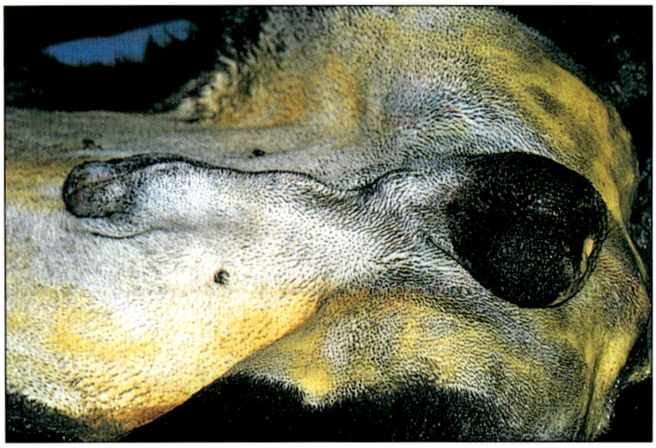

4.115 Terminal urethral strictures as shown above are rare and, more commonly, a scrotal urethrostomy is indicated. In this example, scrotal urethrostomy and penile ablation are required to treat a German shepherd with dysuria associated with a chondrosarcoma of the caudal os penis.

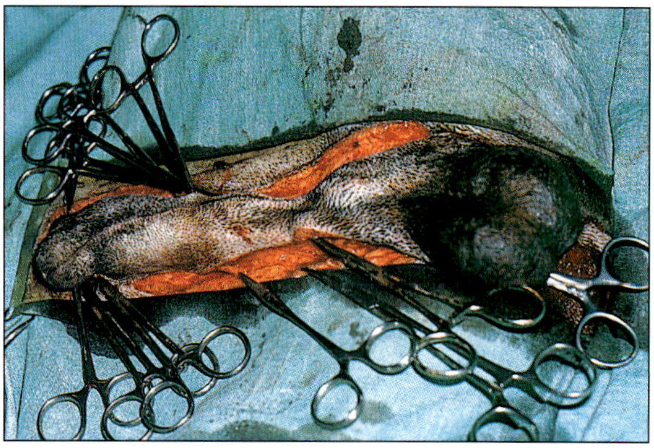

4.116 An elliptical skin incision is made around the penis and scrotum. The branches of the caudal superficial epigastric and external pudendal vessels which supply the prepuce and scrotum are identified, clamped and ligated, along with other subcutaneous vessels.

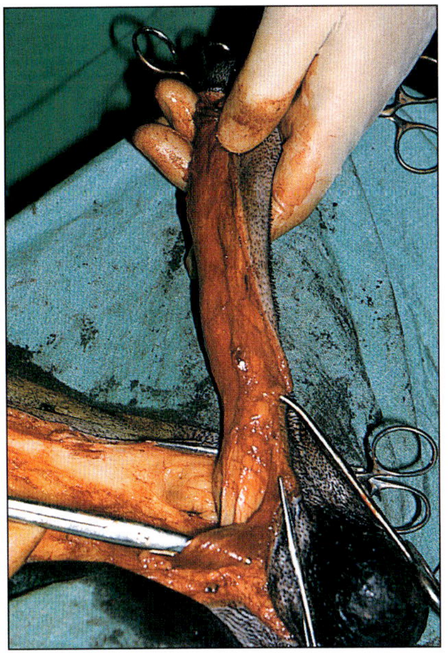

4.117 The penis is freed from subcutaneous fat and fascia by a combination of blunt and sharp dissection, and is elevated.

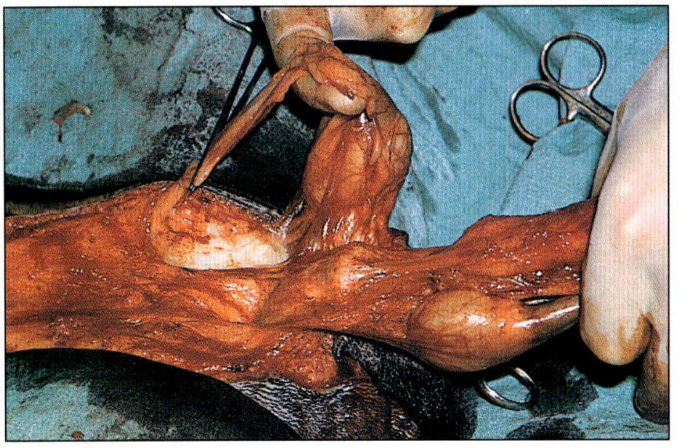

4.118 As the penis is reflected caudally, the spermatic cords can be identified, each covered in its tunic. A closed castration is performed: the cords are ligated individually just outside the external inguinal rings and then clamped and sectioned distal to the ligatures (see **5.2–5.24**). In the photograph, the dog's right spermatic cord has been ligated and sectioned (and is grasped in the nearest hand) and the left cord has been freed from surrounding fascia, prior to ligation.

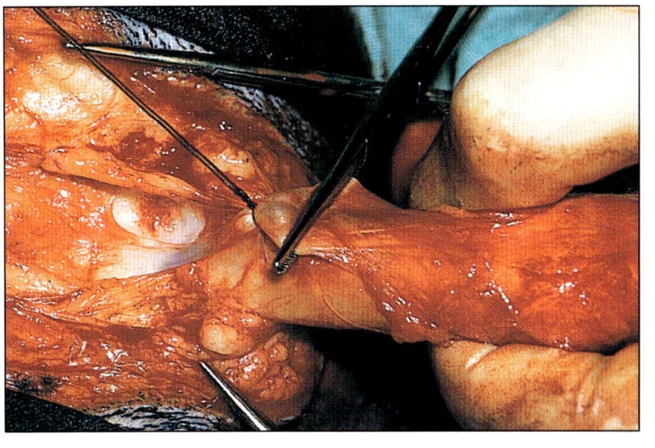

4.119 The dorsal penile artery is identified, ligated and clamped. It is then sectioned between the ligature and clamps.

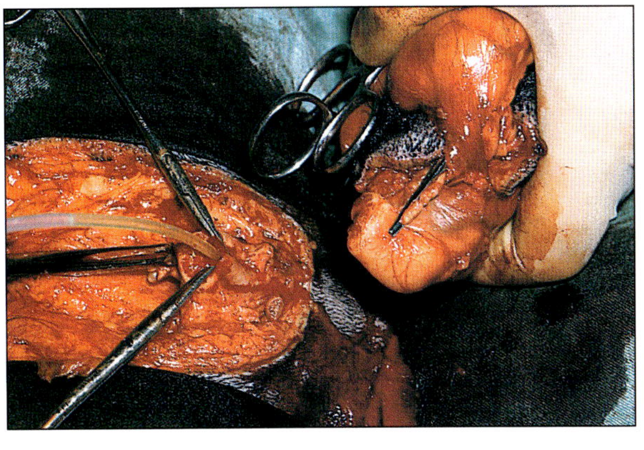

4.120 The penis is transected just distal to the penile artery ligature and the penis, prepuce, testes and scrotum removed. A urinary catheter is inserted into the urethra.

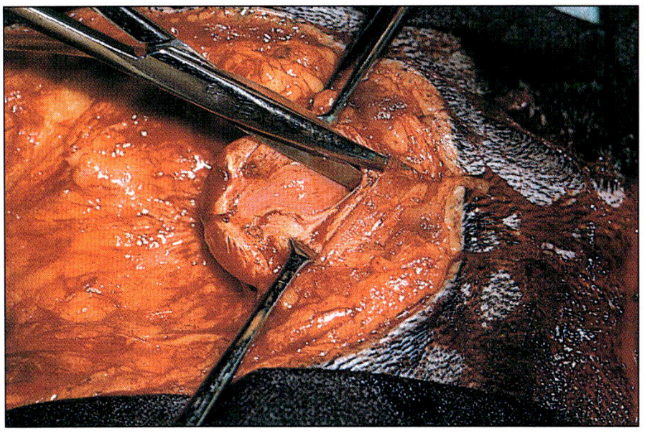

4.121 To reduce the risk of post-operative stenosis of the stoma, the urethra is spatulated by incising it ventrally with scissors.

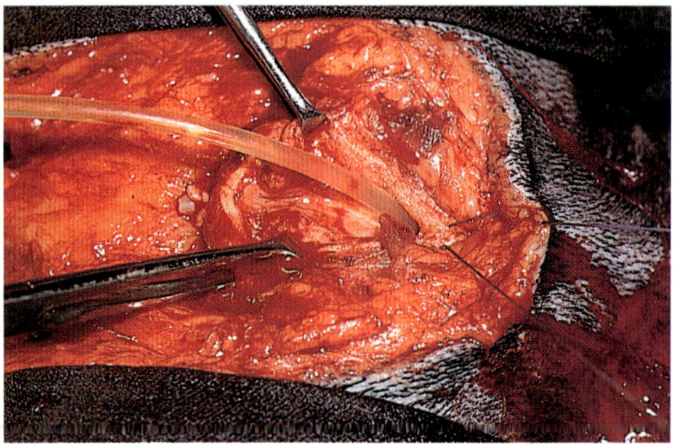

5.122 A suture of no. 2/0 synthetic absorable material is placed between the ventral wall of the urethra at the caudal end of the stoma and the subcutaneous tissues. This is to prevent tension on the suture line after stomatisation.

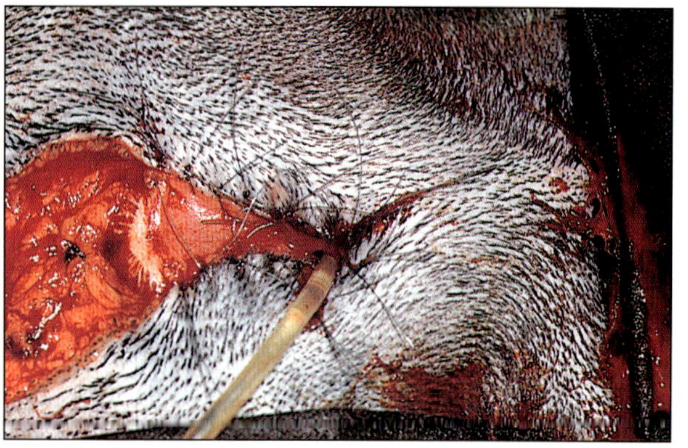

4.123 The urethral urothelium is sutured to the skin with simple interrupted sutures of no. 3/0 monofilament nylon.

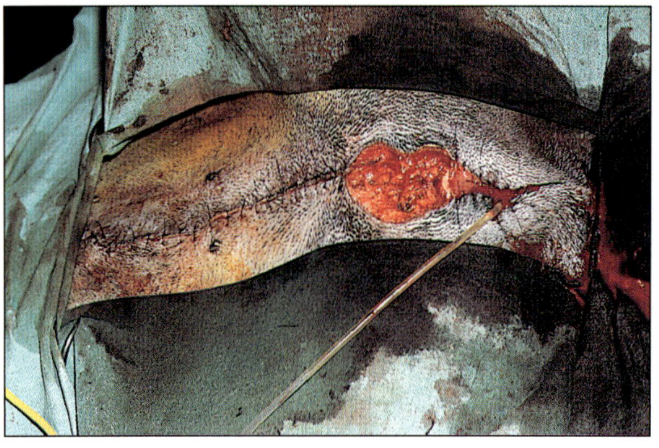

4.124 The ventral abdominal subcutaneous tissues and skin cranial to the stoma are closed in separate layers.

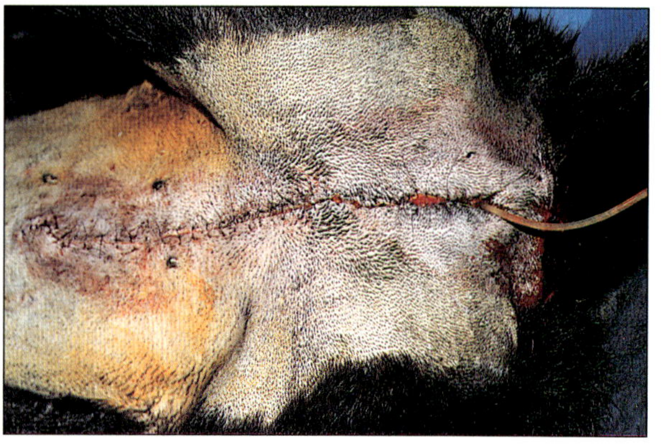

4.125 Closure is completed by suturing the skin to the urethral urothelium at the cranial edge of the stoma.

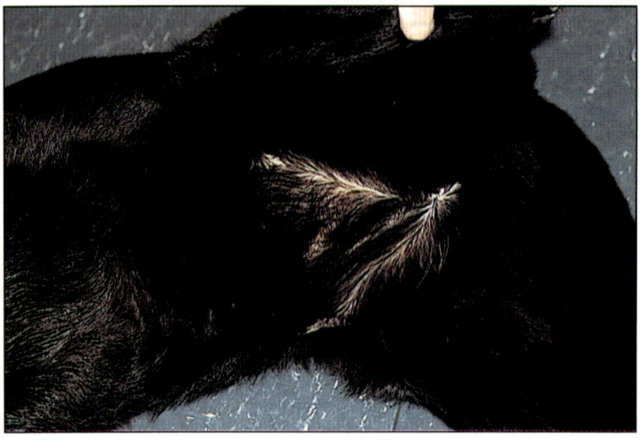

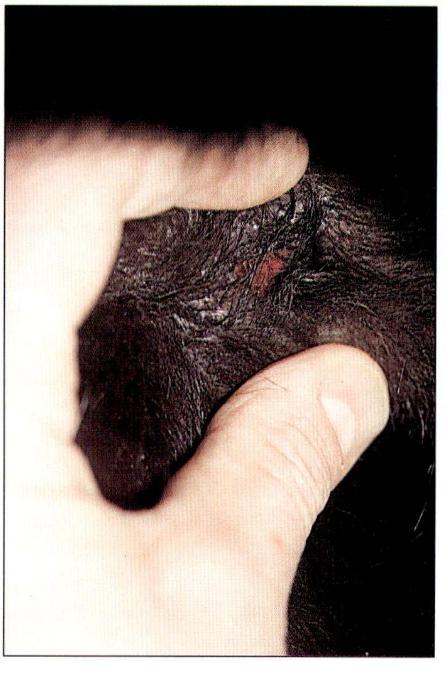

4.126 Although it might not be necessary to excise the penis and scrotum in many cases, the cosmetic effect of this operation is quite good, as can be seen from these follow-up photographs taken three years after surgery.

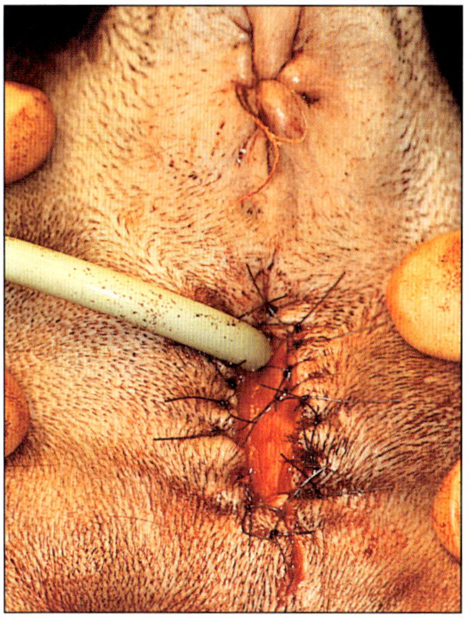

4.127 If a more proximal urethrostomy is required, the perineal site may have to be used. The dog is placed in ventral recumbency with the tail elevated and the hind quarters raised over a sandbag. The anus is closed with a purse-string suture and a perineal urethrotomy performed. The urethral urothelium is sutured to the skin to form a stoma and the urethra immediately distal to the stoma is ligated using no. 1 synthetic absorbable material to ensure that all urine flows through the stoma. A 22Fr Foley catheter has been inserted postoperatively in this animal. This is not usually necessary, but a large catheter was used in this dog to maintain urethral patency after dilation of intrapelvic urethral strictures via the urethrostomy. The radiographs of this dog are shown in **4.137** and **4.141**.

Perineal urethrostomy in the male cat

The technique in male cats is illustrated using diagrams and photographs to facilitate understanding.

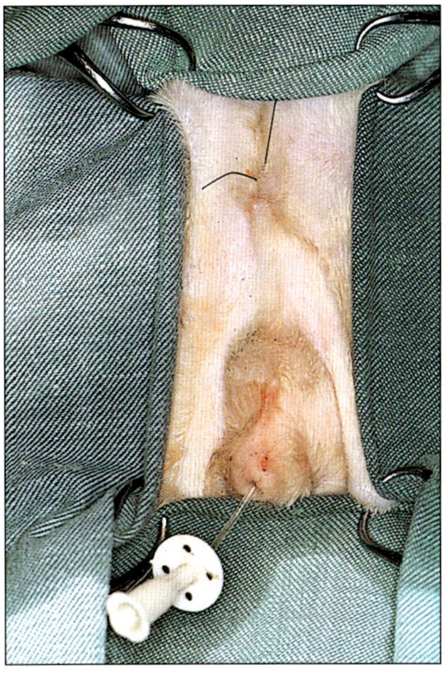

4.128 Perineal urethrostomy in the cat is performed with the animal in the same position as the dog. The operation is best done as an elective procedure rather than at the time of urethral obstruction. Apart from allowing the cat to recover from the systemic and local effects of urethral obstruction, this also means that a 3Fr or 4Fr urethral catheter can be inserted to facilitate identification of the urethral lumen and to empty the bladder of urine. If a catheter cannot be passed, the bladder must be emptied by cystocentesis as a full urinary bladder makes surgery very difficult (its weight tends to pull the membranous urethra cranially). The anus is closed with a purse-string suture.

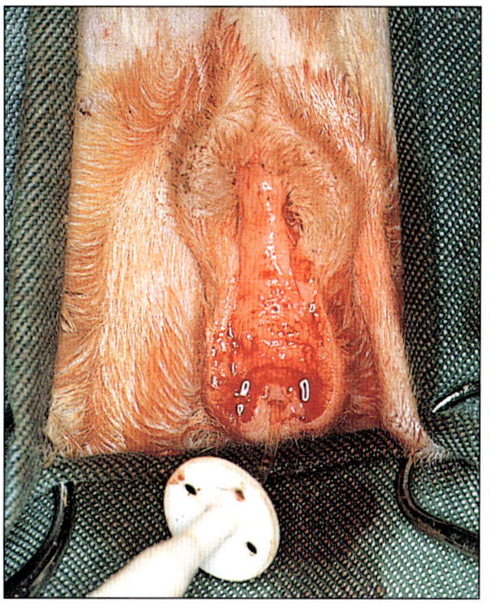

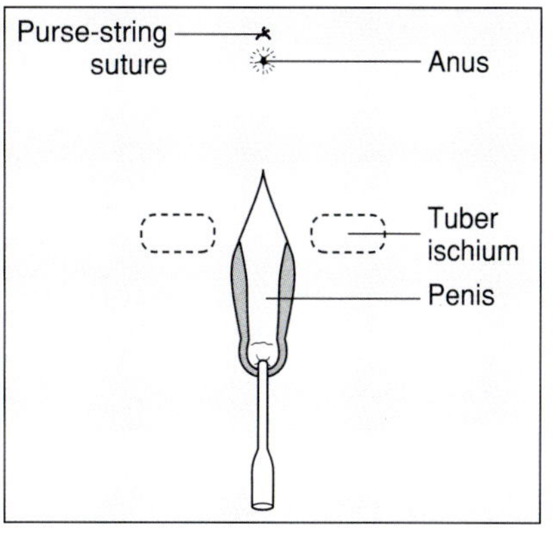

4.129 A vertical skin incision is made from just dorsal to the scrotum to the preputial tip. If the animal is entire, it is castrated. Excess scrotal skin should be excised. The incision is continued ventrally around the tip of the penis, leaving a small amount of preputial mucosa attached to the ventral part of the skin.

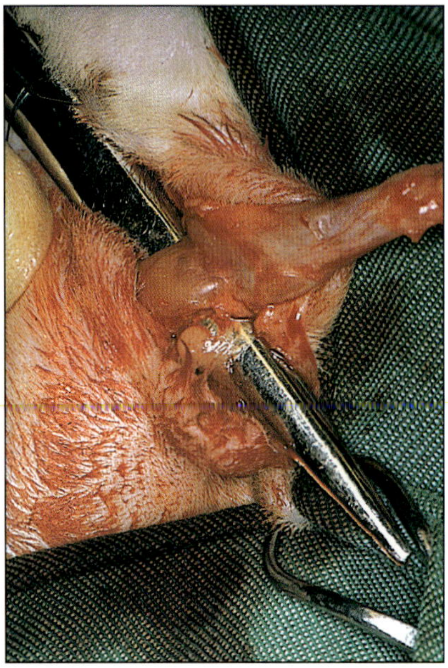

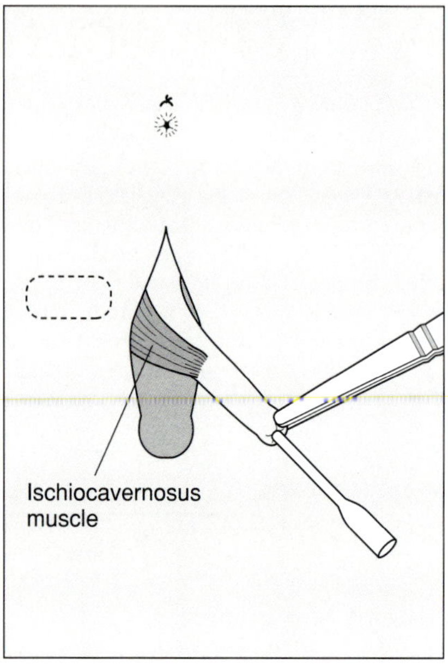

4.130 The penis is freed from surrounding fat and fascia by blunt and sharp dissection and the ischiocavernosus muscles identified. In the photograph , Metzenbaum scissors have been placed behind the cat's left ischio-cavernosus muscle. Each ischiocavernosus muscle is sectioned at its origin on the tuber ischium; haemorrhage is usually minimal and can be controlled with direct local pressure.

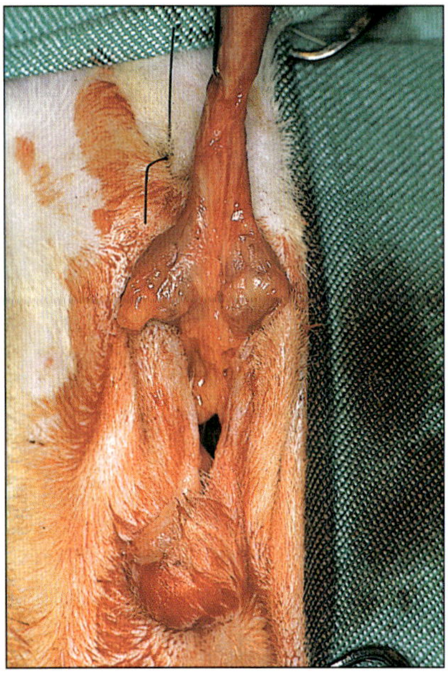

4.131 The penis has been reflected dorsally to demonstrate the two, sectioned ischiocavernosus muscles. The ventral fascial attachments of the penis and urethra to the pelvis are broken down by blunt and sharp dissection to allow mobilization of the urethra in a caudal direction. This is virtually impossible if the bladder is full, hence the need to empty the bladder of urine pre-operatively.

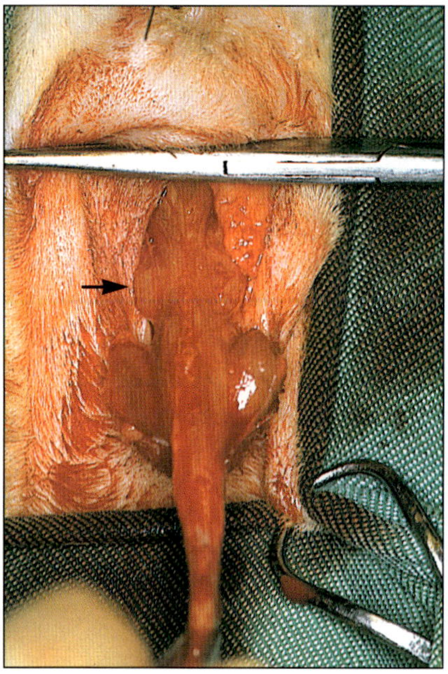

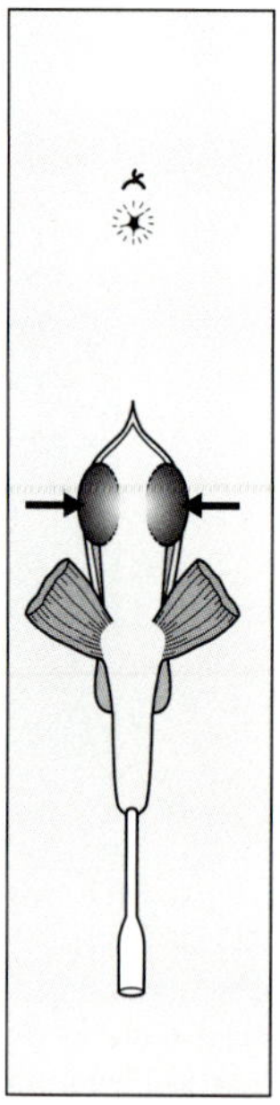

4.132 The penis and pelvic urethra are freed until the paired bulbo-urethral glands (arrowed) can be identified. These can be seen as bilateral bulges on the dorsolateral urethra, proximal to the attachments of the ischiocavernosus muscles.

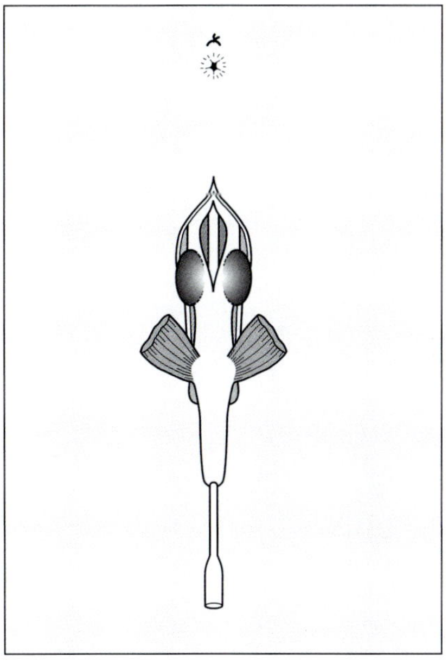

4.133 **At the level of the bulbo-urethral glands the narrow penile urethra widens into the membranous urethra, and so a urethrostomy is performed at, or cranial to, this site and not caudal to it on the penile urethra.** The urethrotomy incision should be as long as possible to allow for the formation of a large stoma.

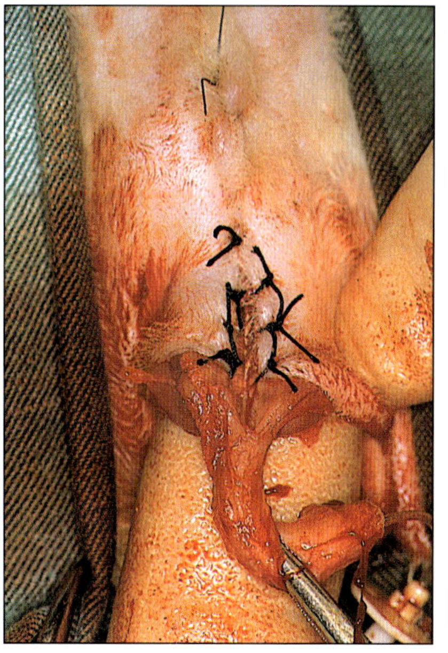

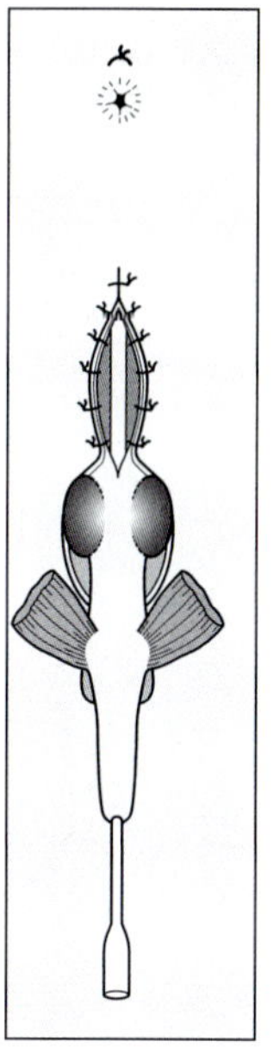

4.134b

4.134 **The dorsal urethral wall at the proximal end of the urethrotomy is sutured to the dorsal end of the skin incision to prevent tension on the suture line post-operatively.** The urethral urothelium is sutured to the skin on both sides of the stoma. As the urothelium is rather delicate, it is necessary to include a small bite into the corpus spongiosum during suturing to prevent the sutures from tearing out of the tissues. Initially, the author used to use absorbable suture material to avoid the necessity of suture removal. This irritated some cats and they licked and traumatized the area sufficiently for local oedema and partial obstruction of the stoma to result. The author then tried silk as a suture material (as shown). Although this proved to be less irritant, it absorbed blood leaking from the stoma postoperatively. This resulted in sutures becoming entangled in dried clots of blood which made suture identification during removal difficult. The author now prefers to use 3/0 or 4/0 monofilament nylon. This leads to minimal reaction and is easily identified. Simple interrupted sutures are used in all cases.

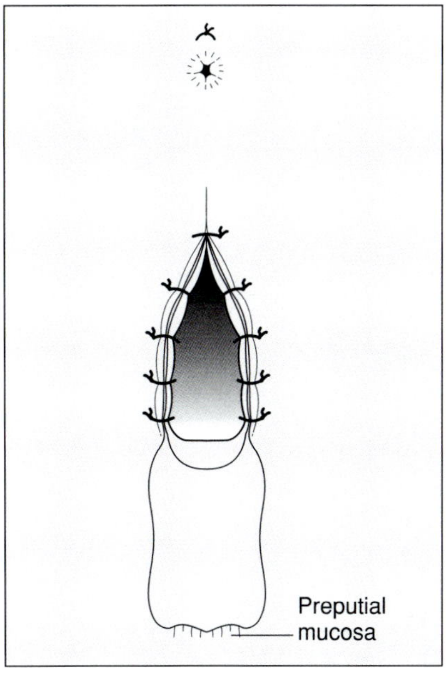

4.135 **The penis is now amputated level with the ventral part of the stoma.**

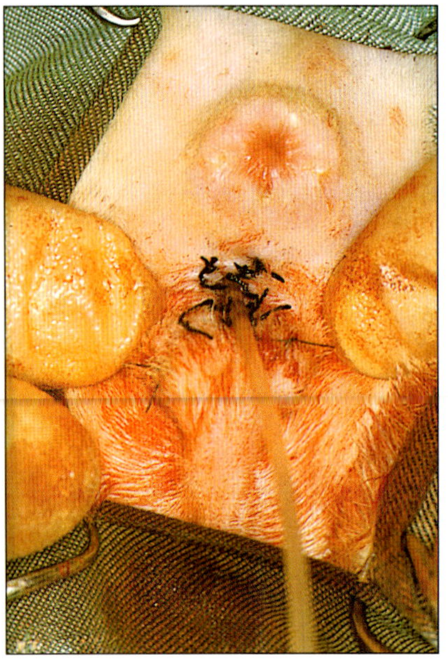

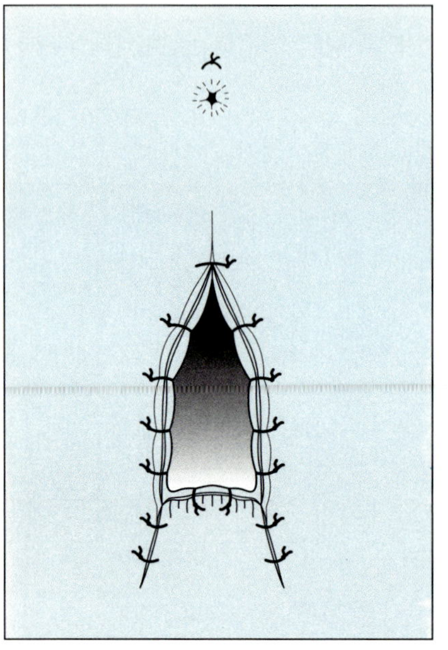

4.136 The urethrostomy is completed by suturing the fascia ventral to the stoma closed from side to side (see 4.111) and then folding the ventral edge of the perineal skin incision (with preputial mucosa attached) dorsally. The preputial mucosa is sutured to the remaining ventral edge of the stoma. This leaves two small open skin wounds at 4 o'clock and 8 o'clock to the stoma which are closed with simple interrupted sutures. The purse-string suture is removed from the anus and the catheter removed from the urethra. It should be possible to introduce a relatively large (6Fr) urinary catheter through the stoma and into the bladder after surgery, as shown. The cat is fitted with an Elizabethan collar to prevent self-traumatization of the stoma or sutures. The skin sutures are removed 10 days after surgery under general anaesthesia.

Urethral repair

Indications

- Urethral trauma.

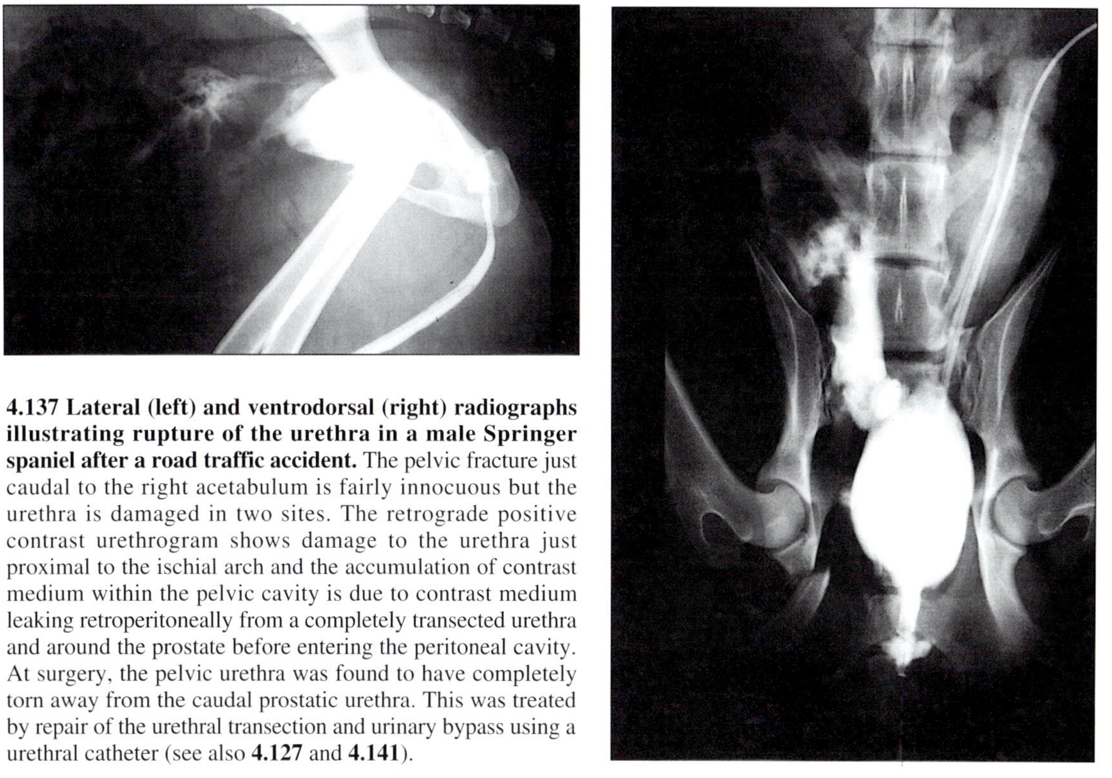

4.137 Lateral (left) and ventrodorsal (right) radiographs illustrating rupture of the urethra in a male Springer spaniel after a road traffic accident. The pelvic fracture just caudal to the right acetabulum is fairly innocuous but the urethra is damaged in two sites. The retrograde positive contrast urethrogram shows damage to the urethra just proximal to the ischial arch and the accumulation of contrast medium within the pelvic cavity is due to contrast medium leaking retroperitoneally from a completely transected urethra and around the prostate before entering the peritoneal cavity. At surgery, the pelvic urethra was found to have completely torn away from the caudal prostatic urethra. This was treated by repair of the urethral transection and urinary bypass using a urethral catheter (see also **4.127** and **4.141**).

Pre- and peri-operative considerations

Urethral (and bladder) rupture should always be suspected in trauma cases, particularly if pelvic injuries are present.

The metabolic effects of urethral rupture are identical to those following bladder rupture. However, as urine frequently leaks predominantly into retroperitoneal fat rather than into the peritoneal cavity, the metabolic signs may be more insidious in the case of the former (the constituents of urine are absorbed less efficiently from retroperitoneal tissues than from the peritoneal cavity). Urine has a necrotizing effect on tissues and early diagnosis and treatment are necessary to prevent widespread tissue necrosis and sloughing (see **3.17**).

The site of rupture should be located accurately, using contrast radiography, to determine the best surgical approach. Access and exposure are often difficult and it may be necessary to split the pelvic symphysis to allow access to pelvic urethral ruptures.

It is suggested that urinary bypass using prepubic and/or urethral catheters may be sufficient to allow urethral tears to heal. Although this is true of small tears, urinary bypass may be insufficient in the case of large tears. The problem is that it is frequently difficult to assess the extent of the urethral damage until the urethra is surgically exposed. However, urinary bypass should be used for between 7 and 10 days following urethral repair.

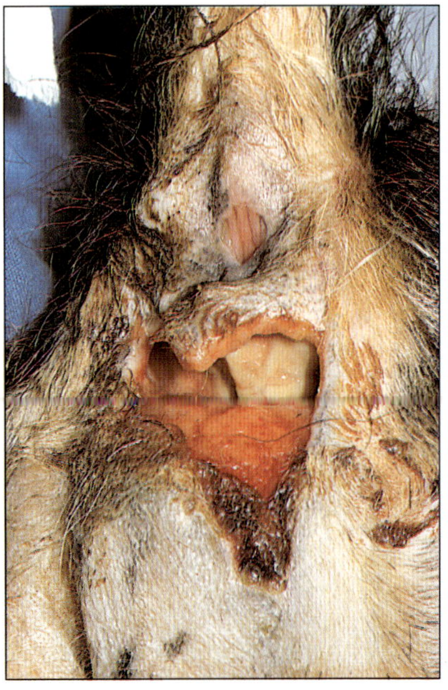

4.138 The necrotizing effect of urine can be seen in this male Dachshund with a rupture of the pelvic urethra. Sloughing of intrapelvic tissues and perineal skin has occurred. This was treated as an open wound until the defect was filled with healthy granulation tissue and then primary skin closure was performed (see also **4.142**).

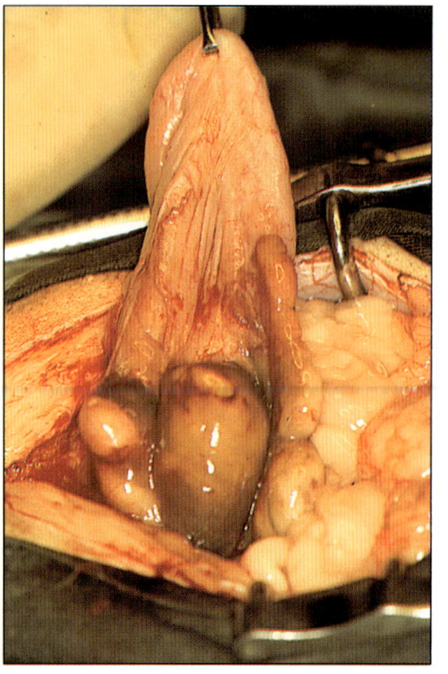

4.139 Identification of the site of urethral rupture during surgery can be difficult because of leakage of urine into surrounding soft tissues. Pre-operative contrast radiography is essential to allow a planned surgical approach and to minimize trauma to the area. In this bitch, contrast radiography had demonstrated a tear in the proximal urethra close to the neck of the bladder. This enabled repair to be performed without the need for pubic osteotomy. The discolouration of the perivesical fat is due to infiltration by urine.

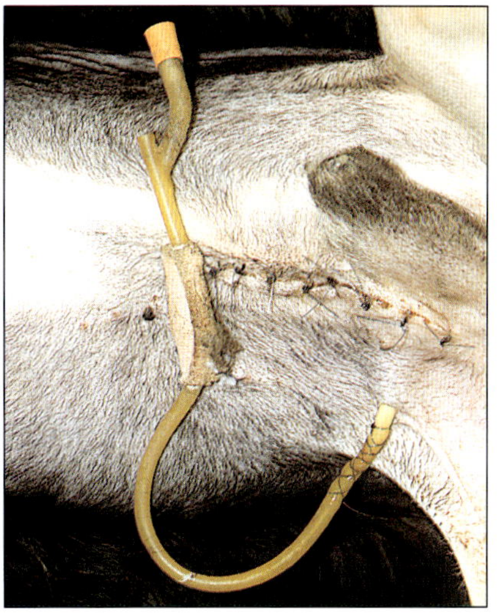

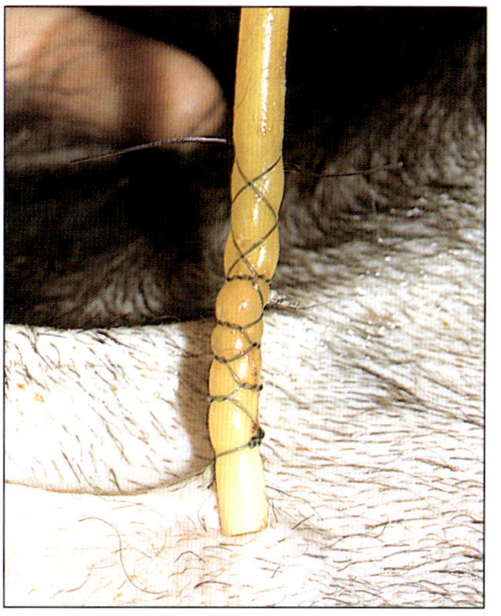

4.140 Urinary bypass alone may be sufficient to allow healing of urethral tears. However, it may not result in a good anatomical repair. In this dog, a pre-pubic catheter **(left)** was used to bypass a ruptured pelvic urethra. The catheter was attached to the skin using a Chinese finger trap suture **(right)**, connected to a closed collecting system and maintained for two weeks. The photograph was taken at the time of catheter removal. Although the urethra healed, the dog remained dysuric due to urethral stricture at the site of rupture and peri-urethral fibrosis of intrapelvic soft tissues after urine-induced necrosis. Part of the problem is that, whereas contrast radiography will usually identify the site of rupture accurately, it often fails to give an accurate indication of the extent of the trauma to the urethra. In cases of severe urethral trauma, urinary bypass alone may not be sufficient. The dilemma is that surgery is often the only method of determining the severity of the trauma and, in the author's opinion, should be performed in cases in which radiography has demonstrated gross urethral trauma or has failed to show that the urethral tear is not extensive. Urinary bypass should always be provided after surgical repair of urethral tears.

Possible surgical/post-surgical complications

Breakdown of the suture line or/and stricture formation may occur. The risks of these complications can be reduced by adequate debridement of necrotic tissue, attention to suturing and the use of an in-dwelling urethral or pre-pubic catheter postoperatively.

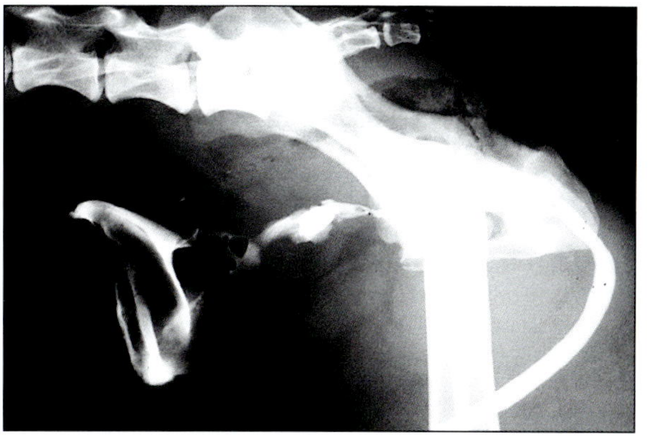

4.141 Follow-up retrograde positive contrast urethrogram in the dog illustrated in 4.137, two months after urethral repair. The dog is dysuric due to urethral strictures at the sites of previous urethral damage and repair (the caudal and cranial pelvic urethra). Urethral stricture is a common complication of urethral trauma. This dog was treated by dilation of the strictures via a perineal urethrostomy (see **4.127**).

4.142 The author is convinced that a cause of urethral stricture after repair is inadequate debridement of the torn ends of urethra before suturing. Devitalized urethral tissues may remain after repair, leading to breakdown of the repair and/or secondary intention rather than primary wound healing. The radiographs illustrated were taken at the time this male Dachshund was presented after a road traffic accident **(right)** and two weeks after surgical repair **(lower right)**. The pelvic urethra of this dog was virtually transected with less than a quarter of the urethral circumference remaining intact. Urine-induced tissue necrosis affected the intrapelvic tissues and perineal skin **(4.138).** A pubic osteotomy provided good exposure of the urethral tear and the torn edges of urethra were debrided back to healthy tissue before repair (this meant resecting up to 1 cm of urethra from each edge). As the follow-up radiograph shows, the urethra has healed in a normal anatomical configuration without stricture formation. This animal remains free from dysuria, three years later.

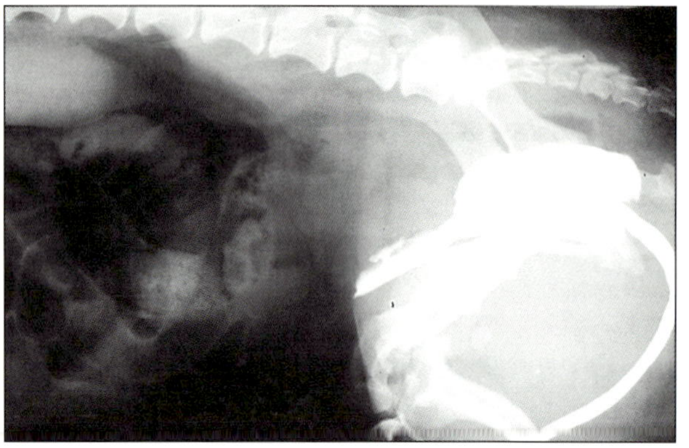

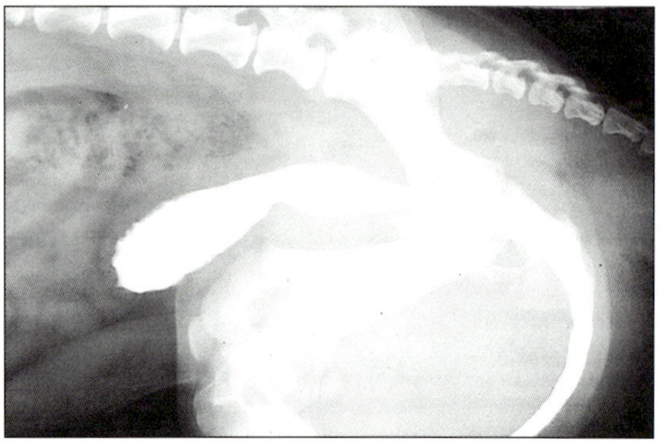

Technique

The urethra is repaired using simple interrupted sutures of fine synthetic absorbable material (see 'Urethral resection' below).

Urethral resection

Indications

- Urethral stricture, neoplasia, gross irreparable trauma.

4.143 Contrast radiographic (a) and urethroscopic (b) appearances of a urethral stricture resulting from urethral trauma and repair in the Cavalier King Charles spaniel bitch illustrated in 4.139. Urothelial polypoid masses, such as the one illustrated just distal to the stricture (**lower right**), are not uncommonly found in the urethra after trauma.

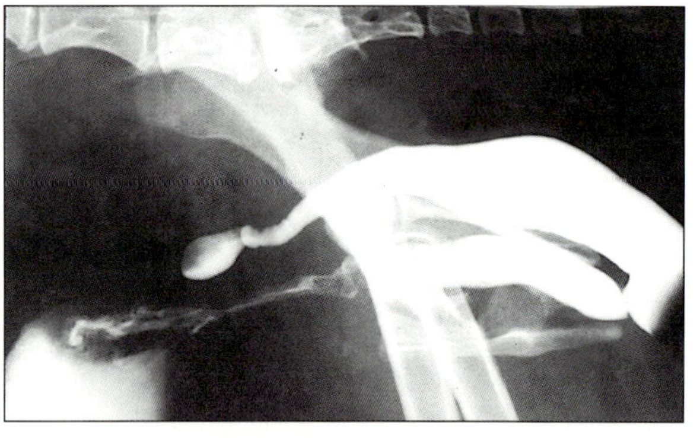

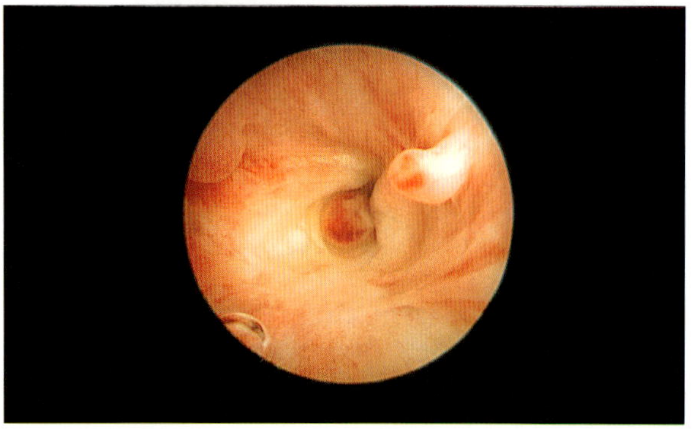

Pre- and peri-operative considerations

As the animal is probably dysuric, the metabolic and local consequences of dysuria should be corrected pre-operatively. This will probably involve bladder emptying by catheterization or cystocentesis and correction of acid–base and fluid disturbances.

Most urethral tumours are malignant and, in view of the poor prognosis associated with urethral malignancy, the justification for surgery must be considered and discussed with the owners. A biopsy should be taken for evidence of malignancy before surgery is contemplated; the catheter biopsy technique (see **3.27**, **3.28**) is ideal for this if the tumour is urothelial in origin or invading the urethral lumen. In the author's view, surgery of extensive urethral malignancy is rarely justified. Local metastasis has usually occurred, rapid recurrence is common after surgery and the quality of life of most animals is not improved by a significant amount and for a significant period of time.

As in the case of urethral trauma, accurate localization of the site at which the urethra requires resection is needed (using vagino-urethrography, urethrography, urethroscopy and biopsy – see Chapters 2 and 3).

If the pelvic urethra is involved, the surgeon should be prepared for pubic osteotomy to obtain adequate exposure.

Possible surgical/post-surgical complications

As can happen with any urethral surgery, wound breakdown and development or recurrence of stricture may occur after surgery. The risks of these can be minimized by attention to the viability of the urethral edges which remain after resection and care in suturing Simple interrupted sutures of fine synthetic absorbable material should be used. Urinary bypass should be provided for 7–10 days postoperatively.

Technique

Resection of the penile urethra was described in **4.115–4.126,** and urethral prolapse amputation is illustrated separately (see **4.148–4.155**). Urethral resection in a bitch with urethral stricture after urethral rupture and surgical repair is described in **4.144–4.147**.

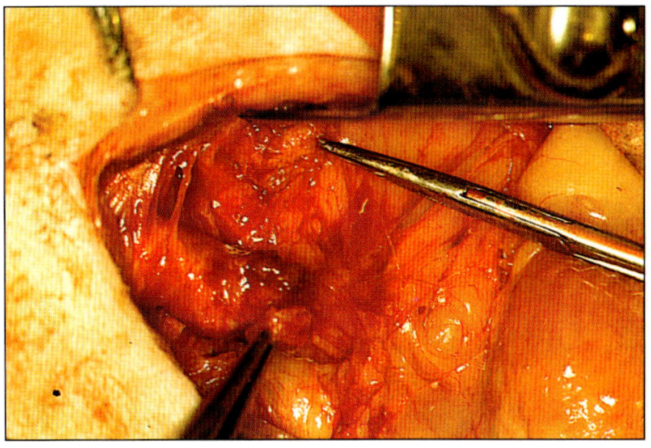

4.144 A pubic osteotomy has been performed on the bitch illustrated in 4.143. The bladder is in the bottom right of the picture and the pelvic fat and fascia ventral to the urethra have been separated to located the urethral stricture (the lower forceps are pointing to the stricture).

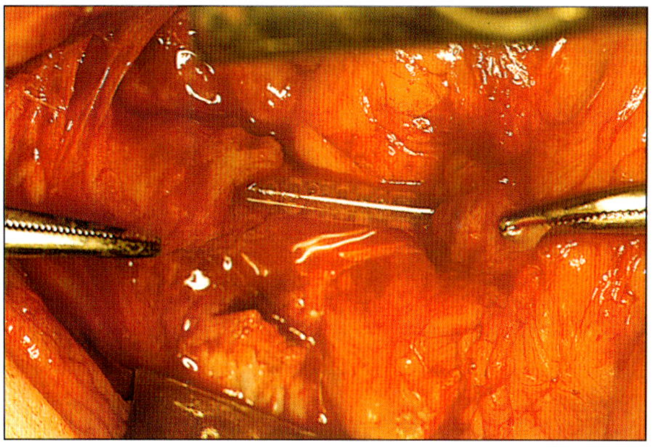

4.145 The strictured length of urethra is resected and a urinary catheter inserted through the external urethral orifice and across the gap between the cut ends of urethra into the proximal urethra and bladder. Bleeding urethral vessels are clamped at the levels of the cut urethral ends, as shown, and subsequently ligated. Initially, it is useful to leave the vascular clamps on the vessels as this facilitates orientation of the urethra, thus preventing rotation of one urethral segment relative to the other during repair.

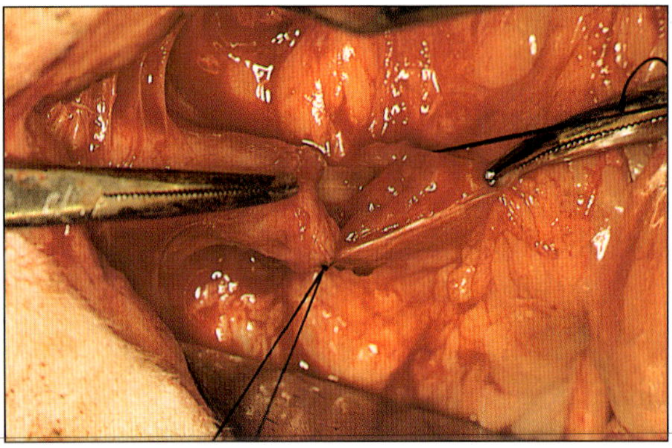

4.146 The first two simple interrupted sutures (in this case, 3/0 polyglactin – Vicryl, Ethicon) are placed 180° apart in the lateral walls of the urethra. This facilitates subsequent suture placement and, if the ends of these sutures are left long as shown, they can be used to rotate the urethra during placement of sutures in the dorsal urethral wall.

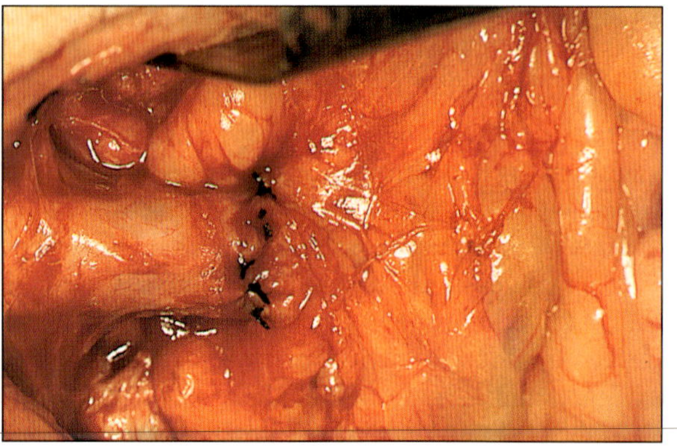

4.147 Suturing is continued around the circumference of the urethra until the urethral ends are joined. Sutures should be placed close together (approximately 2 mm apart) and tied tight enough to achieve apposition without crushing the urethral tissues. Once suturing is completed, the pubic osteotomy and ventral, caudal laparotomy are closed routinely. The catheter can be left *in situ* as an in-dwelling catheter for urinary bypass for 7–10 days.

Urethral prolapse amputation

Indications

- Amputation of urethral prolapse in male dogs.

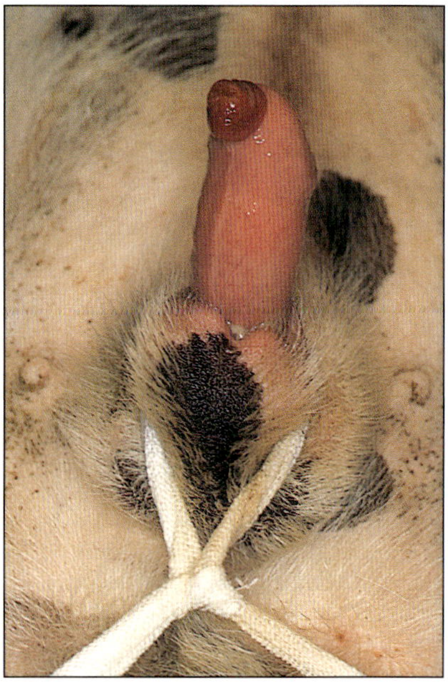

4.148 Urethral prolapse in an English bulldog. The prolapse appears as a 'red pea' on the tip of the penis. During surgery, the prepuce can be retracted and the penis supported by the use of a bandage, loosely tied around the base of the penis and pulled caudally, as shown.

Pre- and peri-operative considerations

This is usually a problem of young, oversexed dogs and may result from trauma to the penile tip during masturbation. It may be necessary, therefore, to treat the dog's oversexuality to prevent postoperative masturbation and possible recurrence.

The prolapse usually bleeds. Although such bleeding has to be differentiated from other causes of preputial, prostatic or urethral haemorrhage, it is usually not severe but may alarm the owner.

If the prolapse is chronic and becomes traumatized, terminal urethral stricture may result.

Possible surgical/post-surgical complications

During surgical resection, it is possible that the urethral urothelium may retract into the penis, preventing suturing. This problem can be overcome by resecting the prolapse in sections, suturing the resected area before a further section is resected, as shown below.

Stricture of the external urethral orifice may occur postoperatively. This is rare and the risks of stricture can be minimized by the use of fine synthetic absorbable suture material, attention to suturing, and prevention of postoperative trauma by the dog. Fine ocular instruments should be used for this technique, if they are available.

Haemorrhage from the penile tip may continue postoperatively, particularly if the dog traumatizes the area by licking and/or becomes sexually excited. Methods of physical and/or chemical restraint such as Elizabethan collars, body braces and sedatives may be required for 7–10 days after surgery.

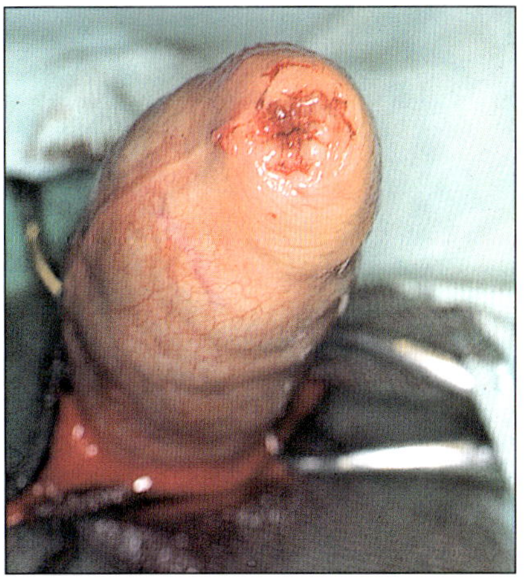

4.149 The risk of postoperative stricture can be reduced by attention to suturing. This is the immediate postoperative appearance of the penis of the dog shown in **4.148**. The urethral urothelium has been sutured to the penile integument using simple interrupted sutures of 5/0 polyglactin (Vicryl, Ethicon) placed closely together. If a continuous pattern is used, it should not be used unbroken around the whole circumference of the repair because, if the sutures are pulled too tight, a purse-string suture may result, leading to stenosis.

Technique

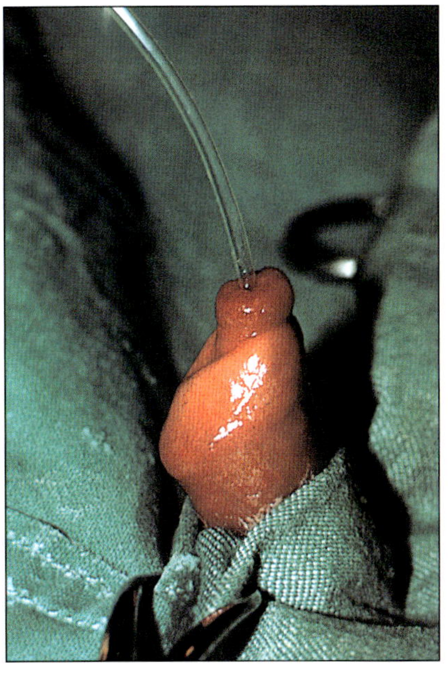

4.150 The penile urethra is catheterized and the penis elevated (as shown in 4.148). The penis is prepared for aseptic surgery using dilute antiseptics followed by sterile saline and avoiding the use of concentrated solutions and irritants such as surgical spirit.

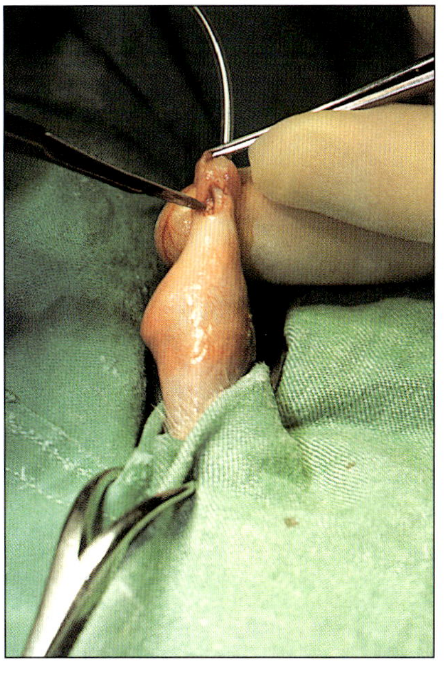

4.151 The prolapse is elevated and the penile integument incised at the base of the prolapse.

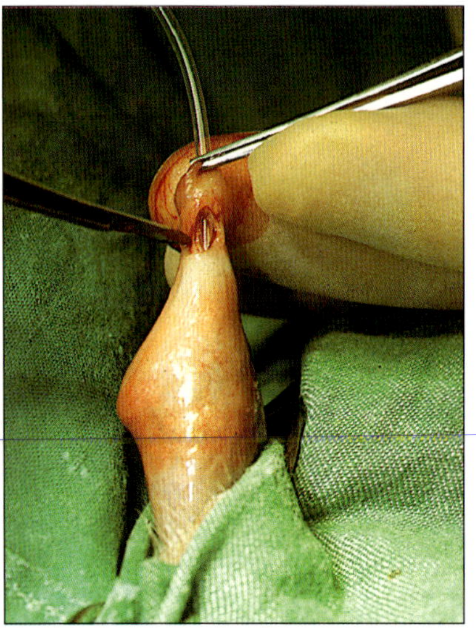

4.152 The incision is continued through the urethral urothelium to expose the catheter in the urethral lumen.

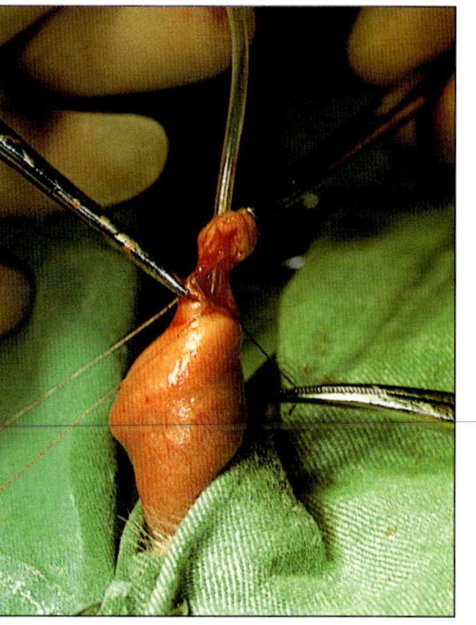

4.153 The urethral urothelium and penile integument are apposed using fine synthetic absorbable sutures. A simple interrupted pattern or continuous suture (as shown) can be used. If a continuous pattern is used, it is advisable to place the suture over a third of the circumference, tie it and then to use two further, separate continuous sutures to complete the remainder of the repair to reduce the risk of stenosis.

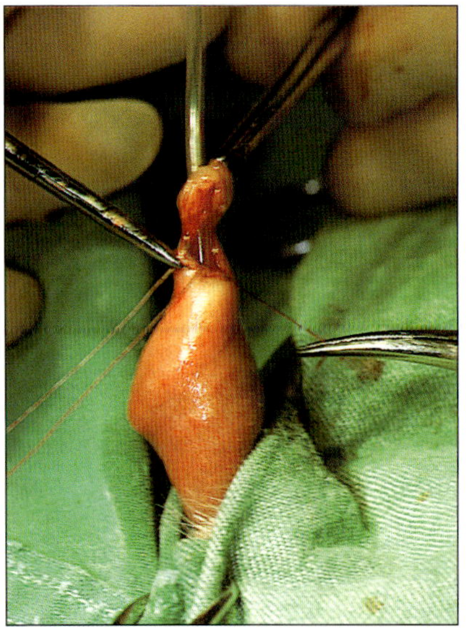

4.154 Once the first incised section is sutured, a further section is incised around the circumference of the base of the prolapse and the urethral urothelium and penile integument apposed as described in 4.153. Eventually, the prolapse will be attached to the penis by only a small section of tissue, as shown.

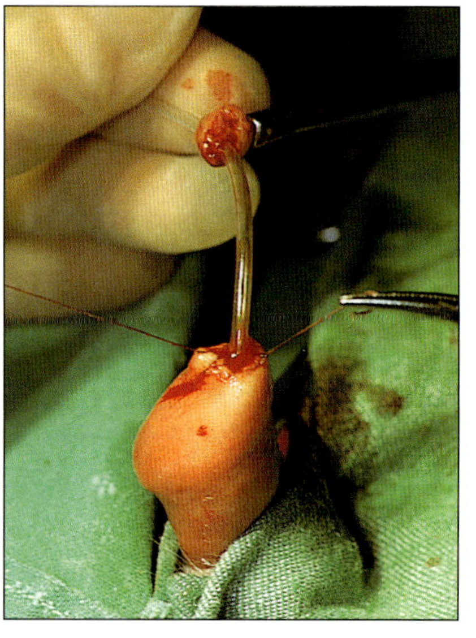

4.155 The final section of tissue is sectioned and the prolapse removed. The remaining defect is closed by apposition of the urethral urothelium and penile integument. The remaining suture ends are cut short after tying. Note the oozing haemorrhage which occurs. This is not serious but may persist as a postoperative problem – and alarm and/or inconvenience the owners if they are not made aware of its possibility. Post-operative haemorrhage can be minimized by prevention of trauma to the surgical site and treatment of the dog's excitement, especially if sexual.

Colposuspension

Indication

- Urinary incontinence due to urethral sphincter mechanism incompetence in bitches.

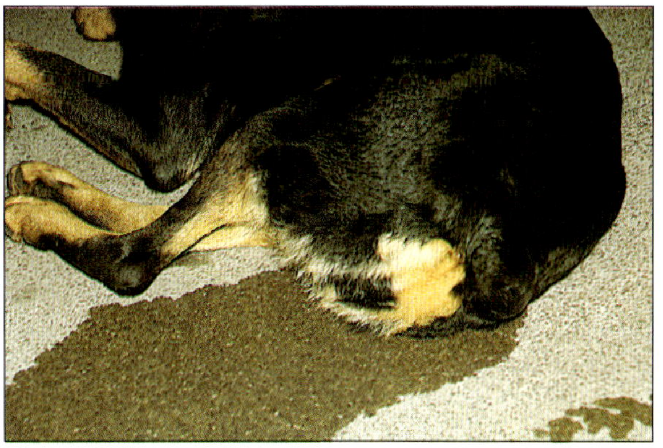

4.156 Urethral sphincter mechanism incompetence is mainly a problem of large breeds of dog. Urine leakage occurs predominantly during recumbency, probably because intravesical pressure rises when a bitch's position changes from standing to recumbency. A number of factors contribute to urine leakage in bitches with urethral sphincter mechanism incompetence. As well as body size and breed, these include poor urethral tone, ovariohysterectomy/ovariectomy, a shorter urethral length than normal (both physical and functional, allowing for body size) and a bladder neck located more caudally than normal.

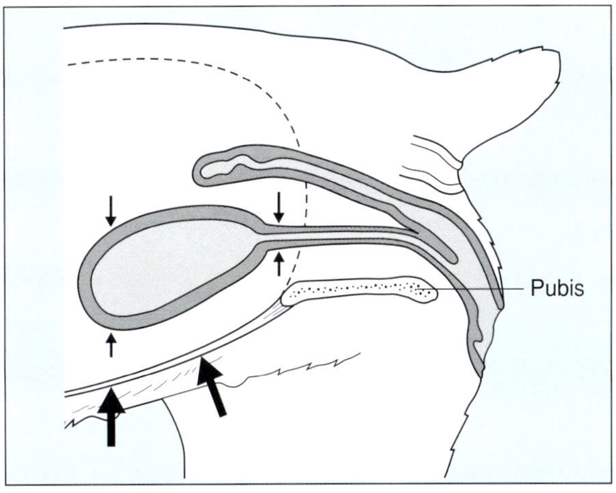

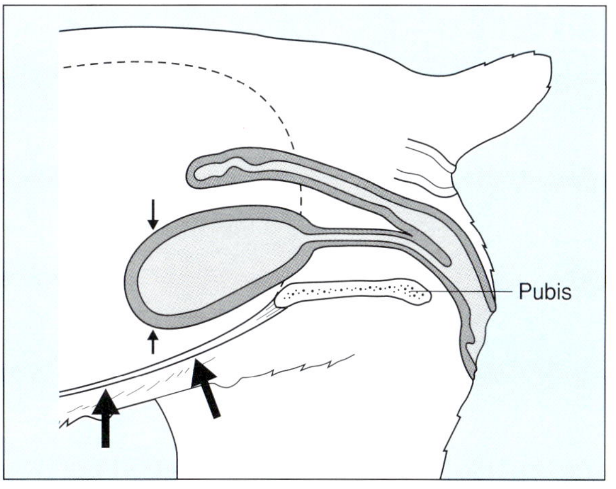

4.157 Colposuspension is intended to correct the position of the bladder neck (although it also has a beneficial effect on urethral urodynamic parameters). The caudal extent of the peritoneal cavity is indicated by the broken line. In animals with an intraperitoneal bladder neck **(left)**, any rise in intraperitoneal pressure resulting from recumbency is transmitted to both bladder and bladder neck/proximal urethra, making leakage of urine unlikely: the increase in intravesical pressure may be counteracted by a simultaneous increase in urethral resistance. In an animal which has a caudally positioned, extraperitoneal bladder neck **(right)**, increases in intraperitoneal pressure are transmitted more efficiently to the intraperitoneal bladder than to the extraperitoneal bladder neck/proximal urethra, which is surrounded by fat and fascia. If urethral tone is adequate, the position of the bladder neck does not matter but, in animals with urethral sphincter mechanism incompetence, a caudally positioned bladder neck may be sufficient to tip the balance in favour of urine leakage.

Pre- and peri-operative considerations

Accurate diagnosis is essential. It is insufficient to assume that a spayed, incontinent bitch is suffering from urethral sphincter incompetence without performing adequate diagnostic investigations to eliminate other possible diagnoses. These should include contrast radiography (Chapter 2), laboratory examinations (Chapter 3) and, if available, urodynamics (Chapter 3).

Colposuspension is not a cure for the condition but, rather, is an attempt to make the best of a bad situation by correction of one of the factors contributing to urinary incontinence due to urethral sphincter mechanism incompetence – the intrapelvic bladder neck. It may also have a beneficial effect on urethral resistance.

Surgery on juvenile bitches with congenital urethral sphincter mechanism incompetence should be deferred until after the bitch's first oestrus period. The first season may result in improvement in urinary continence control and more than half of affected juvenile bitches will become continent after their first oestrus. Animals with severe congenital urethral hypoplasia may be unsuitable cases for colposuspension. In such animals, the bladder neck cannot be returned to an intra-abdominal position by colposuspension. Fortunately, such severe urethral hypoplasia is extremely rare and its treatment is therefore not described here. Details of treatment of these unusual cases can, however, be found in an article by Holt (1993).

In adult bitches, the pros and cons of surgery versus management with drugs (oestrogens, alpha-adrenergics) should first be discussed with the owners. Oestrogens should never be used for long-term control in entire (especially juvenile) bitches because of adverse feedback effects on the pituitary gland. In some juveniles, these effects may be sufficient to prevent the bitch ever having a normal oestrus period. Colposuspension cures 50% of cases and improves most of the remainder, but does nothing for 10%. The author's approach is to treat young adult bitches surgically in the first instance, in the hope that prolonged use of drugs such as oestrogens and alpha-adrenergics can be avoided. Colposuspension is performed on older bitches (greater than 10 years of age) in which drug therapy has failed to control urinary incontinence.

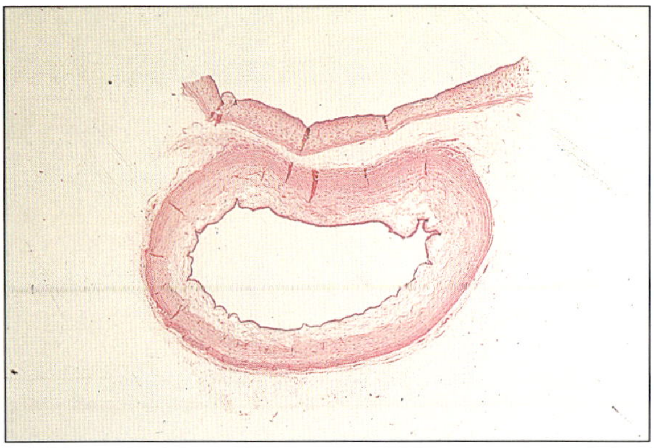

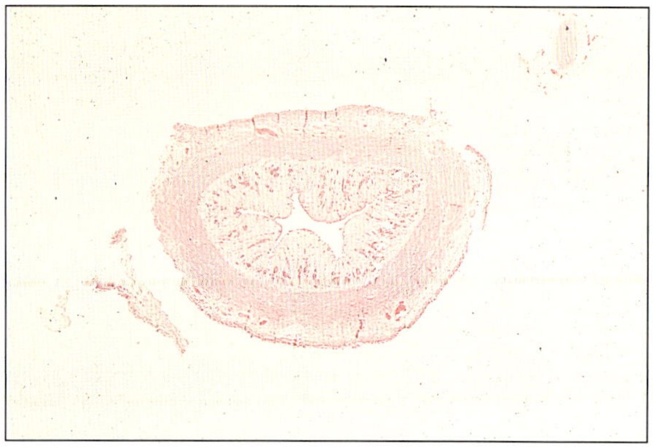

4.158 Non-surgical options for treatment should be considered. As these sections through the mid-urethra of a normal bitch during patency **(left)** and closure **(right)** illustrate, urethral closure depends on a variety of factors. These include urethral tone (both passive and that due to active, neuromuscular function), the efficiency of closure of the urethra by elastic longitudinal folding of the urethral lining and engorgement of suburothelial vascular sinuses (although this makes a minimal contribution to urethral resistance). Oestrogens are frequently used to treat incontinent spayed bitches with urethral sphincter mechanism incompetence. Their beneficial effects are to increase urethral tone by acting directly on urethral smooth muscle, sensitizing smooth muscle to alpha-adrenergic innervation (see **4.159**) and causing engorgement of suburothelial vascular sinuses. In addition, they improve urothelial elasticity, resulting in improved urethral closure. These beneficial effects must be balanced against potential side effects such as bone marrow and liver toxicity and they are not always effective in the long term.

4.159 Sympathomimetics (alpha-adrenergic drugs) are frequently used to attempt to improve the urethral tone of bitches with urethral sphincter mechanism incompetence. As shown in this diagrammatic representation of neuromuscular control of urinary continence, smooth muscle tone is primarily due to sympathetic stimulation. Alpha-adrenergics should, therefore, increase urethral tone by their action on urethral smooth muscle. Alternatively, parasympatholytic agents should be of benefit in reducing intravesical pressure. In practice, alpha-adrenergics are beneficial in many cases of urethral sphincter mechanism incompetence but parasympatholytics have no effect and are best reserved for cases of detrusor instability. In fact, this diagram is a gross oversimplification of neuromuscular control of urinary continence which is still poorly understood. For example, there is sympathetic and parasympathetic innervation of the urethra and bladder, and nerves from both branches meet and interact at the same ganglia on the bladder and urethral walls. In some species, the sympathetic nerves also innervate the urethral striated muscle. This has been shown to be the case in women and cats but not yet the dog. Obviously, the situation is very complex and our attempts to manage the condition are therefore somewhat simplistic. As with oestrogen therapy, alpha-adrenergic treatment is not always successful and potential side effects must be considered. At present, there are no good long-term studies of these side effects and therefore it is difficult to provide sound advice to pet owners.

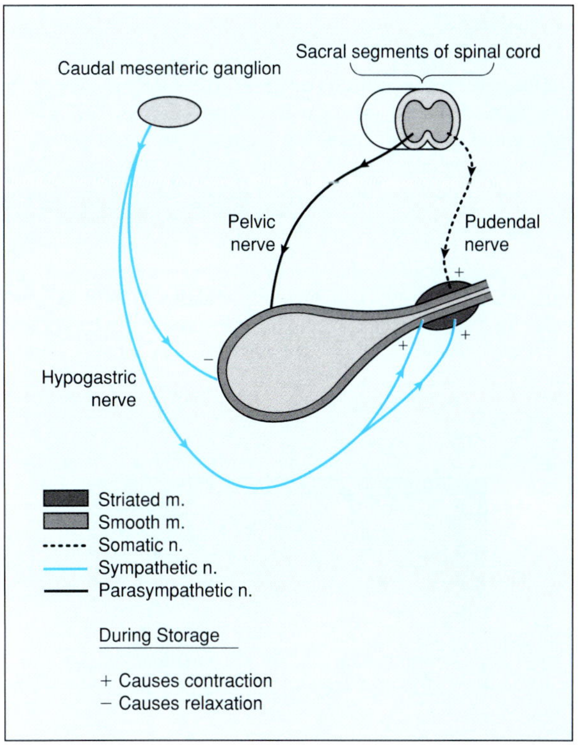

Possible surgical/post-surgical complications

Since the surgery involves trauma to intrapelvic structures, some animals are stimulated to strain, usually immediately after recovery from the general anaesthetic. This can be controlled by the administration of appropriate analgesics such as pethidine pre- and peri-operatively. A further single injection of pethidine after recovery is usually all that is required to prevent straining and relieve any discomfort. Rarely, some bitches find the first defaecation after surgery to be uncomfortable if the faeces are firm and bulky. This can be controlled with stool softeners such as Isogel (Charwell Pharmaceuticals Ltd).

Dysuria may occur immediately postoperatively. This is rare (less than 10% of cases in the author's experience). It may be due to vaginal stimulation by the surgery leading to suppression of the micturition reflex and/or reflex dyssynergia. Clinical observations and the response to diazepam suggest that reflex voluntary dyssynergia is the most likely cause of dysuria after colposuspension. It may be exacerbated by recent oestrogen therapy and so any oestrogen therapy should cease at least one month pre-operatively. Voluntary dyssynergia usually responds to diazepam (Valium, Roche) at a dose of 0.2 mg/kg by mouth two or three times daily. An in-dwelling urinary catheter can be used for a few days if necessary in the minority of animals which are unable to urinate at all. A further potential cause of dysuria is compression of the urethra against the pubis by the vagina. Care should be taken during surgery to avoid placement of vaginal sutures too close to the urethra (see below).

Bitches which are allowed to be very active after colposuspension may tear the sutures from the vagina. This is more likely to happen if they are allowed to run and jump, and owners should be advised of the necessity for restricting the exercise of their animals to only walks on the lead for one month after surgery.

Hymen formation and accumulation of vaginal secretions causing dysuria and/or dyschezia is an extremely rare, longer-term complication of colposuspension. It is due to breakdown of a pre-existing vestibulo-vaginal stricture during the operation and subsequent healing of apposing raw areas of vagina to forming a barrier across the vaginal lumen.

Technique

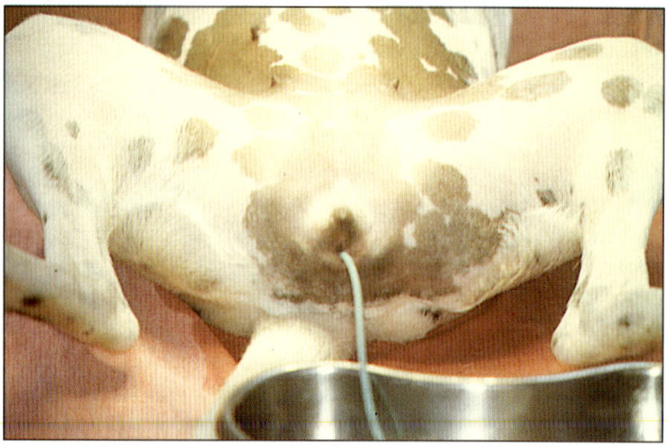

4.160 Under general anaesthesia, the bitch is placed in dorsal recumbency with the hind limbs flexed. The ventral abdominal skin and vagina are prepared for aseptic surgery, the vagina by douching with dilute aqueous povidone iodine solution (Betadine, Napp Laboratories Ltd) or non-ionic quaternary compounds (Trigene, The Hygiene Corporation Ltd). An 8Fr (smaller bitches) or 10Fr (larger bitches) Foley catheter is inserted via the urethra into the bladder and the cuff inflated. The catheter is then gently withdrawn until the cuff rests in the bladder neck. The presence of the catheter facilitates identification of the urethra and bladder neck during surgery.

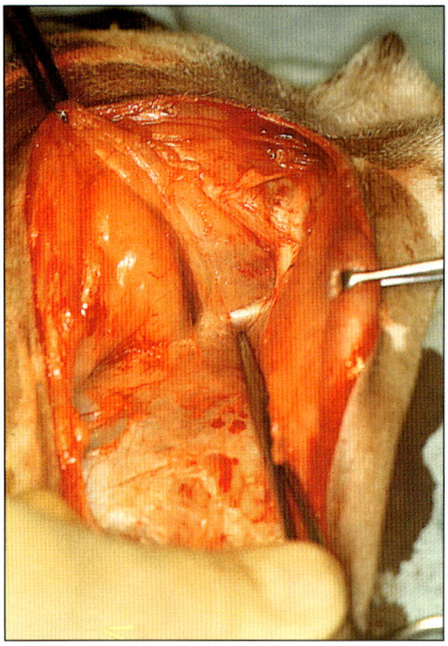

4.161 A mid-line, caudal abdominal approach is made. The prepubic fat and fascia are separated by careful blunt and sharp dissection on both sides of the mid-line and the prepubic tendons and external pudendal vessels identified. In the photograph, the bitch's vulva is in the top right corner and the artery forceps point to the left prepubic tendon. Just lateral to the prepubic tendon, the external pudendal vessels can be seen on the edge of the prepubic fat. These vessels must be identified and avoided during subsequent placement of sutures around the prepubic tendon.

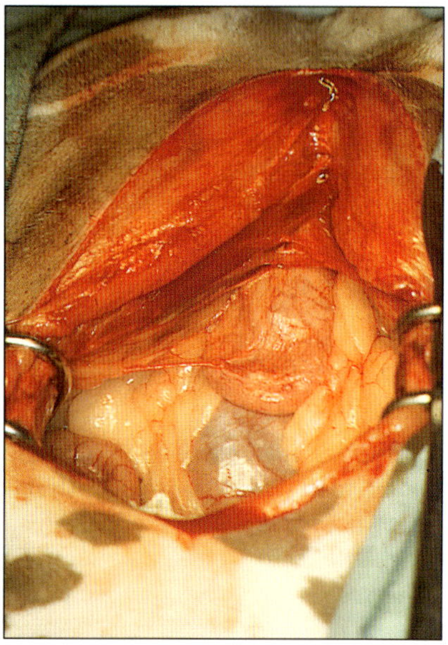

4.162 The mid-line incision is continued through the linea alba of the abdominal muscle wall and extended caudally to the pubic brim. Self-retaining (Gosset) retractors are used to separate the abdominal musculature and the bladder is identified.

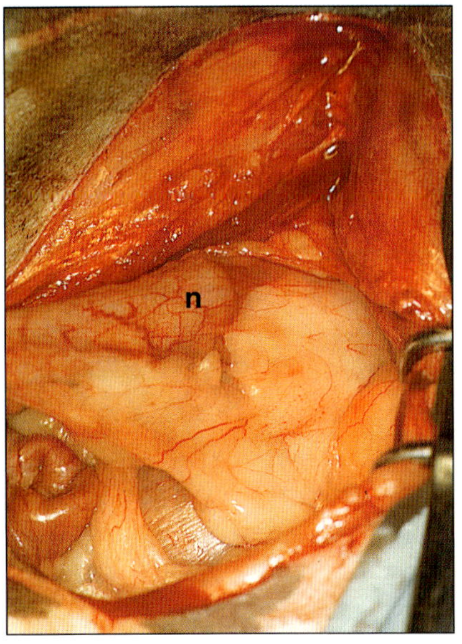

4.163 Cranial traction on the bladder allows the intrapelvic bladder neck (n) to be pulled caudally and identified by the presence of the inflated Foley catheter cuff. Note the presence of the retroperitoneal fat around the bladder neck and urethra.

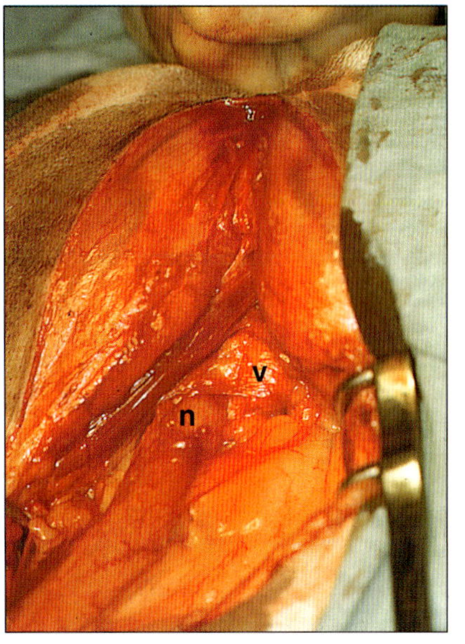

4.164 The vagina is displaced cranially and cleared of fat and fascia on either side of the urethra. This is most easily accomplished by inserting a finger into the vagina. The urethra can be palpated through the ventral vaginal wall and displaced to the bitch's left, while the vaginal wall over the finger tip (**v**) to the right of the urethra is pushed cranially and ventrally towards the caudal end of the incision. The vaginal wall can then be exposed by pushing off the overlying fat and fascia in a caudal direction using a dry swab. The bladder neck can be seen as a swelling due to the presence of the Foley catheter cuff in the bladder (**n**). The vaginal wall is grasped with tissue forceps. The technique is repeated on the other side of the urethra. The surgeon then changes his/her gloves and the vulva is covered with a large sterile swab or surgical drape throughout the remainder of the procedure. In bitches in which one's finger and the vagina are of incompatible sizes (very large or very small bitches or those with gross vaginal strictures or septae), the vagina has to be located by blunt and sharp dissection of the overlying fat and fascia on either side of the urethra, grasped with tissue forceps and then pulled cranially. This is more difficult than the use of a finger in the vagina and, fortunately, most bitches with urethral sphincter mechanism incompetence are of a size which is usually compatible with one's finger – depending on the size of one's finger, of course!

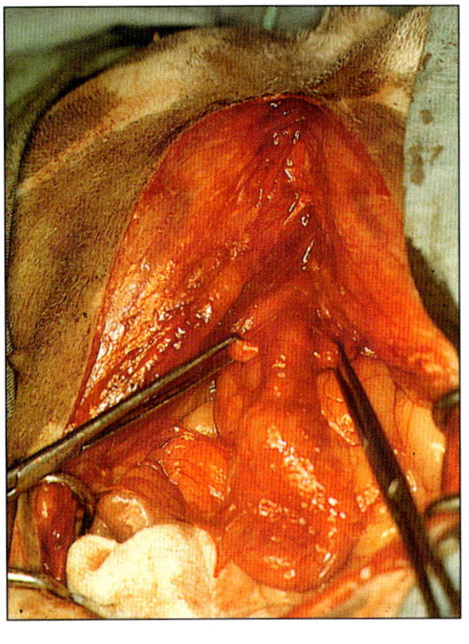

4.165 In this illustration, the vagina on either side of the urethra has been grasped with Allis tissue forceps and pulled cranially. As can be seen, this results in movement of the bladder neck and proximal urethra from an intrapelvic to an intra-abdominal position. (The swab in the abdomen is not essential and was used to prevent small intestine from obscuring part of the photographic field).

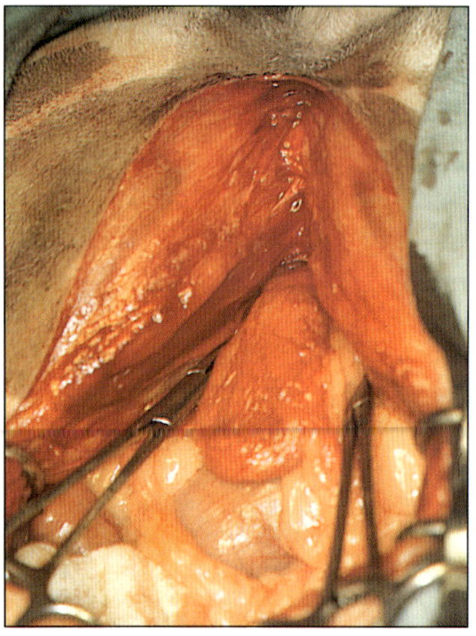

4.166 If the tension on the tissue forceps is released, the cranial vagina and bladder neck move back to an intrapelvic position. The vagina must therefore be anchored cranially to maintain the bladder neck in an intra-abdominal position.

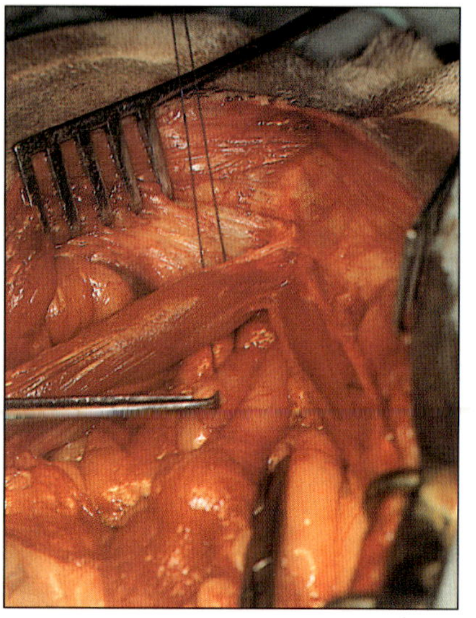

4.167 The vagina is sutured to the prepubic tendon on each side of, and approximately 1–1.5 cm away from, the mid-line. The sutures (monofilament nylon) are taken through the abdominal wall caudal to the tendon, in and out of the vaginal wall (as far laterally as possible) and back out of the abdominal wall cranial to the tendon. The placement of a suture attaching the left vaginal wall to the left prepubic tendon is illustrated. It is possible that the sutures may enter the vaginal lumen during this procedure, hence the need for preparation of the vagina for aseptic surgery.

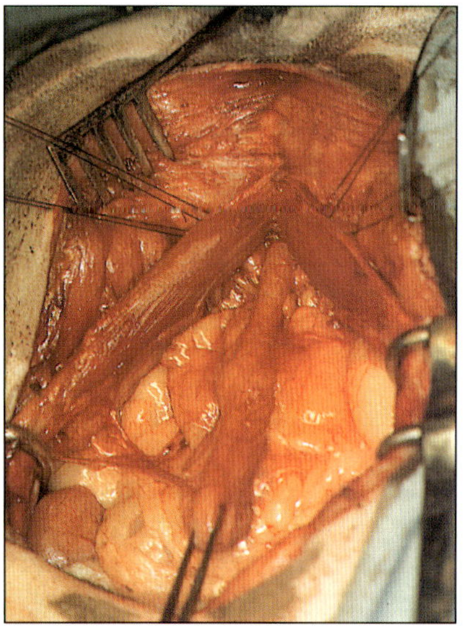

4.168 The number of sutures which can be placed around the prepubic tendon depends on the size of the bitch and is limited by the external pudendal vessels laterally. Most bitches are medium to large breeds and the optimum number of sutures is two on each side, as illustrated. No. 0 nylon is suitable for most bitches but no. 1 nylon should be used in very large breeds. On the rare occasions when colposuspension is performed in small or toy breeds, it may be possible only to place one suture through the vagina and around the prepubic tendon on either side of the mid-line. Once the sutures have been placed, they are pulled tight to ensure that, after they are tied, the urethra will not be compressed against the pubis by an arch of vagina as this may result in postoperative dysuria. It should be possible to insert the tip of a blunt-ended instrument – such as Mayo scissors or Kilner needle holders – alongside the urethra between the vaginal arch and pubis. If the urethra is compressed the sutures should be repositioned, but this is not usually necessary if the sutures have been placed as laterally on the vagina as possible. If all is well, the sutures are tied, the Foley catheter removed and the abdomen closed routinely.

Prostatic cyst/abscess drainage

Indications

- Drainage of non-removable para- or intraprostatic cysts or abscesses.

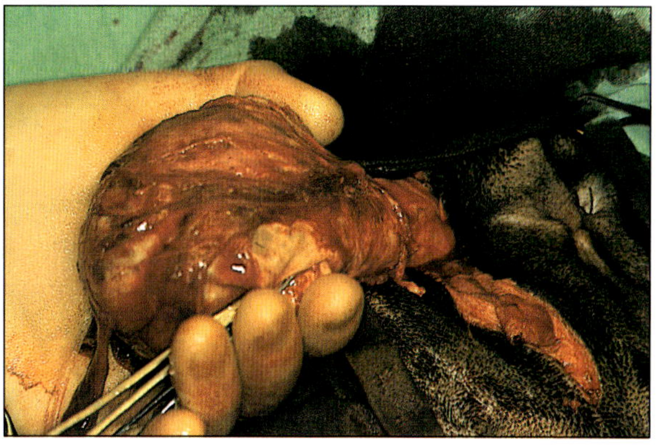

4.169 This paraprostatic cyst in the perineum of a Great Dane had a mineralized wall and was attached to the prostate by a narrow pedicle. It was therefore possible to excise the cyst across the pedicle. Unfortunately, this situation is uncommon and drainage procedures are usually required.

Pre- and peri-operative considerations

The systemic and metabolic effects of any dysuria /toxaemia should be treated with appropriate fluid and antimicrobial therapy. The choice of antibiotic should be governed by bacteriological examination of cyst/abscess fluid obtained by centesis (see Chapter 3). If this is not possible, trimethoprim sulphonamide is a useful antibiotic in the first instance as it is usually active against the organisms commonly found in prostatic abscesses, such as *Escherichia coli*, and enters prostatic secretions in high concentrations. Temporary drainage by centesis may significantly improve the animal's condition until surgery can be performed. In a few instances of small intraprostatic cysts and abscesses, drainage by centesis, castration and antimicrobial therapy may be sufficient to resolve the situation. More often, however, a more radical procedure is required.

A variety of techniques have been described for the treatment of prostatic cysts and abscesses. These include excision, drainage using Penrose and other drains, marsupialization and partial or total prostatectomy. None of these techniques gives consistently good results in every case and the choice of method, therefore, depends on the experience and preference of the surgeon. The author prefers to excise paraprostatic cysts if these are attached to the prostate by a pedicle. Unfortunately this is rare. For the treatment of non-excisable cysts or abscesses, the author employs marsupialization or Foley catheter drainage.

Accurate diagnosis is essential and small cysts or abscesses require ultrasonography for accurate localization and sampling of contents (see Chapter 3). Cyst and abscess contents should be submitted for cytological as well as bacteriological examinations as carcinomas may be found in the lining of a proportion of prostatic cysts and abscesses. For this reason, caudal abdominal and thoracic radiographs should be examined for evidence of malignancy (local and distant metastases). In addition, an attempt should be made to determine if the cyst/abscess cavity communicates with the prostatic urethra, using retrograde positive contrast urethrography (see Chapter 2) and ultrasonography. Any communication between the cyst/abscess and the prostatic urethra is a contraindication for marsupialization because of the risk of postoperative urethrocutaneous fistulation (see below). In addition, drainage using Penrose drains in such cases is hazardous because of the risk of leakage of urine from the urethra into the peritoneal cavity. Such a communication may be detected by contrast radiography and ultrasonography but should also be assumed to be present in dogs with prostatic abscessation which have a purulent urethral discharge (e.g. **1.7**). However, it is not always possible to detect this communication and owners should be warned of the fact before surgery is performed on their animals. In dogs with a communication between the cyst/abscess cavity and the urethra, the author prefers to perform a more temporary drainage using a Foley catheter.

Ultrasonography will demonstrate if multiple cysts or abscesses are present and, often, whether the lumina of these communicate with each other. This information is useful during the subsequent surgical technique as the surgeon is prepared for the possibility of breaking down septae between non-communicating intraprostatic cavities.

The site for drainage is prepubic (unless the cyst/abscess is perineal) and the side is determined by the location of the fluid-filled swelling. A separate laparotomy is required (on the opposite side to the drainage site) to facilitate surgical manipulations and so the ventral abdominal skin on both sides of the prepuce should be prepared for aseptic surgery.

If the cyst/abscess has extended caudally into the perineum through a perineal rupture, the options are to drain it by centesis through the perineum, return it to the abdomen and drain it prepubically, or to marsupialize it through the ventral perineum.

It may not be possible to marsupialize an intra-prostatic cyst or abscess if the prostate is insufficiently mobile. It is advisable to be prepared for the possibilities of tube (Foley catheter) or Penrose drainage, if necessary.

There is some controversy about the role of castration in prostatic cysts/abscesses. However, hormonal imbalances may contribute to the aetiology of prostatic cysts and abscesses. For example, excessive oestrogens may lead to squamous metaplasia of the lining epithelium of prostatic ducts. This may result in duct blockage, accumulation of prostatic secretions (+/– bacteria) and intraprostatic cyst/abscess formation. In addition, castration has been shown to have a beneficial effect in cases of bacterial prostatitis, which may precede abscessation. In the author's view, the owners of dogs with prostatic cysts/abscessation should be advised to have their animals castrated.

A proportion of dogs have a persistent discharge from the stoma after marsupialization. This is rare but owners should be advised of the possibility before surgery is performed.

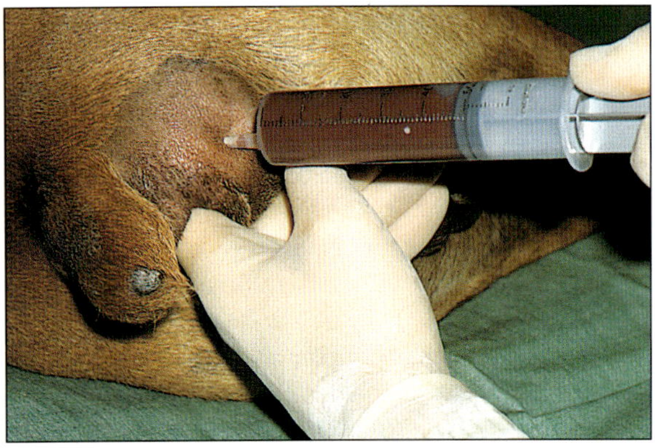

4.170 Drainage of prostatic cysts and abscesses by centesis may temporarily alleviate the signs while the dog is stabilized. This Boxer has a prostatic abscess extending into the perineum. Drainage of the abscess fluid contents relieved the dysuria and dyschezia which were present and, along with antibiotic therapy, allowed the animal to be stabilized so that surgery could be performed as an elective procedure a few days later rather than as an emergency technique in a toxaemic patient with metabolic disturbances secondary to dysuria. This also enabled the abscess fluid to be examined bacteriologically and cytologically for the identification (and antibiotic sensitivities) of the causal organisms and presence or abscence of malignant cells before surgery. The presence of malignant cells is a contra-indication for surgical intervention as such cases are associated with a hopeless prognosis.

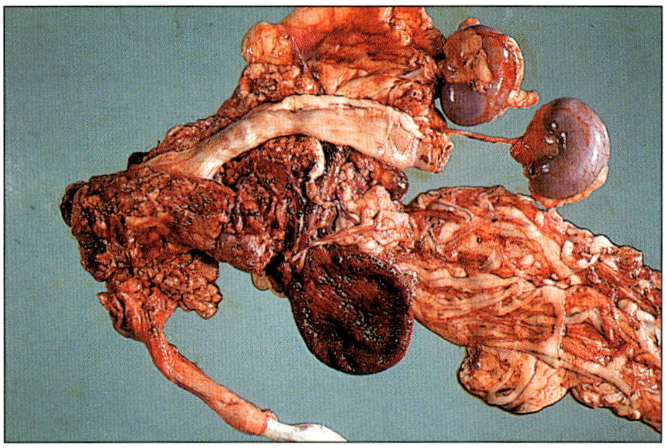

4.171 Widespread local malignancy associated with a carcinoma of the lining of a prostatic cyst (demonstrated *post mortem*). The tumour had extended within the pelvis to involve the rectum and urethra, resulting in clinical signs of dyschezia and dysuria. The effect of urine retention on the bladder can be appreciated. The malignancy is not usually as apparent as this and so a biopsy of the cyst/abscess lining during surgery is mandatory (see also **4.181**).

4.172 Prostatic cysts and abscesses which extend caudally into a perineal rupture may be treated in two ways. The first is to drain the cyst/abscess by centesis and return it to the abdominal cavity during perineal rupture repair. The cyst/abscess can then be drained prepubically in the usual way. However, the degree of surgical intervention can be reduced by draining the cyst/abscess through the ventral perineum and then repairing the perineal rupture dorsal to it. This is illustrated in this figure, in which a fenestrated polyurethane tube has been inserted into the marsupialized cyst. The perineal rupture dorsal to the stoma has been repaired and all that remains is to close the subcutaneous tissues and skin. A purse-string suture can be seen in the anus in the top left side of the photograph and some inspissated cyst material is present on the surgical drape ventral to the stoma. It is advisable to leave a drainage tube in the stoma in these cases for the first 4–5 days after surgery The cranial portion of the cyst/abscess may extend ventral to the pubis (in the abdomen) and thus be lower than the stoma in the perineum. The tube is used to ensure adequate drainage by flushing until the cyst/abscess cavity reduces in size.

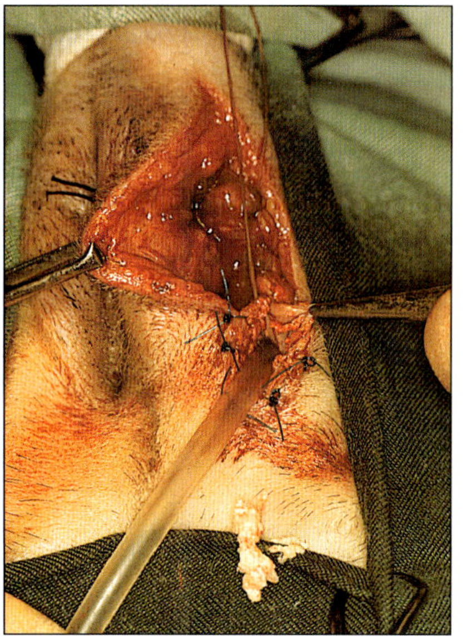

Possible surgical/post-surgical complications

Peritonitis may result from spillage of pus into the abdomen during surgery. This is unusual and the risk can be minimized by a number of basic precautions. The abscess/cyst should be drained by needle aspiration during the laparotomy. This facilitates manipulation of the cyst/abscess wall (particularly if it is to be drawn through the abdominal wall during marsupialization) and reduces the risk of contamination once the cyst/abscess is incised. The area around the cyst/abscess should be packed off with sterile swabs during surgery. Once the abscess/cyst has been marsupialized or the drain inserted, local suction and peritoneal lavage (using sterile normal saline) should be employed to remove any contaminating fluids before closure of the laparotomy.

Urethrocutaneous fistulation may follow marsupialization if the cyst/abscess was draining into the prostatic urethra pre-operatively. This is very difficult to treat although it may close spontaneously if it is detected in the early postoperative period and an in-dwelling urethral catheter used. Prevention by detection of a communication between the cyst/abscess cavity and urethra before surgery is preferable so that an alternative technique to marsupialization, such as Foley catheter drainage, can be used.

If Foley catheter drainage is used, there may be problems in maintaining the catheter *in situ* for at least 10 days. These can be minimized by attention to suturing techniques (see below). The use of omentum between the cyst/abscess and abdominal walls reduces the risk of contamination of the peritoneal cavity by cyst/abscess contents leaking around the catheter or after catheter removal.

If the sutures used to appose the wall of the cyst/abscess to the abdominal wall break down, a ventral rupture may occur. It is best, therefore, to use a simple interrupted pattern (rather than continuous) of a synthetic absorbable material which retains its strength for a reasonable period of time rather than, say, chromic catgut.

Persistence of the stoma and discharge may be a long-term problem after marsupialization. This problem may persist for the remainder of the dog's life and, in the author's experience, is more frequently associated with marsupialization of cysts than abscesses. It is not usually a major problem and is often manifest as a slight, tacky discharge from a small stoma but, as mentioned previously, it is prudent to warn owners of its possibility before surgery.

Serious postoperative problems may result from the presence of malignant change in the lining of the cyst or abscess (see **4.171** and **4.181**). This may not always be detected by pre-operative cytology and so it is essential to biopsy the lining of the cyst or abscess during drainage procedures. The prognosis is always guarded after prostatic cyst/abscess drainage procedures because of the possibilities of complications or/and recurrence or development of further cysts/abscesses. Even this prognosis cannot be given to the owners, however, until the results of the biopsy are known as the presence of malignancy is associated with a hopeless prognosis.

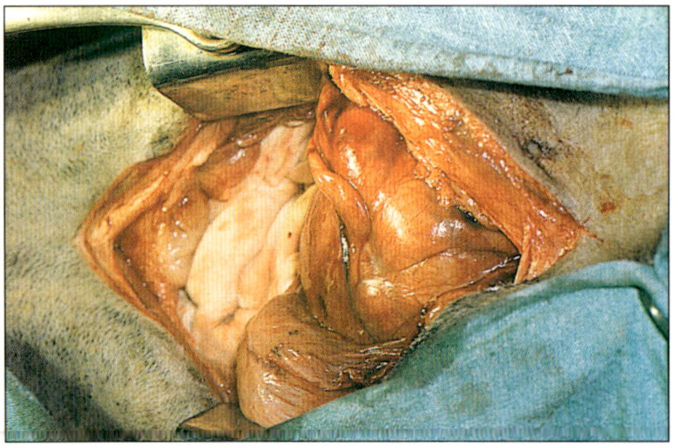

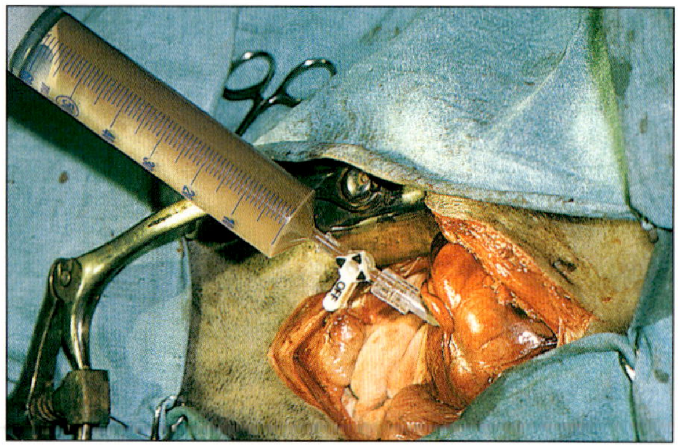

4.173 **A tense prostatic cyst to the left of the dog's bladder (left).** Apart from the risk of contamination of the peritoneal cavity with cyst fluid during surgical drainage, it is impossible to grasp the tense cyst wall and draw it through an abdominal incision during marsupialization. The cyst (or abscess) should be drained by needle centesis **(right)**, after which its wall is easily grasped **(middle)** and can be exteriorized through the abdominal wall incision (see **4.178–4.181**).

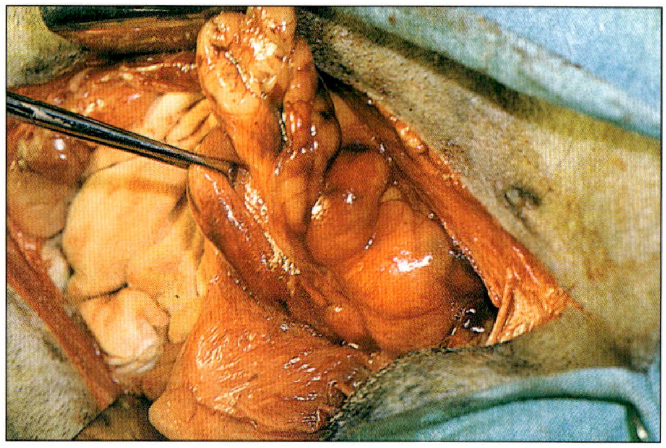

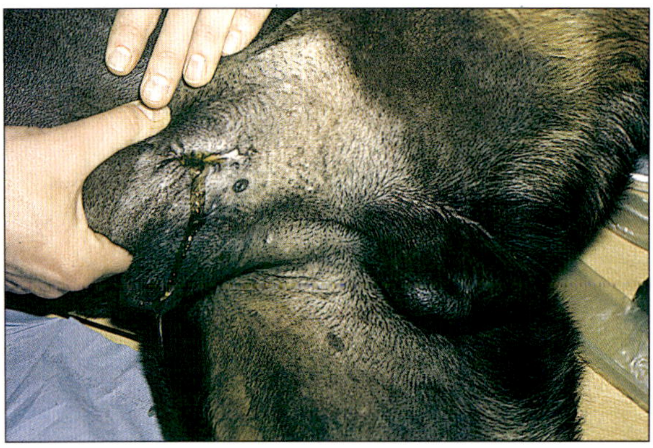

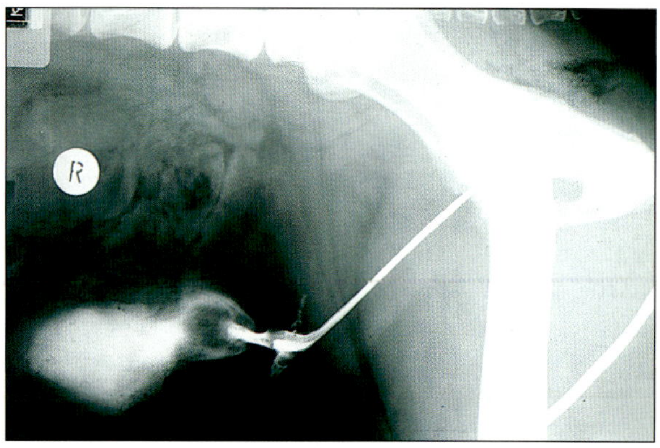

4.174 Urethrocutaneous fistulation may occur after marsupialization if the cyst/abscess communicates with the prostatic urethra. The pre-operative radiograph of this Rottweiler is illustrated in **2.49**. The dog, which was dysuric pre-operatively, responded well to surgery but began to urinate through the marsupialization stoma **(left)**. When urethrography was repeated **(right)**, communications between the prostatic urethra and cyst cavity were obvious but these were not clearly defined on the pre-operative radiograph, possibly because the high intracyst pressure prevented contrast medium from entering the cyst from the urethra. It may be useful, in the investigation of cases in which urethra–cyst/abscess communication is suspected, to repeat urethrography after drainage of the cyst by centesis. Fortunately, this particular dog lived under a caravan on a fairground and thus was not a problem to the owners. Although he was continent, he tended to smell of urine unless he was washed frequently and, about twice yearly, developed cystitis which responded to antibiotic treatment. He continued to urinate predominantly through his stoma for the next five years until he died of old age.

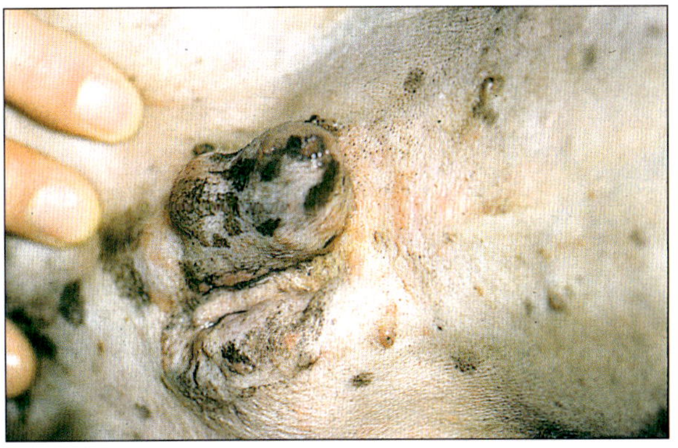

4.175 The swelling adjacent to this dog's marsupialization stoma was a ventral rupture associated with breakdown of the chromic catgut sutures which were used to appose the cyst and abdominal walls. Simple interrupted sutures of synthetic absorbable material are preferable. The swelling on the ventral prepuce was a mast cell tumour which was subsequently excised.

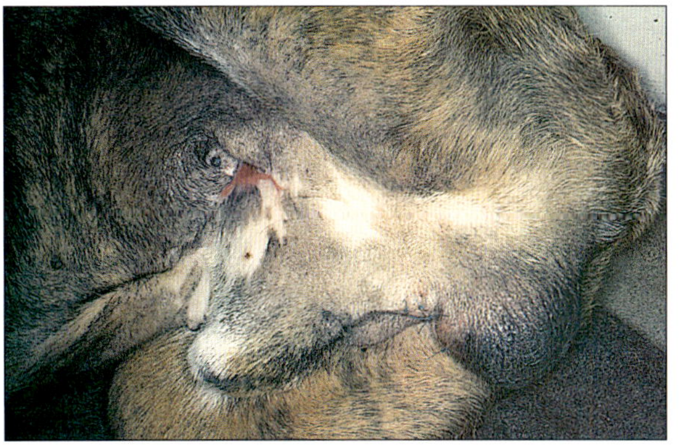

4.176 The appearance of the stoma in a Boxer, two weeks after marsupialization of a prostatic abscess. Drainage from the abscess cavity has ceased and the stoma is healing by secondary intention. Occasionally, this does not happen and the stoma remains patent and continues to discharge serous fluid. Owners should be made aware of this possibility before surgery is performed.

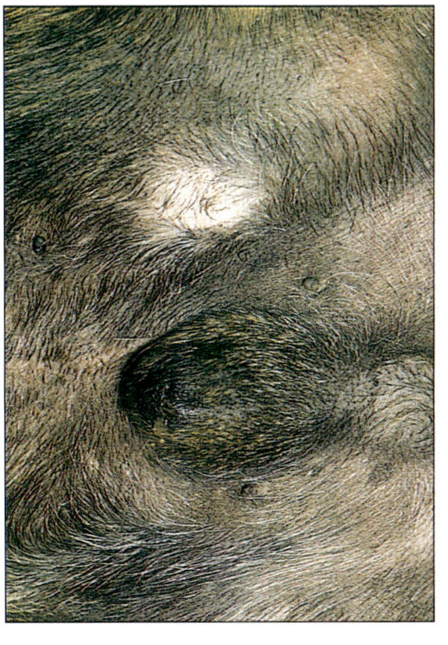

4.177 The appearance of a prostatic abscess stoma in another Boxer, four months after marsupialization. The stoma has healed.

Techniques

Marsupialization

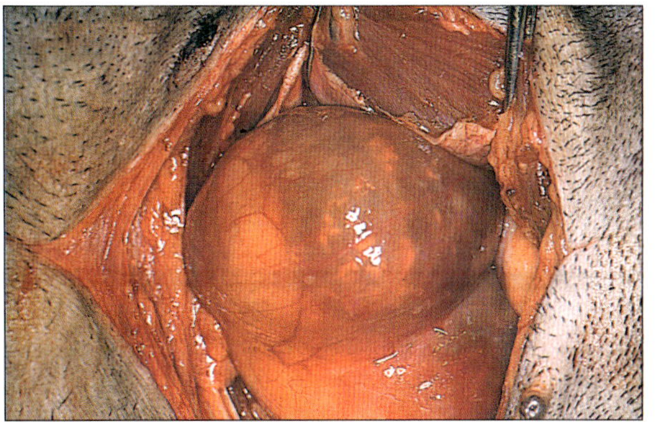

4.178 With the animal under general anaesthesia and a urethral catheter in place, the cyst/abscess is approached via a caudal paramedian laparotomy on the side opposite to the stoma site. The latter can be judged by palpation of the ventral abdomen when the dog is anaesthetized and in dorsal recumbency. The cyst/abscess should be drained by centesis to facilitate handling (see **4.173**). A paramedian incision is made through the abdominal wall at the stoma site and the cyst/abscess pulled through the abdominal muscle incision, as shown.

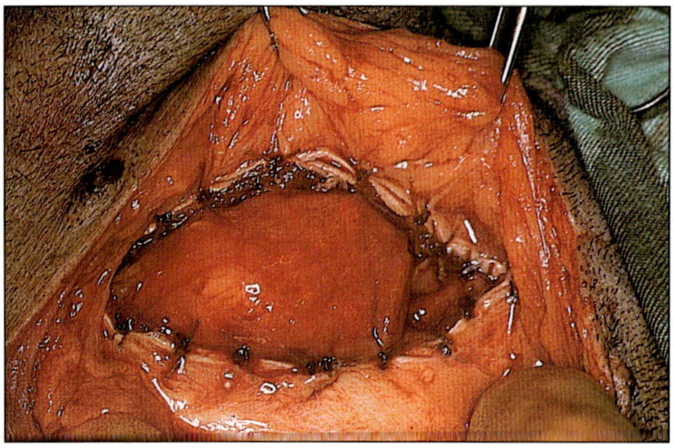

4.179 The cyst/abscess wall is sutured to the abdominal muscle wall and external rectus sheath with simple interrupted synthetic absorbable sutures. The cyst/abscess wall is now incised and the remaining contents drained by suction. The opening in the cyst/abscess wall should be large enough to allow insertion of a finger to break down septae between adjacent cysts/abscesses so that all drain into the cavity being marsupialized. Care should be taken to avoid damage to the urethra which can be palpated (if the cavity is close to it) by the presence of the catheter. A biopsy of the cyst/abscess lining should be taken.

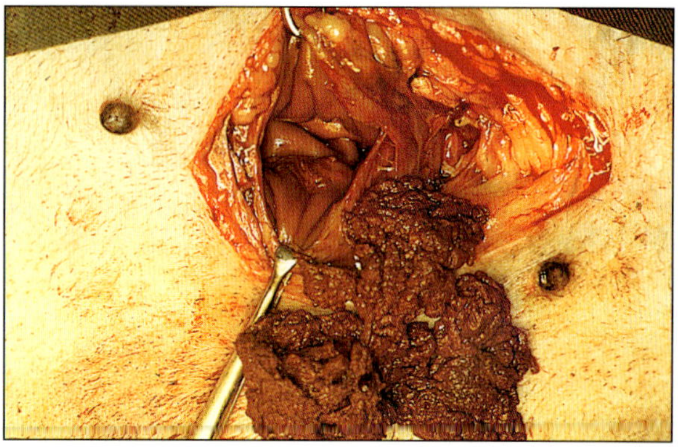

4.180 In some cases, the contents of the cyst/abscess may be inspissated, making their removal more difficult. (This is a different dog to that illustrated in **4.178, 4.179** and **4.181.**)

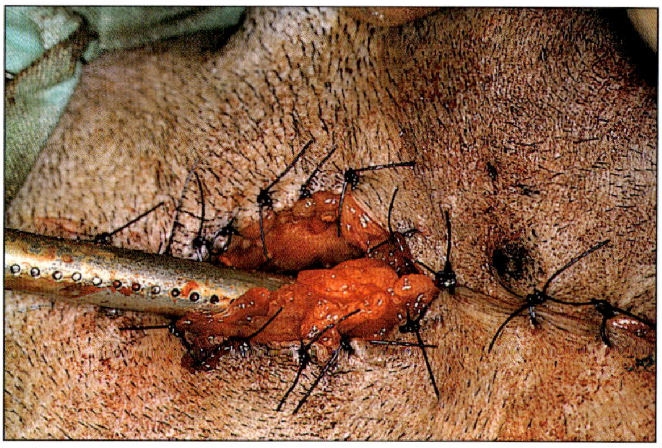

4.181 Marsupialization is completed by suturing the opening in the cyst to the skin incision using simple interrupted sutures of monofilament nylon. The laparotomy is closed routinely. After marsupialization, the stoma should be kept clean and barrier creams applied to the surrounding skin until drainage stops. The cyst/abscess cavity should be flushed twice daily using sterile saline (+/– antibiotics based on bacteriological sensitivities) administered via a syringe, the nozzle of which can be inserted into the stoma. Parenteral antibiotics based on bacteriological sensitivities should be continued for at least three weeks postoperatively. A metal suction probe has been inserted through the stoma. Note the appearance of the cyst lining below the suction probe; a biopsy of this tissue revealed that a carcinoma was present. Local metastases soon became apparent, necessitating euthanasia three months post-operatively. This dog had undergone bilateral perineal rupture repair (see **5.29**), castration and prostatic cyst marsupialization with a poor result. Unfortunately, malignant cells could not be detected on cytological examinations pre-operatively. If they had been, the animal could have been spared ineffective surgical intervention.

Foley catheter drainage

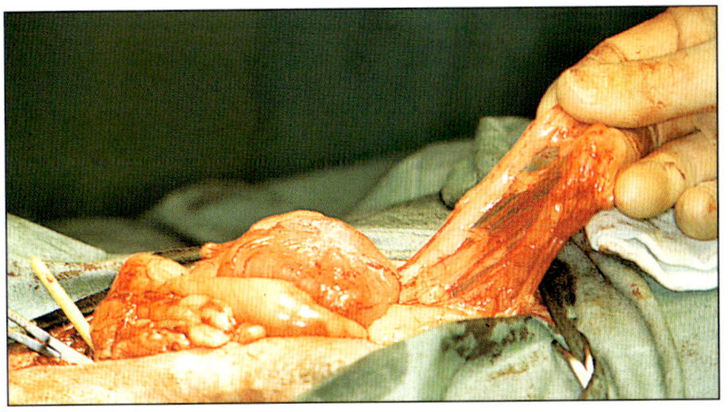

4.182 In cases in which the cyst/abscess is known to communicate with the urethra, marsupialization is contra-indicated. In such cases, the author prefers to perform Foley catheter drainage. Under general anaesthesia, a laparotomy is performed and the cyst/abscess drained, as described in **4.173**. The tip of a 16–20Fr Foley catheter is passed through a stab incision in the abdominal wall on the side of drainage (the opposite side to the laparotomy). A section of omentum which will easily reach the cyst/abscess is located.

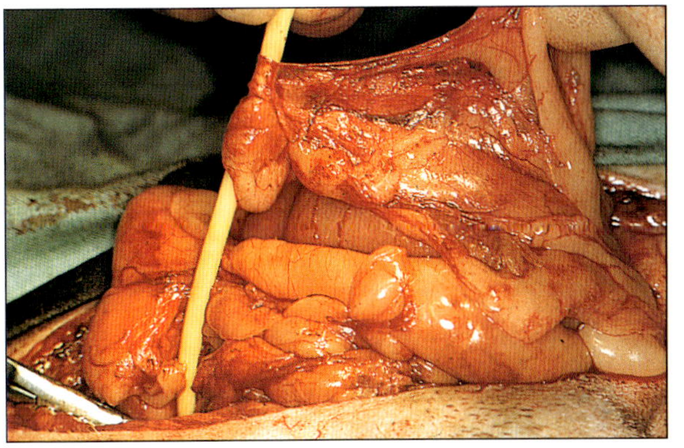

4.183 The Foley catheter tip within the abdomen is passed through the omentum.

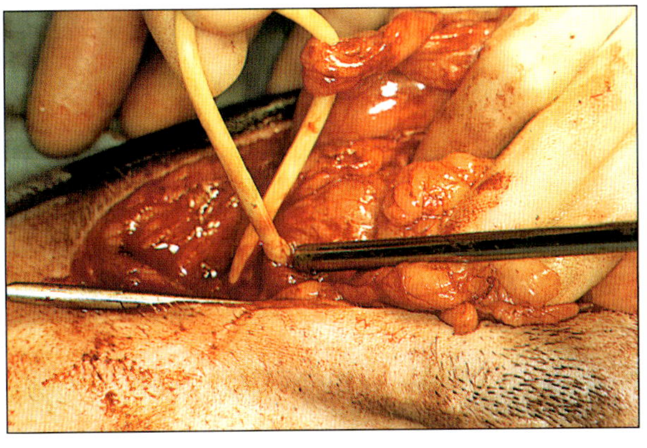

4.184 A stab incision is made into the cyst/abscess cavity and the contents, which remained after drainage by centesis, removed. A biopsy is taken of the cyst/abscess lining. The tip of the Foley catheter is inserted into the cyst/abscesss cavity and the catheter cuff inflated. Diluted iodine-based positive contrast medium can be used to inflate the cuff in case it is necessary to determine the site of the catheter tip radiographically after surgery. The volume used depends on the size of the cavity into which the catheter tip has been introduced, but the degree of inflation of the cuff should be sufficient to prevent withdrawal of the catheter from the cyst/abscess cavity.

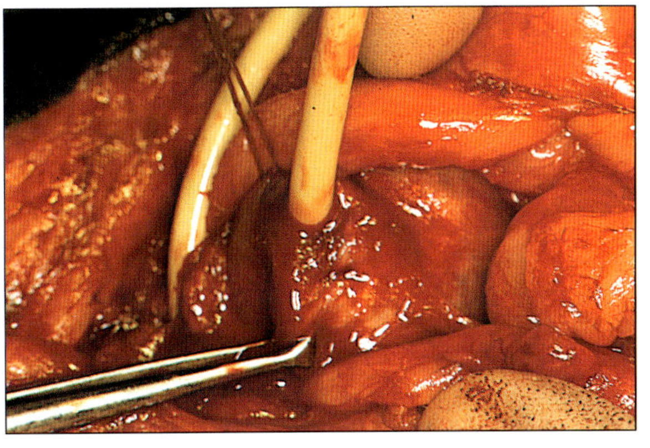

4.185 A purse-string suture of synthetic absorbable material is placed within the cyst/abscess wall around the Foley catheter as it enters the cavity. This is to prevent the catheter exiting from the cyst/abscess cavity and to reduce the risk of contamination of the abdomen by cyst/abscess contents. The presence of a layer of omentum around the Foley catheter and between the cyst/abscess and abdominal wall is intended to prevent peritoneal cavity contamination and provide lymphatic drainage in the event of minor spillage from the cyst/abscess cavity.

4.186 Traction is applied to the Foley catheter outside the abdomen until the cyst/abscess wall lies against the ventral abdominal wall and a purse-string suture of monofilament nylon is placed through the skin around the Foley catheter as it exits the abdomen. The ends of this suture are then tied around the catheter before being cut. The catheter is attached to the ventral abdominal skin at a number of points, as shown, using simple interrupted sutures of monofilament nylon. Alternatively, a Chinese finger trap suture could be used (see **4.140**). The laparotomy is closed routinely. Attempts to maintain a closed drainage system are often unsuccessful. Suction drainage tends to result in occlusion of the catheter tip by prostatic tissue and it is difficult to maintain the drainage bag of a closed system below the level of the cyst/abscess. As there is little pressure within the cyst/abscess cavity, this may result in reflux of material back into the cyst/abscess. The author has experienced no problems leaving the Foley catheter as an open drain, as long as the drain is flushed three times daily with sterile normal saline. In the presence of infection, water-soluble antibiotics, to which the organisms are sensitive, can be added to the saline. In any event, parenteral antibiotic cover should be given, especially if the cyst was infected or an abscess was present. As in this case, the dog should be castrated. Ideally, the Foley catheter should be left *in situ* for 10 days, after which the cuff is deflated, nylon sutures removed and the catheter pulled from the cyst/abscess. In practice, despite the inflation of the catheter cuff and the use of a purse-string suture in the cyst wall, it is not uncommon for the inflated catheter cuff to appear in a subcutaneous position after 4–5 days. This can be confirmed radiographically. Under these circumstances, the catheter should be removed as it is impossible to re-introduce it into the cyst/abscess without further surgical intervention and, in most instances, the cyst/abscess will still resolve.

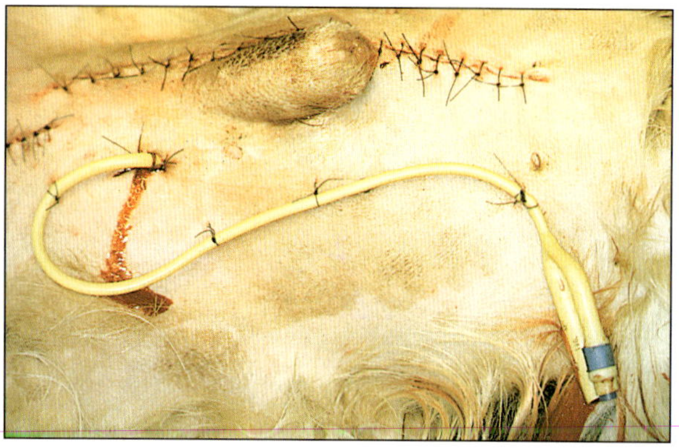

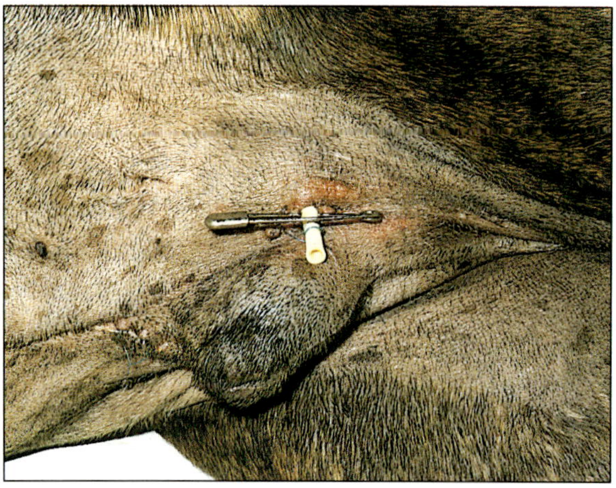

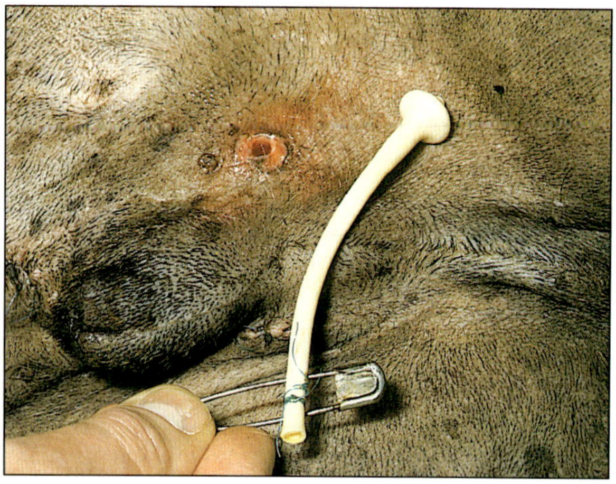

4.187 Recently, the author used a mushroom-tipped catheter as an alternative to a Foley catheter for the drainage of prostatic cysts and abscesses. These photographs were taken just before (**left**) and after (**right**) removal of a mushroom-tipped catheter (Depezzer catheter, Rusch UK Ltd) from the prostatic abscess of a boxer dog. The safety pin is advisable, because even a Chinese finger- trap suture is not enough to prevent the catheter inverting through the skin wound to a subcutaneous position as the tissues swell postoperatively, if the catheter is cut too short. The safety pin is covered with a padded dressing (not shown) to prevent trauma to the skin. The catheter can be cut short (unlike the Foley catheter) and appears to remain in the cyst/abscess cavity better than a Foley catheter. It is, however, more difficult to move.

5 Other Surgical Procedures

In this chapter, other surgical procedures which may be required in animals with urological signs are described under the same subheadings as those in Chapter 4.

Castration

Indications

There are a variety of indications for castration in small animals. Those which relate to urological disorders are primarily conditions affecting the male dog. These include benign prostatic disease, perineal rupture and inguinal/scrotal hernia.

Pre- and peri-operative considerations

Scrotal skin is very sensitive and should therefore be prepared for surgery with care, particularly if scrotectomy is not to be performed. The hair should be clipped without trauma to the scrotal skin and surgical spirit should not be used to disinfect the skin as it may induce a severe scrotal dermatitis. The author prefers to use diluted povidone–iodine (Betadine, Napp Laboratories Ltd) or non-ionic quaternary compounds (Trigene, The Hygeine Corporation Ltd) alone for scrotal skin disinfection.

If the scrotum is left *in situ*, it may swell postoperatively with oedema fluids, blood or, if asepsis is poor, pus. Such swelling can be minimized by attention to atraumatic surgical technique, adequate haemostasis and good aseptic technique. However, owners should be prepared for these possibilities before surgery is performed. Castration involving scrotal excision eliminates this problem. Although it is more time-consuming, it is the method of choice if the scrotum is involved in the disease process (e.g. testicular neoplasia or inflammation with extension into the surrounding tissues).

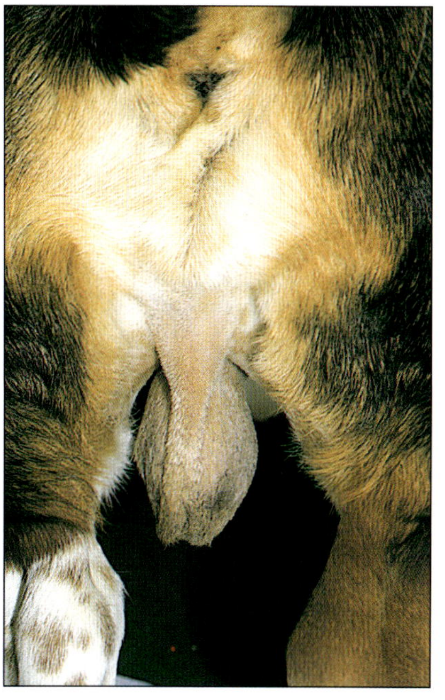

5.1 Oedematous scrotal swelling three days after castration. The owners should be made aware of the possibility of such swelling if the scrotum is not excised during castration.

Possible surgical/post-surgical complications

Scrotal swelling after castration has already been mentioned. The most serious potential postoperative complication is haemorrhage from the spermatic vessels and these should be ligated with care (see below).

Inguinal herniation may be present pre-operatively and may occur after surgery with disastrous results if an open castration technique is used. This is less of a problem in small animals than in large animals such as horses but, even so, in the author's opinion castration should always be performed using a 'closed' technique (see below).

Techniques

Castration with retention of the scrotum

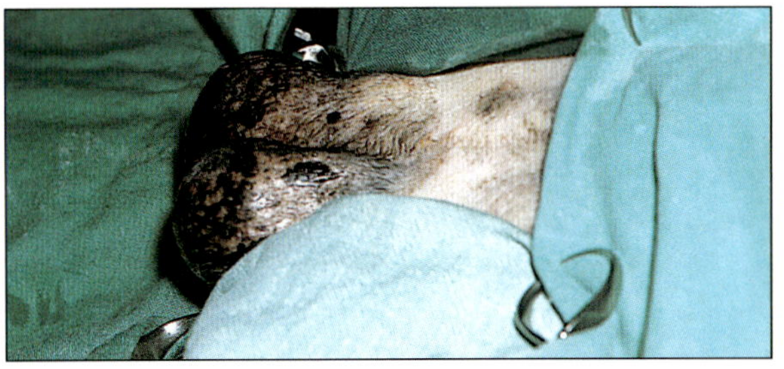

5.2 The anaesthetized dog is positioned in dorsal recumbency, with the hind limbs abducted. The scrotum and surrounding skin are prepared for aseptic surgery, avoiding the use of strong antiseptics such as surgical spirit if the scrotum is to be retained. The area is draped (caudal is to the left in this photograph).

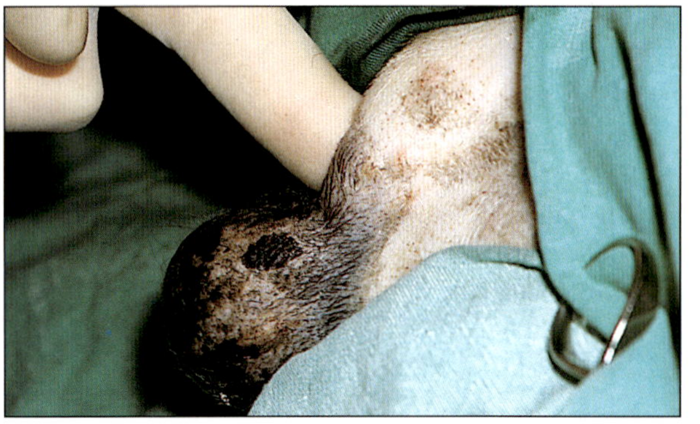

5.3 To avoid postoperative scrotal skin irritation, the skin incision is made prescrotally. The second finger of the left hand (if one is right-handed) is used to push one of the testes to a prescrotal position.

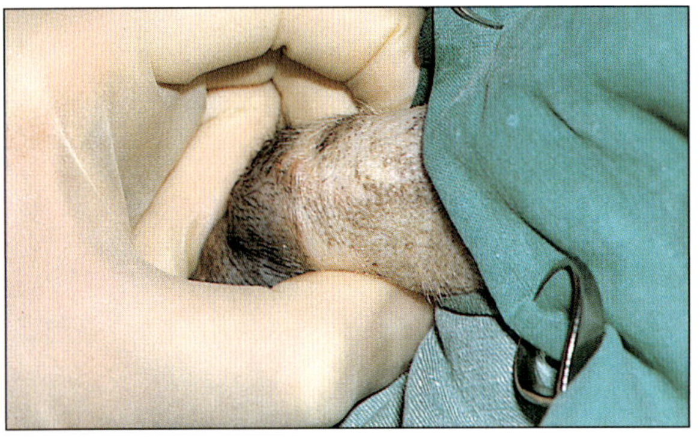

5.4 While the second finger maintains the testis in that position, the first finger and thumb are used to tense the testis upwards and immobilize it against the prescrotal skin.

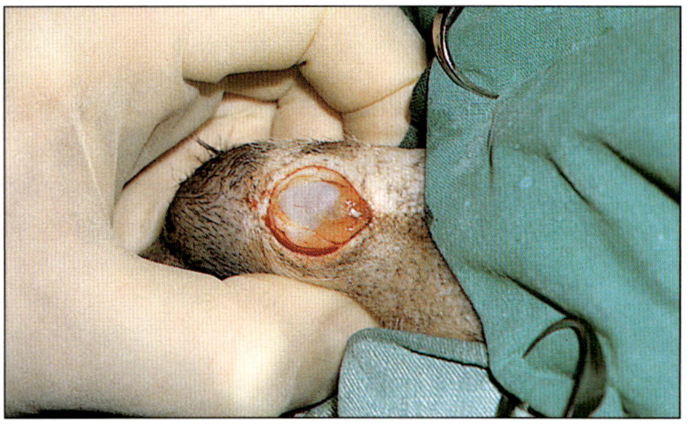

5.5 The skin and subcutaneous fascia are incised to expose the tunica vaginalis over the testis. Usually, a small amount of fat (external to the tunic) appears in the incision site when the incision has reached the required depth. The fat can be seen at the cranial end of the incision.

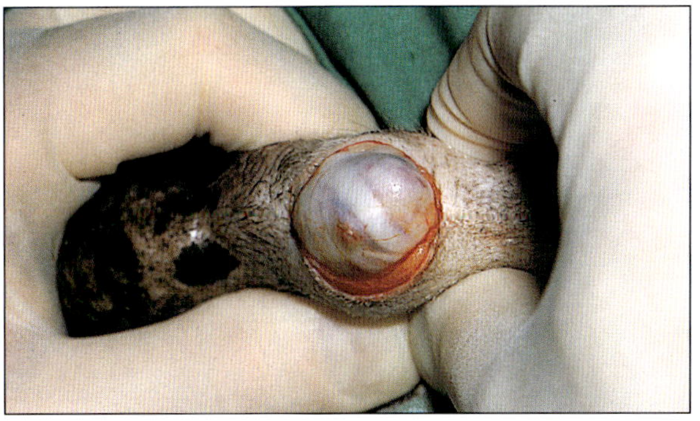

5.6 The thumb and index finger of both hands are used to apply pressure beneath and thus exteriorize the testis.

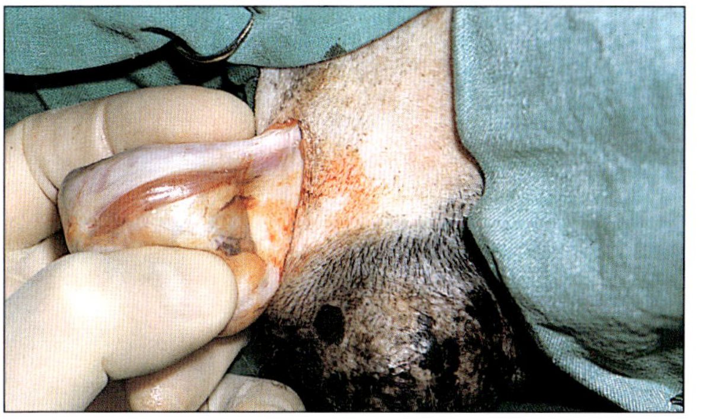

5.7 The testis is grasped firmly in the left hand and the cremaster muscle and tunic-covered vas deferens and pampiniform plexus identified at the cranial end of the testis.

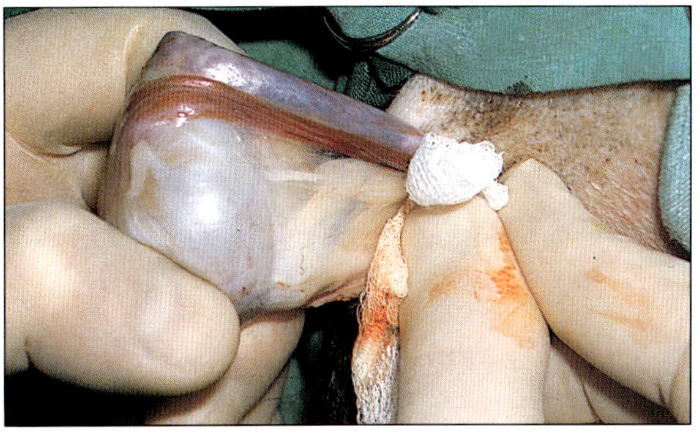

5.8 A dry swab is used to push fascia proximally from the lateral side of the testis.

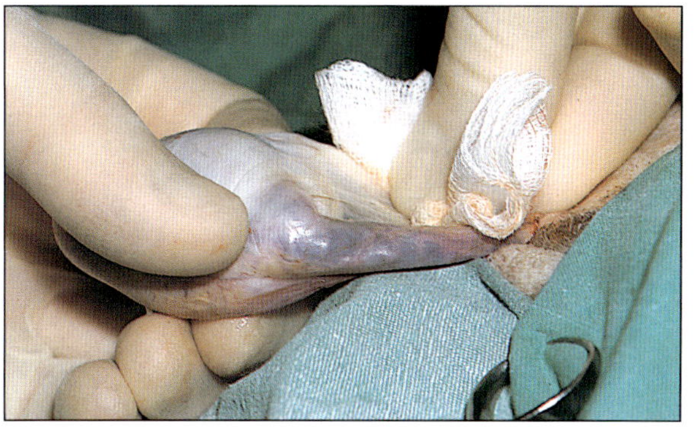

5.9 The same procedure is used to debride the medial side of the testis.

5.10

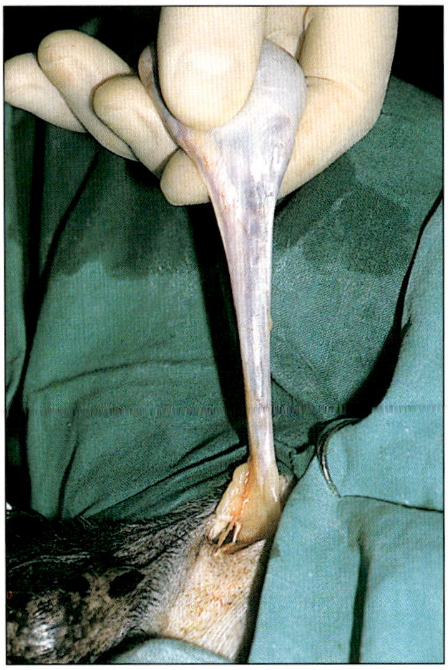

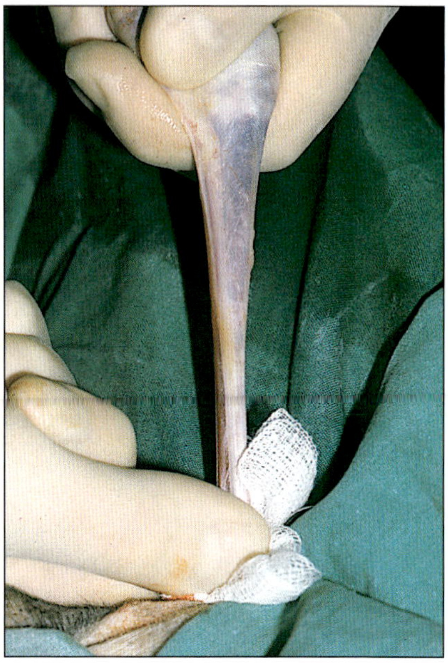

5.10 The gubernaculum can now easily be broken down and the testis and spermatic cord exteriorized, as shown.

5.11 Any remaining fascia is cleared from the tunic over the spermatic cord by wiping with a swab from distally to proximally.

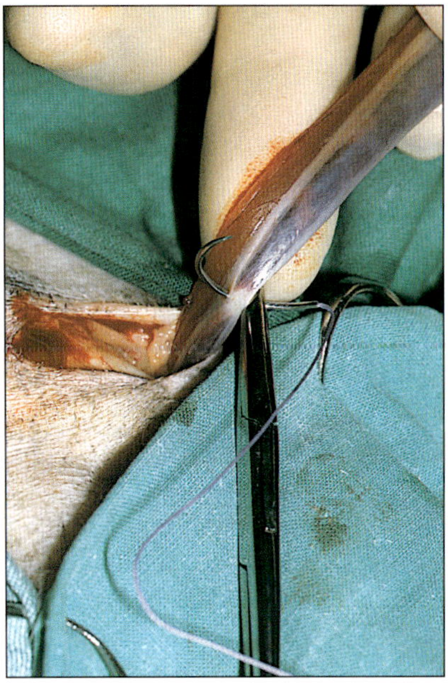

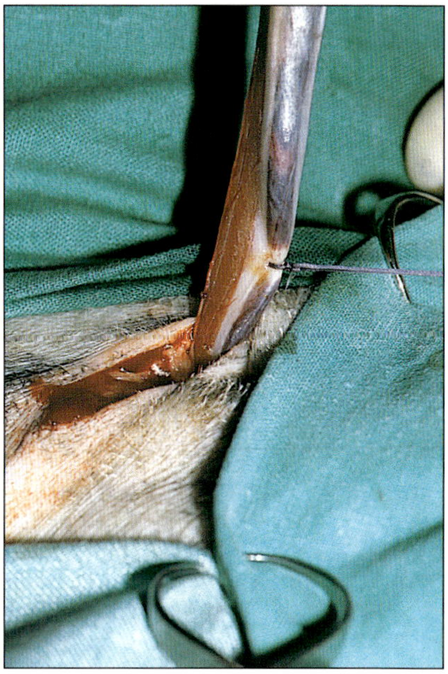

5.12 The spermatic cord is now ligated. The author prefers to use a transfixing ligature of no. 2/0 or 0 polyglactin (Vicryl, Ethicon). It is important that transfixing ligatures do not enter hollow viscera such as, in this case, the vas deferens if the risk of granuloma formation is to be avoided. The ligature is therefore taken through the tunic and between the spermatic vessels (cranially) and the vas (caudally), as illustrated.

5.13 The ligature is tied cranially to ligate the spermatic vessels.

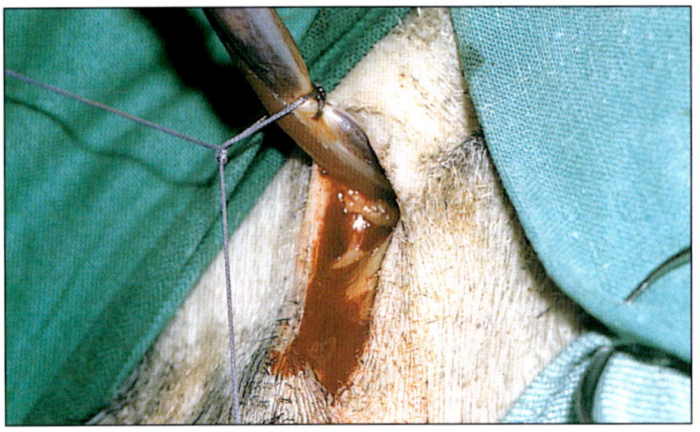

5.14 The ends of the ligature are then taken caudally, around each side of the spermatic cord, and again tied.

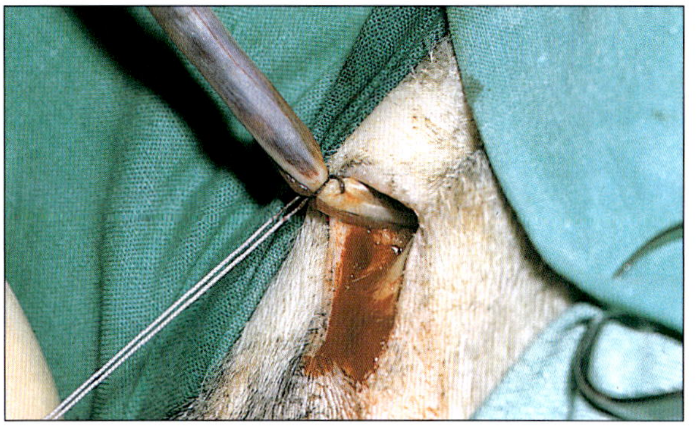

5.15 The result is that, during placement of the transfixing ligature, the vascular component of the spermatic cord is ligated twice, thus minimizing the risk of haemorrhage.

5.16

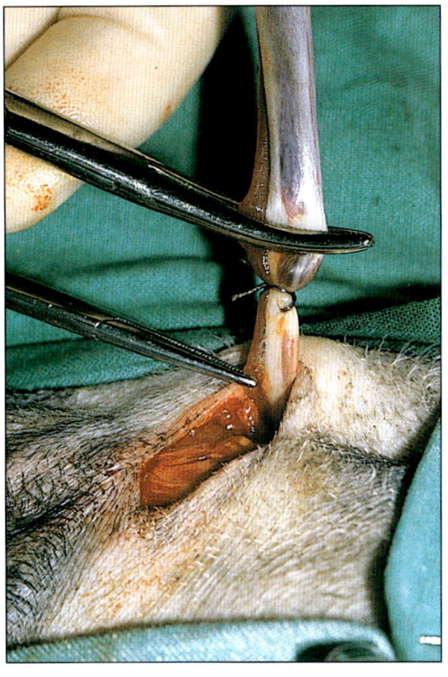

5.16 Vascular clamps are applied to the spermatic cord just distal to the ligature. A second pair of clamps is used to grasp a caudal, non-vascular part of the spermatic cord (in this case the cremaster muscle). The spermatic cord is sectioned between the ligature and the first pair of clamps and the testis is removed.

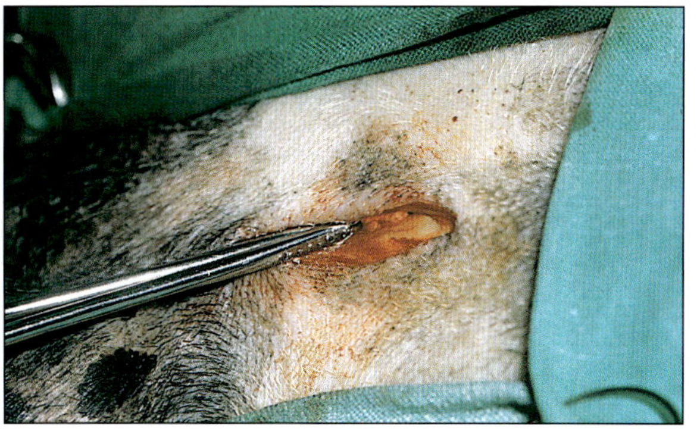

5.17 The ligated spermatic cord is allowed to retract through the incision towards the external inguinal ring. The adequacy of the ligation is unknown until this stage as, even if the ligature has not been placed tight enough, the tension on the spermatic vessels while the testis is exteriorized may prevent haemorrhage from occurring. If haemorrhage does occur when the tension on the spermatic cord remnants is released, the cord can be re-exteriorized using the forceps and religated. If, as should happen, no haemorrhage occurs, the forceps are removed. Castration is completed by displacing the remaining testis cranially to the skin incision, incising the overlying fascia and repeating the procedure described above. The skin is then closed routinely (the subcutaneous fascia is not usually closed).

Castration including scrotectomy

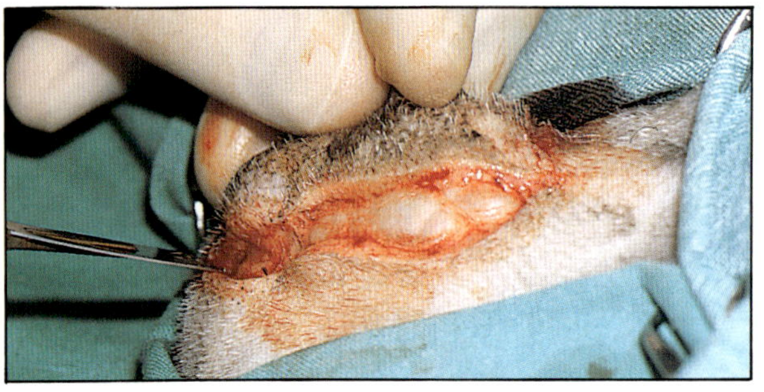

5.18 The dog is positioned and the surgical site prepared as in 5.2. An eliptical skin incision is made around the base of the scrotum.

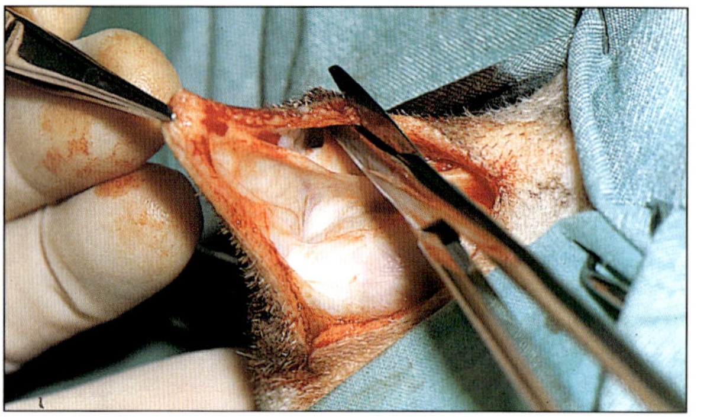

5.19 The subcuticular fascia is undermined and incised, freeing the edges of the scrotal skin.

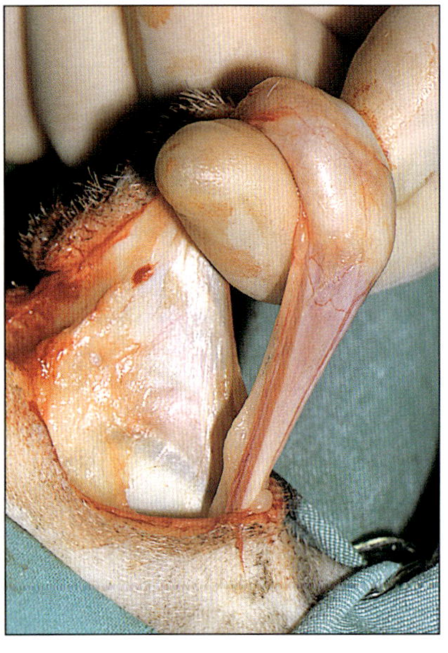

5.20 Each testis is identified within its tunic. Its spermatic cord is cleared of extraneous fascia, ligated and sectioned, as described above.

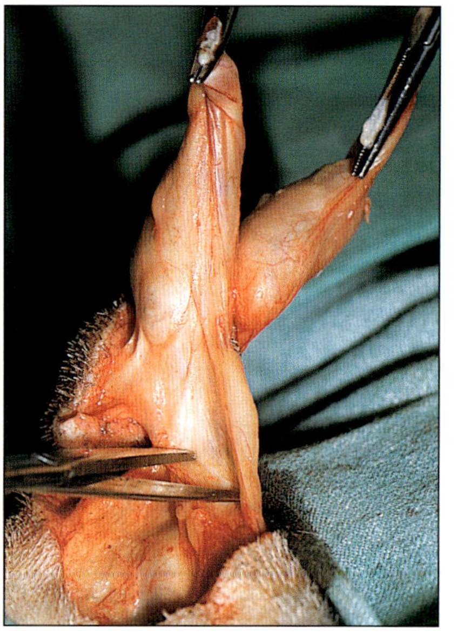

5.21 After both cords have been ligated, the remaining fascia is separated by blunt and sharp dissection.

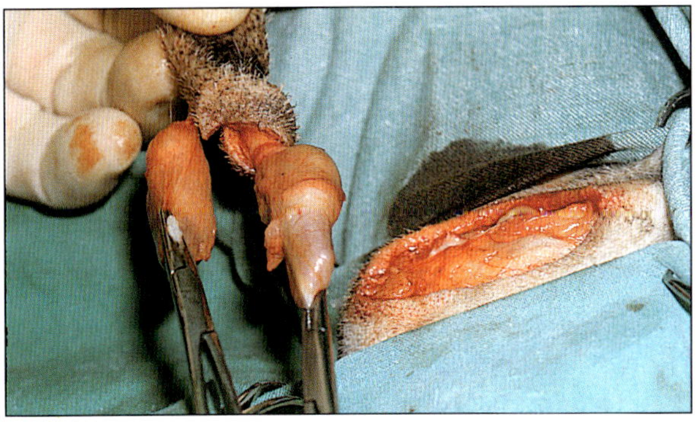

5.22 The testes and scrotum can now be removed.

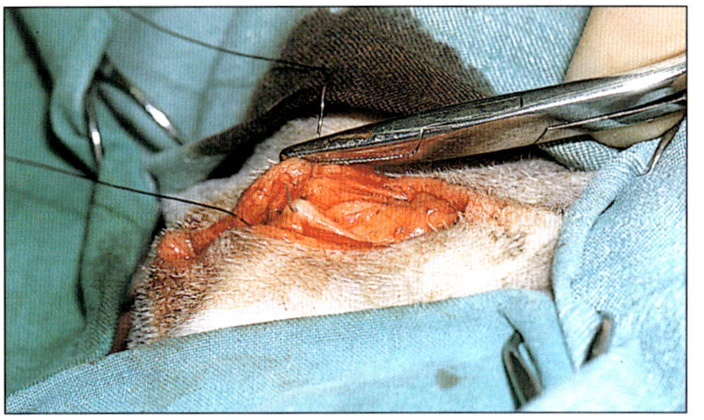

5.23 The subcutaneous fascia is closed using a simple continuous suture pattern of synthetic absorbable material.

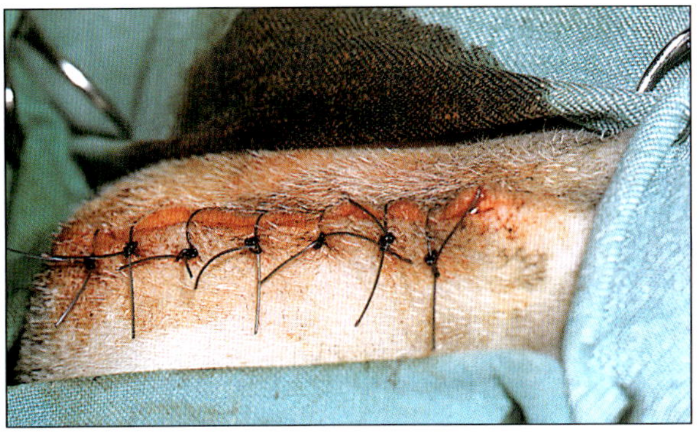

5.24 The skin wound is closed routinely, in this case with simple interrupted monofilament polypropylene sutures. A subcuticular suture of synthetic absorbable material would also be suitable.

Perineal rupture repair

Indications

In urological cases, perineal rupture in the dog or cat with retroflexion of the urinary bladder, prostatic cyst/abscess and/or prostate into the perineum.

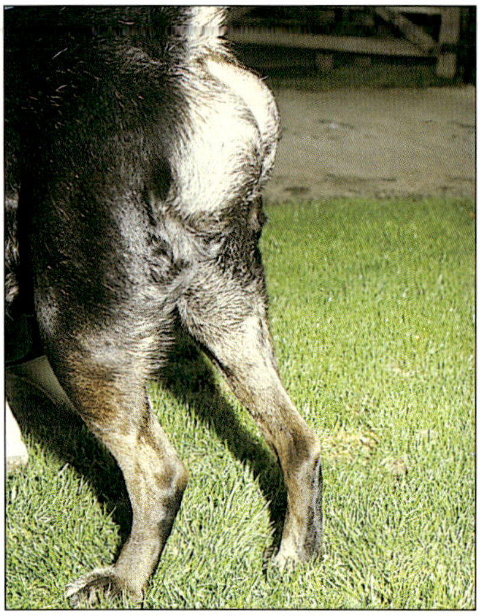

5.25 In urological cases, perineal rupture repair is indicated if there is caudal displacement of the urinary bladder, prostatic cyst/abscesss and/or prostate gland into the rupture. This may or may not lead to dysuria and/or urinary incontinence. The fluid swelling in the perineum has to be differentiated from those associated with displacement of other viscera (see **5.26–5.29**). In addition, rectal abnormalities may be present, resulting in dyschezia (see **5.30–5.36**).

Pre- and peri-operative considerations

A fluid-filled swelling in a perineal rupture may not be the urinary bladder. Prostatic cysts and seroma formation secondary to necrosis of pelvic fat can lead to similar swellings and these must be differentiated from bladder retroflexion by clinical, radiographic, laboratory and/or ultrasonographic examinations (see Chapters 1–3).

A variety of rectal abnormalities may develop as a result of perineal rupture and lead to dyschezia.

Perineal rupture repair should be postponed in dysuric dogs with bladder retroflexion until the animal has been stabilized. These dogs are suffering the metabolic consequences of urinary obstruction (uraemia, acidosis and hyperkalaemia) and may be poor anaesthetic risks. Bladder wall ischaemia, stretching and breakdown of tight junctions may be occurring and the priority in these cases is the dysuria, rather than the perineal rupture itself. In addition, the inflammatory response to the presence of a distended bladder within the pelvic cavity and perineum makes tissue identification even more difficult than usual. In such cases, the bladder should be decompressed, returned to the abdomen, and an in-dwelling catheter used for 3–5 days until the animal's metabolic condition has been stabilized by appropriate fluid and electrolyte therapy.

A detailed knowledge of local anatomy is imperative. It is rare to operate on a perineal rupture and to be able to see the anatomy frequently depicted in drawings in surgical texts. The surgeon's familiarity with perineal and pelvic anatomy should be such that he/she is aware of where structures to be avoided or located *should be*, even if these are not directly visible. Often, the surgical field resembles nothing more than a cavity, apparently lined by fat and fascia. The surgeon should be aware of the locations of the following: the external anal sphincter muscle and its innervation (the caudal rectal /haemorrhoidal nerves); the levator ani, coccygeus and internal obturator muscles; the internal pudendal vessels; the sciatic nerve, sacrotuberous ligament and caudal gluteal vessels; the rectum; the anal sacs; pelvic fat; the urethra. It is necessary to be able to palpate some of these structures (e.g. pulses in arteries, sacrotuberous ligament). Great care should be taken to identify the locations of the sciatic nerve, internal pudendal and caudal rectal/haemorrhoidal vessels and nerves, and the caudal gluteal vessels, because trauma to these structures can lead to limb paralysis, faecal incontinence and/or severe haemorrhage. If pelvic fat has to be removed, it must be ligated first as it has a copious blood supply. It should be noted that the cat has no sacrotuberous ligament.

During surgery, the dog should be positioned in ventral recumbency with the hind quarters elevated over a sandbag and the tail raised. Docked breeds pose particular problems (see below).

The rectum should be emptied of faeces and the anus closed with a purse-string suture to prevent contamination. Enemas are usually contra-indicated as dogs with perineal ruptures are frequently dyschezic due to rectal abnormalities such as deviations, dilatations and diverticula. Faeces are best removed digitally under general anaesthesia. This should be performed with care because of the risks of rupturing a rectal diverticulum; such rupture is usually fatal.

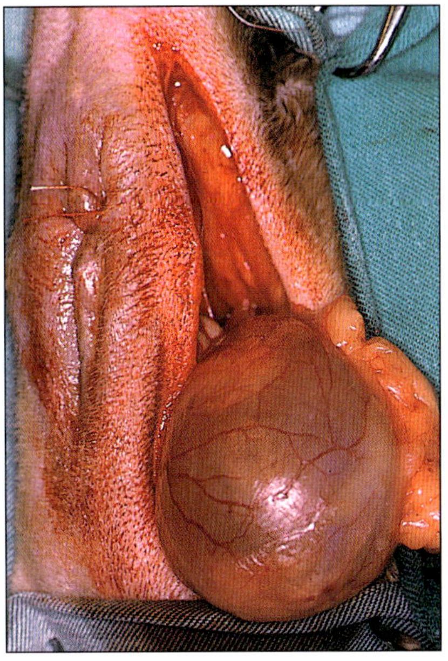

5.26 Retroflexion of the urinary bladder into a perineal rupture is not always associated with dysuria. The only sign in this dog was unilateral perineal swelling, which reduced in size during micturition.

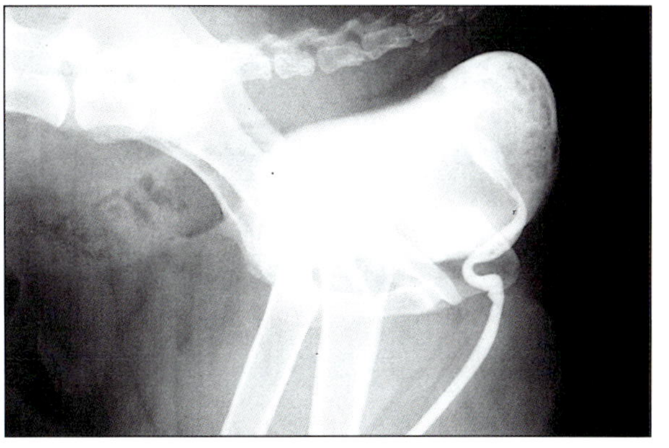

5.27 Retrograde positive contrast urethrocystography is the best way of confirming retroflexion of the bladder into a perineal rupture.

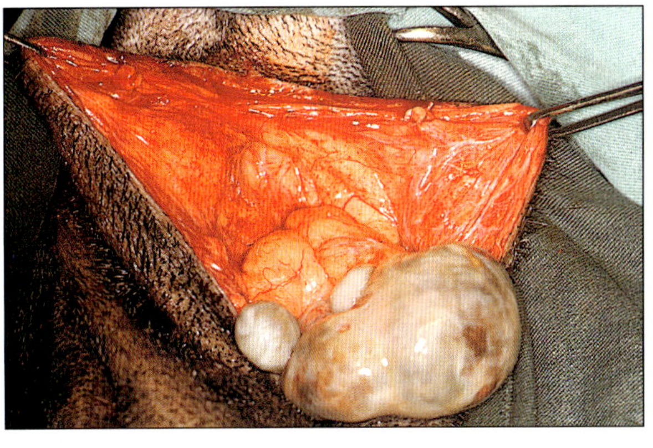

5.28 Prolapse and necrosis of pelvic fat in a perineal rupture leads to transudation of serum and can result in a fluid-filled swelling. This fat is highly vascular and should be ligated before removal, if this is indicated. (This is the same animal as that illustrated in **5.25**.)

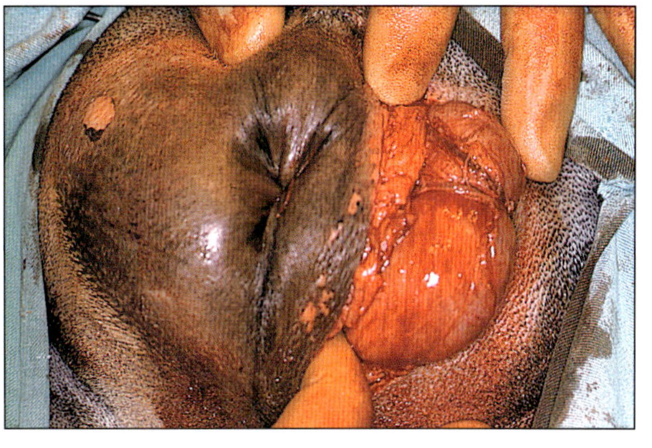

5.29 The third cause of a fluid swelling in a perineal rupture is the presence of a prostatic cyst. Such cysts can be drained by needle centesis, pushed cranially and the perineum repaired. If so, the cyst is likely to refill, requiring a prepubic drainage procedure (see Chapter 4). An alternative is to marsupialize the cyst through the perineum (see **4.172**). The first method of treatment was used in this dog, a Rottweiler. The cyst refilled and was treated by prepubic marsupialization. Unfortunately, a carcinoma was present in the lining of the cyst but was detected only when the cyst lining was biopsied during marsupialization; this case is also illustrated in **4.178, 4.179** and **4.181**.

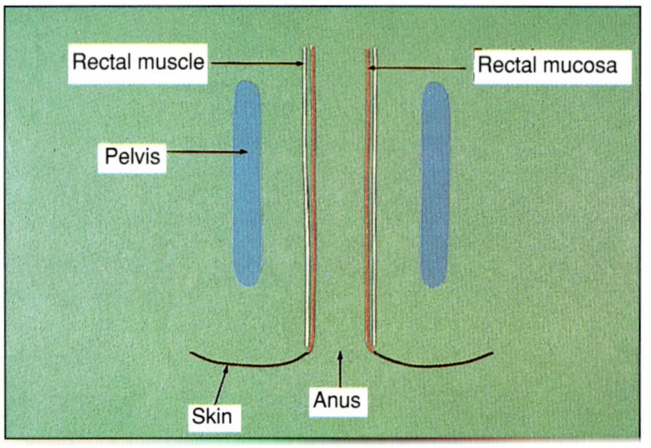

5.30 Perineal support is essential to maintain the rectum as a straight tube to facilitate defaecation. If the support is lost, three types of rectal complications may develop, either individually or in combination.

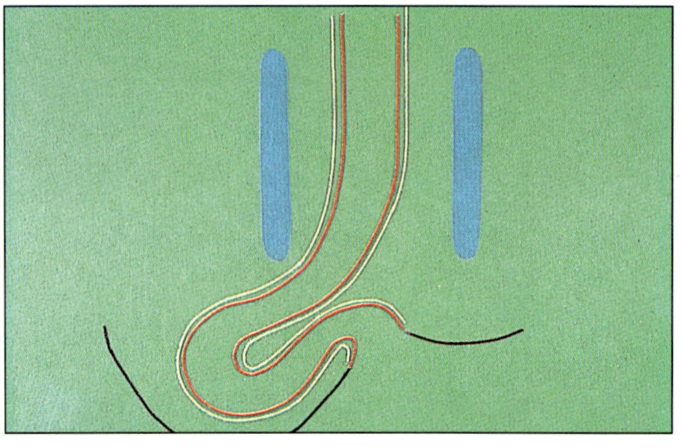

5.31 The rectum may deviate to one side. This deviation is worsened during tenesmus and so the animal's attempts to defaecate only exacerbate the situation and lead to faecal impaction which in turn may result in rectal dilatation.

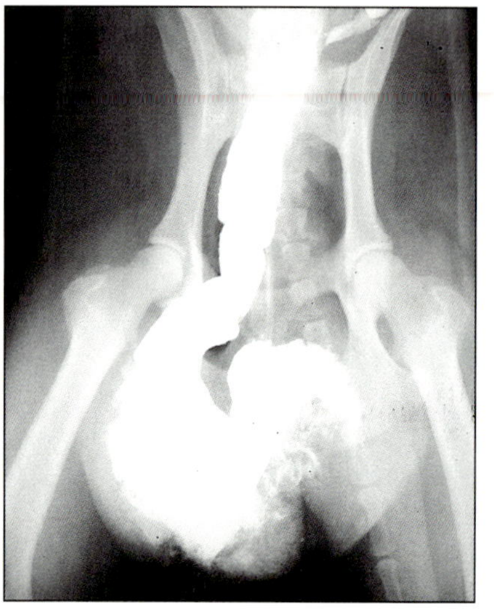

5.32 Rectal deviation can be demonstrated by means of a barium enema but this is not usually necessary. Digital rectal examination is normally sufficient to diagnose this and other rectal abnormalities.

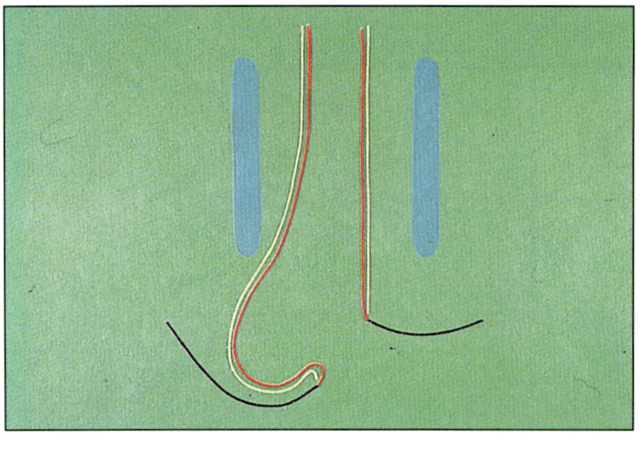

5.33 Rectal dilatation can occur alone but is often found in association with deviation.

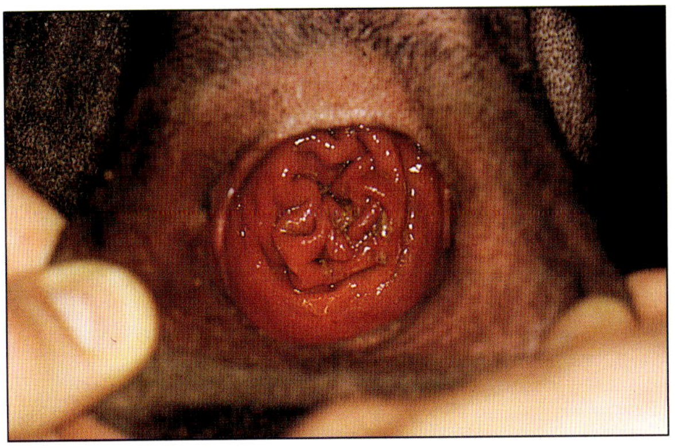

Fig. 5.34 The folds of the dilated rectum can be appreciated in this Great Dane, after removal of faeces from the rectum. One of the problems of rectal dilatation is that the stretched, atonic rectum may prolapse pre- and/or postoperatively. Rectal tone usually returns once the perineal support has been reconstituted. If not, affected animals may benefit from a colopexy – which is also useful if rectal prolapse persists as a postoperative problem.

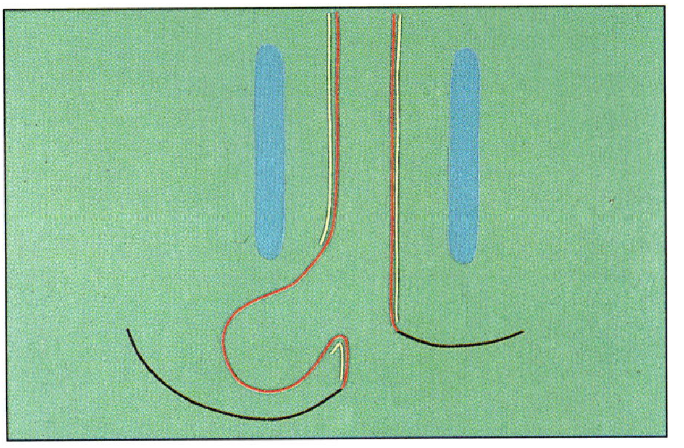

5.35 A very rare complication of perineal rupture is a rectal diverticulum in which the rectal wall muscle is breached, allowing mucosa to prolapse through.

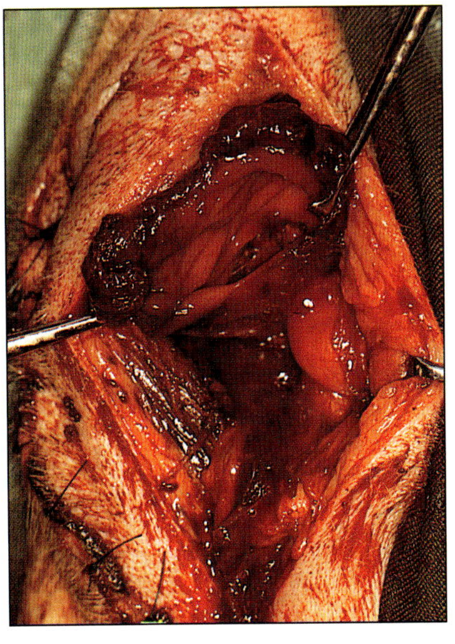

5.36 The prolapsed mucosa of a rectal diverticulum is very fragile. This dog ate a meal of bones the day before presentation. The bones passed into the diverticulum and tore the wall, allowing faeces to pass into the pelvic cavity. Despite intensive therapy, the dog developed severe peritonitis and euthanasia was carried out on humane grounds 24 hours later. Rectal examination of dogs with perineal rupture should always be performed with care!

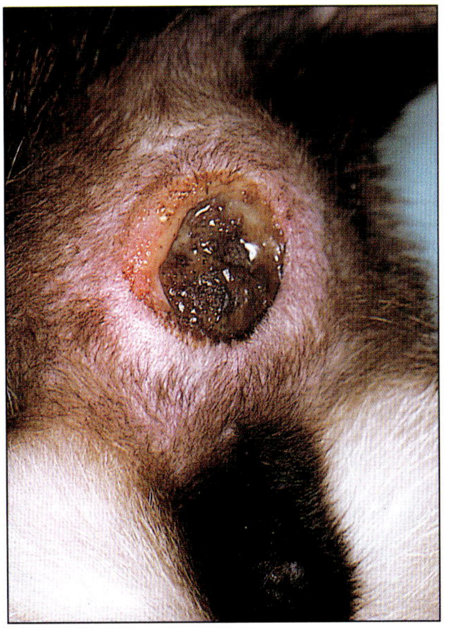

5.37 Perineal rupture is rare in cats but, when it does occur, usually results in rectal dilatation.

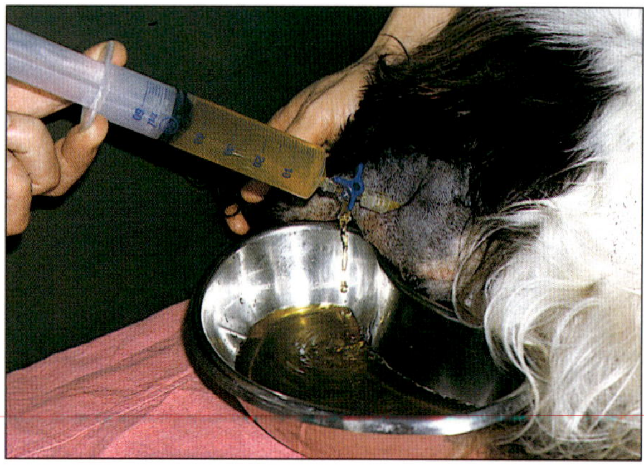

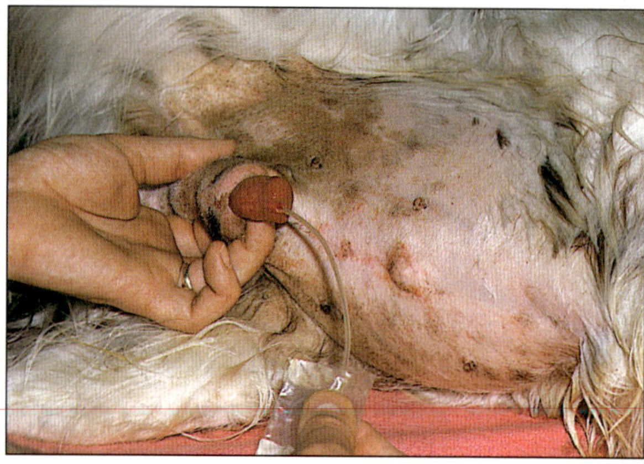

5.38 If retroflexion of the bladder into a perineal rupture results in dysuria, the priority for treatment is relief of the dysuria. It is dangerous to attempt forceful catheterization of the bladder; the tortuous course of the urethra (see **5.27**) means that iatrogenic trauma by the catheter is highly likely. Initially, therefore, the bladder should be drained by needle centesis through the perineum **(left)**. A catheter is then inserted gently *per urethram* to the level of the ischial arch of the urethra **(right)**. After drainage by centesis, the bladder can then usually be returned to the abdomen by direct digital pressure through the perineal defect **(middle)** and the catheter advanced into it. The catheter is retained as an in-dwelling catheter for 4–5 days. This allows the bladder and perineum to recover from the effects of bladder entrapment and distension while the animal is treated for the metabolic effects of dysuria. In addition, the use of a polyurethrane catheter, which is soft but stiff, tends to prevent the bladder from returning to the perineum.

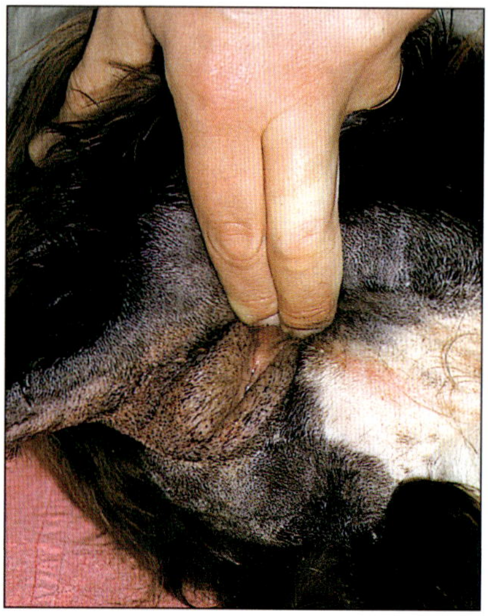

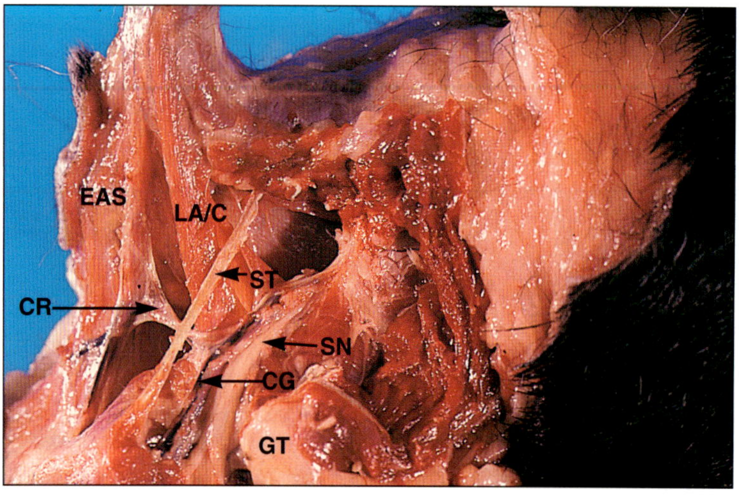

5.39 A knowledge of local anatomy is imperative. In this dissection of a dog, the gluteal musculature has been removed from the caudal, right lateral pelvis. The tail has been elevated. Note the position of the following structures and their relationships to each other: EAS, external anal sphincter muscle; LA/C, levator ani (caudomedial)/coccygeus (craniolateral) muscles; CR, caudal rectal (haemorrhoidal) vein, artery and nerve; ST, sacrotuberous ligament; SN, sciatic nerve; CG, caudal gluteal artery and vein; GT, greater trochanter of proximal femur. The breakdown of the perineum usually occurs at the junction between the external anal sphincter and the levator ani muscles (separated on this dissection). Rarely, breakdown occurs between the levator ani and coccygeus muscles.

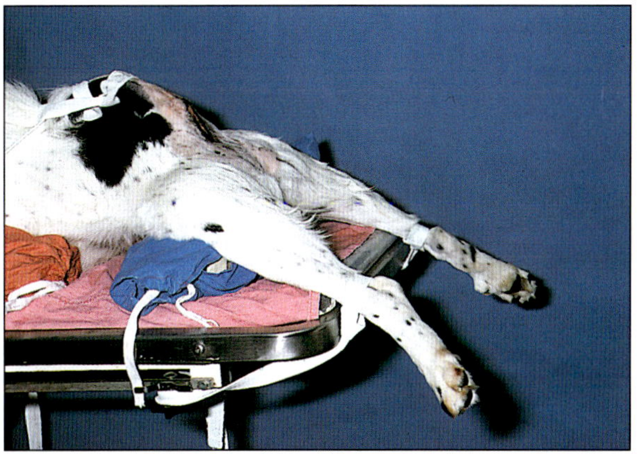

5.40 The dog should be positioned for surgery in sternal recumbency with the hind quarters raised by extending the back legs over a sandbag placed under the proximal thighs. The tail should be elevated using tapes.

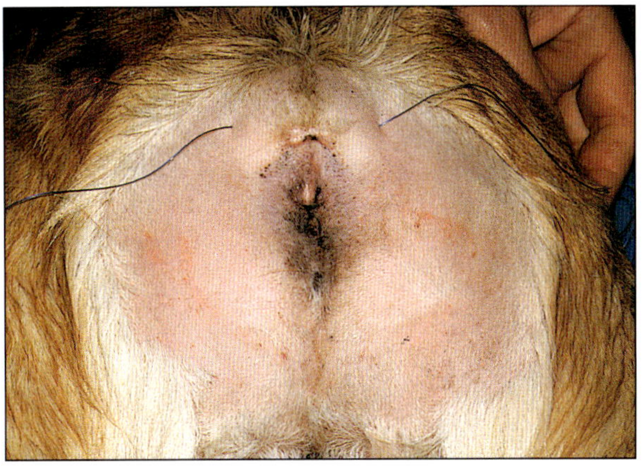

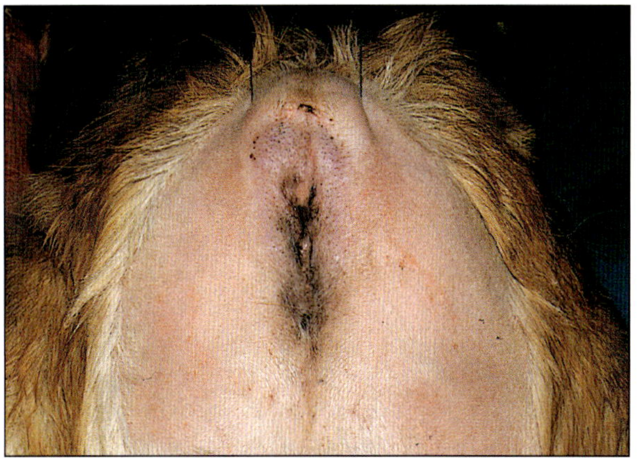

5.41 The tails of short-docked breeds are difficult to elevate. In these animals, a large cutting needle can be used to pass no. 2 monofilament nylon ventral to the tail, as illustrated **(left)**. The nylon is then tied to itself as a loose loop. Tapes are placed through this loop and used to elevate the remnants of the tail **(right)**.

Possible surgical/post-surgical complications

These include neurological damage, trauma to intrapelvic and perineal soft tissues, and recurrence.

Damage to the sciatic nerve may cause hind limb paresis or paralysis and is usually associated with placement of sutures around the sacrotuberous ligament. The location of the sciatic nerve (and its distance from the sacrotuberous ligament) can be judged by its proximity to the caudal gluteal artery, the pulse of which can be palpated cranial and lateral to the sacrotuberous ligament during palpation of the latter (see **5.39**). Sutures should be placed as closely as possible around the ligament.

Damage to the internal pudendal or caudal rectal/haemorrhoidal nerve may lead to paralysis of the external anal sphincter muscle and postoperative faecal incontinence. This can be avoided by identification of the nerves by observing the pulses in their accompanying arteries and avoiding them when placing sutures through the external anal sphincter and internal obturator muscles (see **5.39**).

Haemorrhage may be a problem if the caudal gluteal vessels are traumatized during placement of sutures around the sacrotuberous ligament. This can be avoided by location of the caudal gluteal artery by palpating its pulse and placing sutures close to the ligament. If haemorrhage does occur, haemostasis can be achieved only by direct digital pressure to the area as these vessels (like the sciatic nerve and sacrotuberous ligament) are buried in the soft tissues of the lateral pelvic region.

Trauma to other soft tissues is rare but care must be taken to avoid placing sutures into the rectum or urethra. Sutures placed in the rectum may fix the bowel wall laterally and prevent resolution of existing rectal abnormalities such as deviation/dilatation. In addition, if such sutures allow spillage of rectal contents, fatal peritonitis or, in the long term if the animal survives, rectocutaneous fistulation may occur. If sutures penetrate the wall of the urethra, dysuria and/or leakage of urine into the pelvic cavity may result. Urethral trauma is avoided if sutures are placed in the internal obturator muscle in a cranio caudal rather than a latero–medial direction (see **5.48**).

Tenesmus may occur during the recovery period after surgical repair. If so, it is probably due to irritation of the rectal wall during rectal evacuation pre-operatively (many animals also have a pre-existing proctitis) and/or stimulation of stretch receptors in the pelvic diaphragm during surgery. It may predispose to breakdown of the repair or rectal prolapse, the latter particularly if rectal dilatation is present. Tenesmus can be prevented by the use of analgesics, locally and parenterally. Local analgesia of the rectum can be achieved by inserting 3–5 ml of lignocaine in a water-miscible base (Xylocaine 5% ointment, Astra) into the rectum at the end of surgery, using a syringe. In the rare instance of tenesmus which is not prevented by parenteral and local analgesia, epidural analgesia may be required. However, this is extremely rare. In the longer term, it is important to prevent undue straining during defaecation throughout the healing period. This can be achieved by the addition of stool softeners such as Isogel (Charwell Pharmaceuticals Ltd) to the dog's diet for at least four weeks postoperatively.

Recurrence of the rupture occurs in a proportion of cases. The recurrence rate appears to bear little relationship to the technique which is used but does vary between different surgeons apparently using the same technique. It is lower if the dogs are neutered at the time of surgery and, in the author's opinion, this should always be advised.

Technique

A variety of surgical techniques have been described for correcting perineal ruptures in dogs. This is a reminder that no single technique has a 100% success rate. Whichever technique is used, there will be a proportion of animals in which the repair breaks down and the rupture recurs.

In the standard technique, the cranial edge of the external anal sphincter muscle is sutured to the levator ani muscle cranially and the internal obturator muscle ventrally. This is associated with a fairly high recurrence rate (up to 50%), probably because the pelvic diaphragm muscles are often atrophied in these cases, making them both difficult to identify and also poor anchoring tissues for sutures. Alternative techniques are to include the sacrotuberous ligament in the repair or to close the perineal defect using superficial gluteal or/and internal obturator muscle flaps, synthetic or collagen meshes. The author's preferred method is to perform repair using the sacrotuberous ligament.

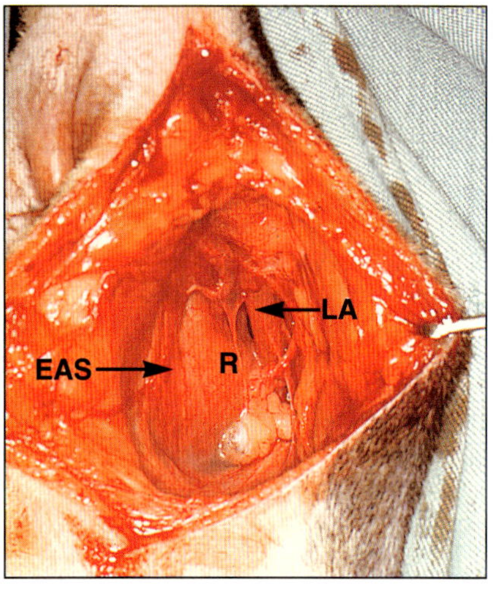

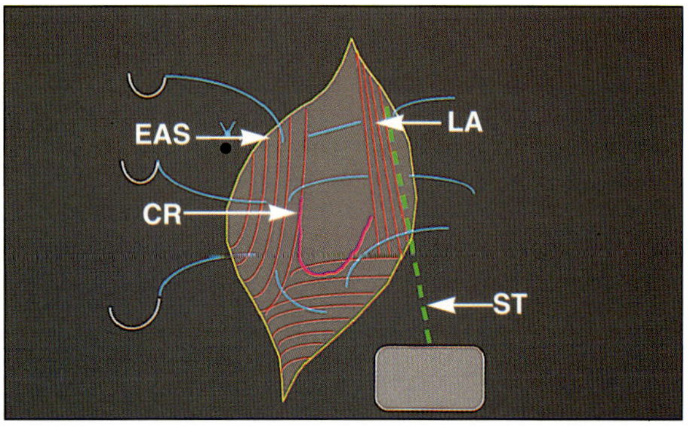

5.42 (top) The 'best' example of a perineal rupture. The right perineum has been opened revealing the defect between the external anal sphincter (EAS) and levator ani (LA) muscles into which a rectal deviation (R) protrudes (refer to **5.39**). White, lobulated pelvic fat can be seen on the floor of the pelvis and beneath this fat is the internal obturator muscle. It is extremely unusual to be able to see this much anatomy and so the technique of perineal rupture repair is illustrated on the type of case likely to be encountered by the reader. The author prefers the technique of re-apposing the external anal sphincter to the levator ani cranially (but including the sacrotuberous ligament in the sutures) and to the internal obturator muscle ventrally. This is summarized in the diagram **(bottom)**, although only three sutures are shown in this figure.

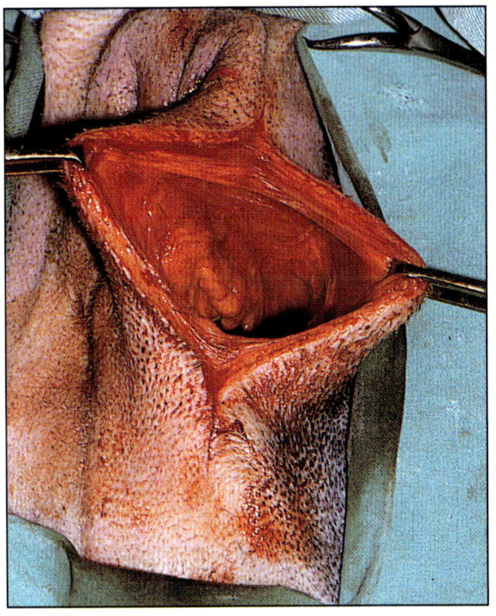

5.43 This is a more typical case. The animal has been anaesthetized, its rectum evacuated of faeces and the anal sacs emptied. The dog is positioned for surgery in ventral recumbency with the hind limbs extended caudally over a sandbag and the tail elevated (see **5.40**). A temporary purse-string suture is used to close the anus. After routine aseptic skin preparation and draping, an incision is made just lateral to the region of the external anal sphincter muscle. This can frequently be judged by palpating the defect in the perineum but, if not, the skin is incised just lateral to the lateral margin of the glandular circumanal skin which corresponds to the lateral edges of the external anal sphincter muscle. The incision is extended ventrally to a level just above the pelvic floor (this can be judged by palpating the tuber ischium on the affected side. The subcutaneous fat and fascia are separated by blunt dissection and the perineal defect exposed. This dog has a right-sided perineal rupture with no anatomy visible apart from fat and fascia. This is fairly typical.

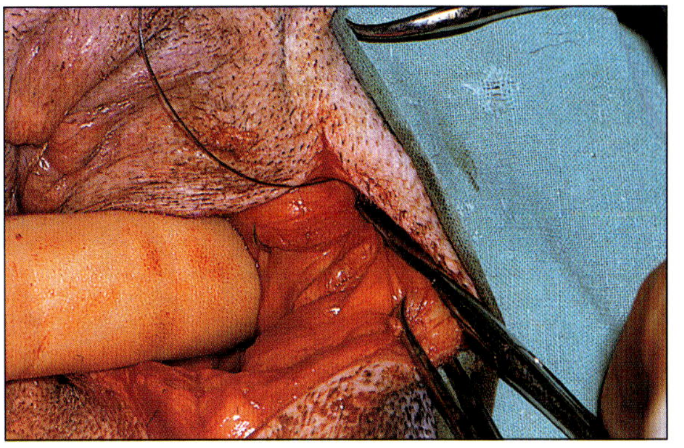

5.44 Here, an index finger has been inserted into the defect, medial to the levator ani muscle. The sacrotuberous ligament is palpated through the muscle; this is always possible, even when the muscle is not visible, as in this case. With the ball of the finger on the ligament, the finger tip is bent slightly ventrally and laterally into a small depression. A pulse should now be palpable by the tip of the finger. This pulse is in the caudal gluteal artery and gives an indication of how close the sciatic nerve and caudal gluteal vessels are to the ligament (see **5.39**). A curved round-bodied suture needle with swaged-on no. 0 monofilament polyamide is inserted dorsally, lateral to the ligament. The needle is curved cranially around the ligament, staying as close to the ligament as possible. Automatically, the tip of the needle exits medially through the levator ani muscle remnants. The needle tip is palpated as it emerges from the levator ani muscle and is braced against the finger tip. This is to prevent the needle point from damaging the rectum and also to avoid losing it in the lateral pelvic soft tissues when the needle holders are released. The needle holders are now used to grip close to the point of the needle, which is then withdrawn and the suture is pulled around the sacrotuberous ligament.

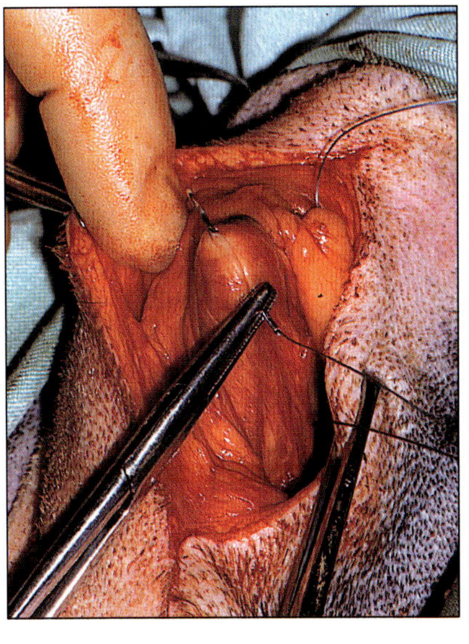

5.45 The external anal sphincter muscle is now identified beneath the medial part of the skin incision. The muscle is usually visible but, if not, its position can be determined by placing an index finger on the lateral wall of the rectum and curling it caudally until a thickening is appreciated. This is the cranial edge of the external anal sphincter muscle. A bite is then taken through the cranial edge of the muscle, as shown.

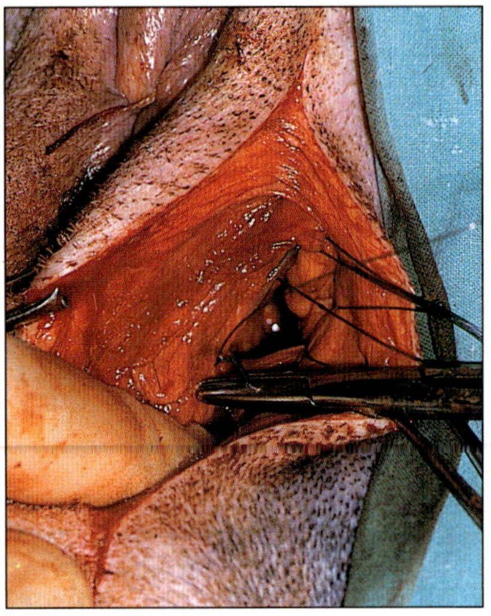

5.46 Sutures continue to be pre-placed between the sacrotuberous ligament and the external anal sphincter muscle, as described above. However, care should be taken to avoid placing sutures around or through the caudal rectal nerve as it enters the external anal sphincter muscle. The location of this nerve can usually be identified by detecting the pulse in its adjacent artery; but if not it should be assumed to be entering the sphincter at the '8 o'clock' (left side) or '4 o'clock' (right side) positions on the cranial edge of the sphincter muscle. The nerve is not apparent in this dog but the needle holders are being used to point to the location of its entry into the sphincter. This area must be avoided during suture placement, as illustrated by the position of the middle of the three sutures in **5.42b**.

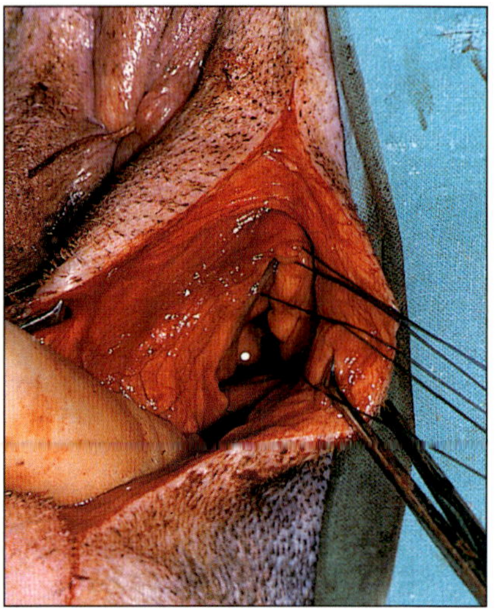

5.47 When the last suture has been placed between the ventral end of the sacrotuberous ligament (close to its insertion into the tuber ischium) and the external anal sphincter muscle, a defect remains in the ventral perineum, as shown. This can be closed by suturing the external anal sphincter muscle to the internal obturator muscle.

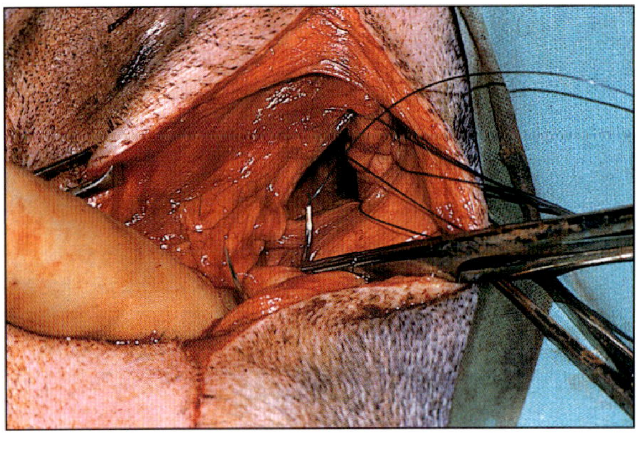

5.48 A suture is placed in the internal obturator muscle, as shown. The suture enters the muscle caudal to the internal pudendal vessels (the pulse in the artery can be palpated on the pelvic floor overlying the internal obturator muscle). It is preferable to insert the needle in a craniocaudal direction, as illustrated. This is slightly more difficult than passing the needle lateromedially but greatly reduces the risk of trauma to the urethra. If the muscle cannot be seen, the needle is passed ventrally until it contacts the bone of the ischium and is then continued caudally and dorsally to exit the muscle. In doing so, it has to have passed in and out of the internal obturator muscle.

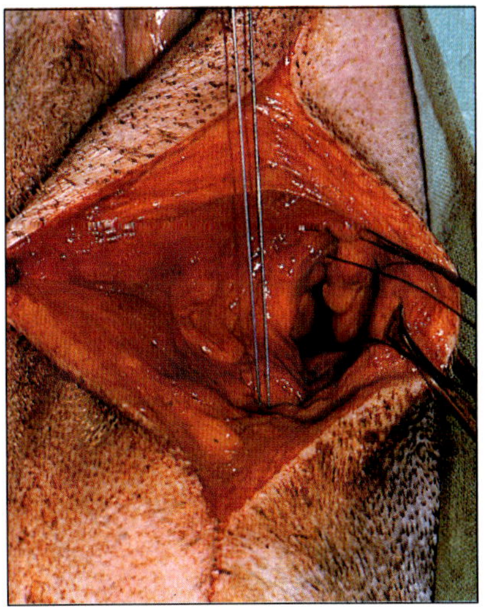

5.49 If one is unsure of the suture placement in the internal obturator muscle, tension should be applied to the suture, as illustrated. If the suture has passed through fat and fascia only, it will tear out and should be replaced.

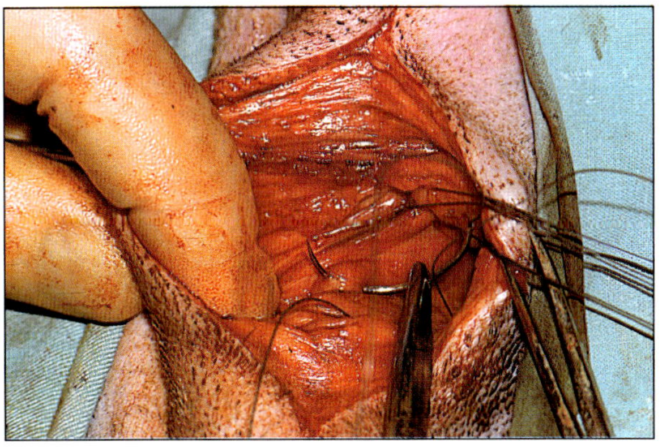

5.50 The suture is then taken through the ventral part of the cranial edge of the external anal sphincter muscle, care being taken to avoid the caudal rectal nerve.

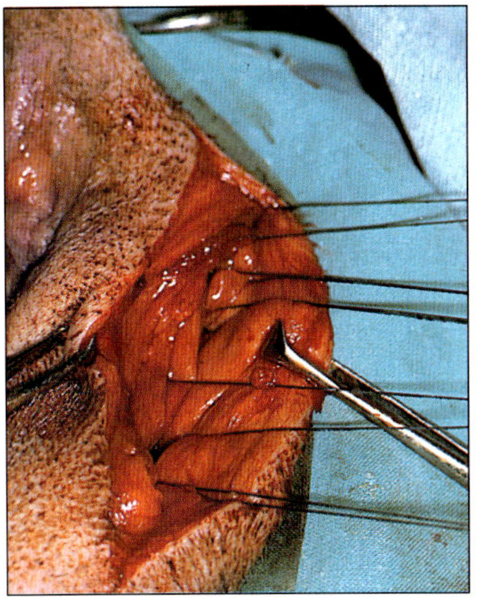

5.51 When all the sutures have been placed, they can be tied. The author prefers to commence at the ventral part of the defect as this tends to prevent viscera such as pelvic fat from prolapsing through the defect while the remaining sutures are being tied.

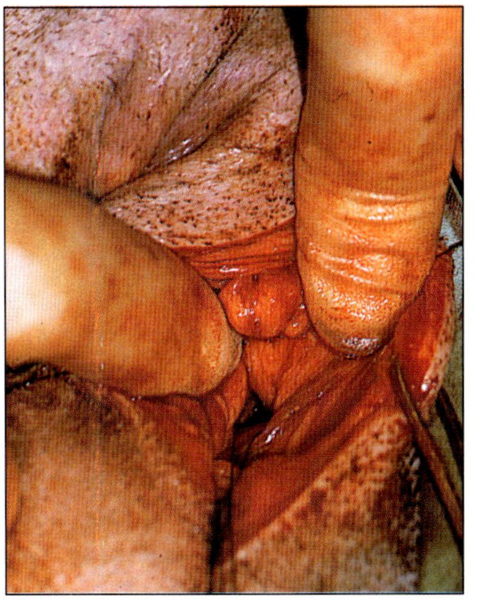

5.52 Care should be taken to tie all sutures tight. The dorsal-most sutures in a large dog will be tied some 6–8 cm from the perineal skin wound edges and so finger tip tightening of the suture knots at this depth is required, as shown.

5.53 Once the defect has been closed, the return of perineal support can be appreciated by local palpation. The remaining tissues are apposed. The fascia is closed with a simple continuous absorbable suture. The author prefers to use no. 0 chromic catgut in the hope that any resultant fibrosis of perineal fascia may contribute to perineal support. Frequently, there is little fat and fascia medially. In this case, the lateral fat and fascia are sutured to the superficial fibres of the external anal sphincter muscle. The skin is closed routinely and the purse-string suture removed from the anus. The dog can now be repositioned and castrated (see **5.2–5.24**).

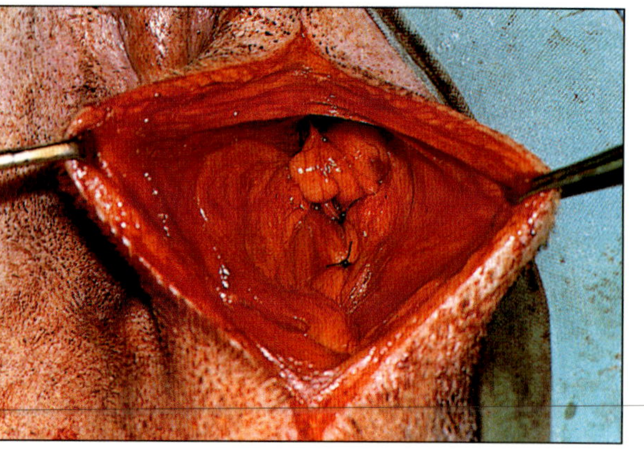

Inguinal/scrotal hernia repair

Indications

In urological cases, inguinal/scrotal hernia repair is usually indicated because of displacement of the urinary bladder (see **2.55**) or extension of a prostatic cyst into the hernia.

Pre- and peri-operative considerations

Displacement and entrapment of the bladder within the hernia may lead to dysuria, as may the presence of a prostatic cyst or abscess (see Chapter 4). As in the case of perineal rupture with bladder retroflexion, it is the dysuria which requires urgent treatment rather than hernia repair. The bladder should be drained and returned to the abdomen, if possible, as described under 'Perineal Rupture Repair' (see **5.38**). Similarly, a prostatic cyst/abscess can be drained by centesis, temporarily to relieve the signs whilst the animal's condition is stabilized (see **4.170**).

There is a hereditary predisposition to inguinal herniation and the owners should be informed that affected animals should not be used for breeding. In male animals, closed castration is usually a necessary component of surgical repair. In some dogs, however, the condition is not apparent until the hernia contents enlarge later in life. Such enlargement may follow an increase in size of the hernia ring and contents due to tenesmus (e.g. the dog with perineal rupture – see **2.55**) or enlargement of herniated viscera such as bladder, prostatic cyst or uterus.

Inguinal hernias are often classified as 'direct' or 'indirect'. This is an extrapolation from human terminology and the definitions are the opposite of what one might expect. A direct hernia involves passage of abdominal viscera into a dilated peritoneal sac just distal to the external inguinal ring, whereas in indirect herniation the viscera pass distally, within the vaginal tunic itself. Both types occur in small animals. An example of a direct hernia is shown in **2.55,** while an indirect hernia is present in the dog illustrated in **5.55–5.60.** The hernia type makes no difference to the clinical management of the case.

Possible surgical/post-surgical complications

Postoperative oedematous swelling is common but is not usually of any significance. However, severe swelling can occur if there is trauma to the inguinal blood and lymphatic vessels. These are located at the caudal end of the external inguinal ring. Trauma can be avoided by identifying the external pudendal vessels and ensuring that a space is left for these (and the adjacent lymphatics) during closure of the external inguinal ring.

Haemorrhage can be minimized by avoidance of trauma to the external pudendal vessels and adequate ligation of the spermatic vessels (see **5.12–5.17**).

Breakdown of the repair and evisceration are possible postoperative complications but are extremely unlikely if closed castration and adequate closure of the external inguinal ring are performed.

Technique

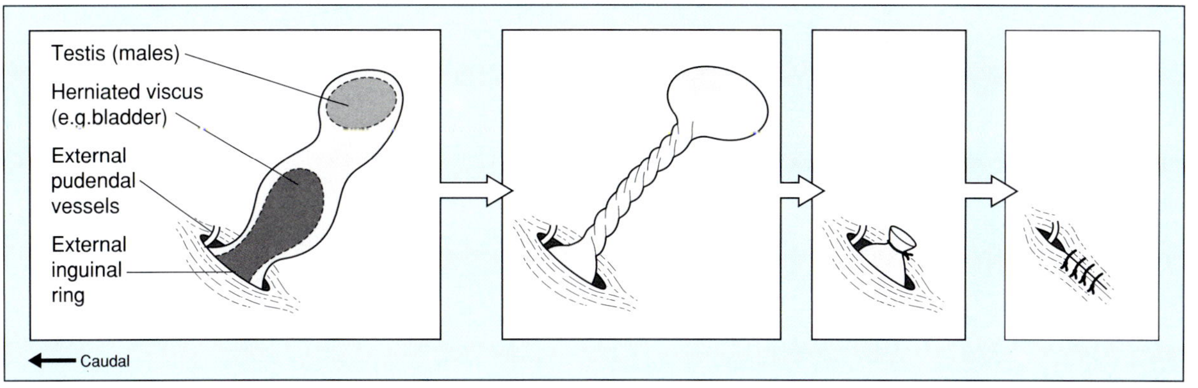

5.54 Diagrammatic representation of inguinal hernia repair. Although twisting of the vaginal tunic during reduction of hernia contents is often recommended (to prevent viscera from re-herniating during reduction and repair), it is not always necessary.

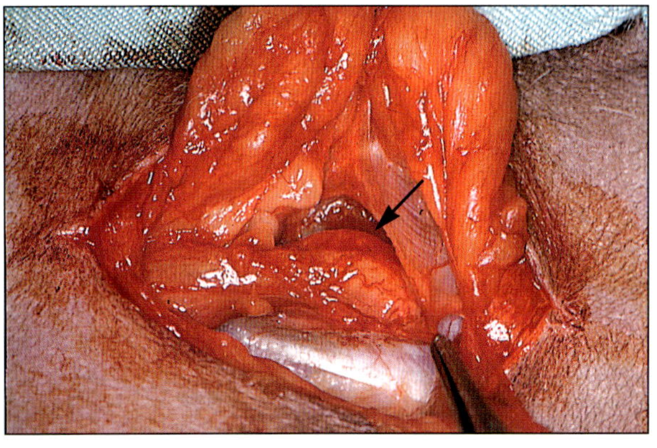

5.55 A skin incision is made directly over the hernia and the cod fat bluntly separated and reflected medially. In this male Dandie Dinmont, the dog's head is to the right and the penis is covered by the upper surgical drape. The cod fat has been reflected medially (upwards in the illustration) to expose the external inguinal ring. The craniomedial part of the ring is formed by the edge of the external abdominal oblique muscle (arrowed). Most of the hernia has been reduced but some omental fat can still be seen through the vaginal tunic, just to the left of the point of the forceps.

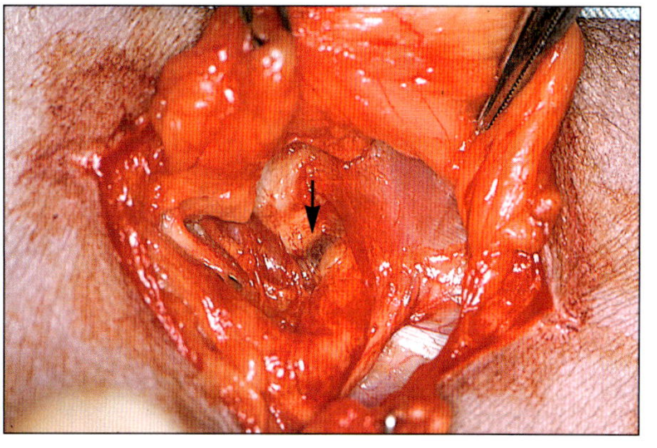

5.56 When the vaginal tunic is displaced craniolaterally, the large external pudendal vessels can be seen (arrowed). These and their adjacent (invisible) lymphatics must be avoided.

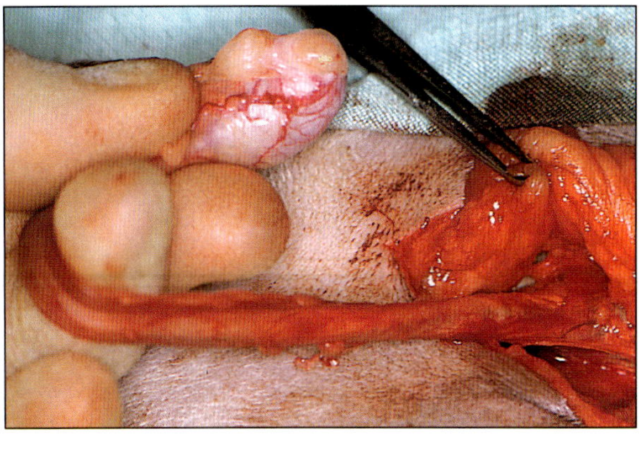

5.57 The tunic-covered testis and spermatic cord are exteriorized by blunt dissection of fascial attachments and the hernia contents returned to the abdomen (if this has not already been carried out). In the bitch, the vaginal tunic sac is freed from surrounding fascial attachments by blunt dissection. In both sexes, care is taken to avoid the external pudendal vessels and their branches, including caudal epigastric vessels. If the viscera are incarcerated and non-reducible, it may be necessary to incise the proximal vaginal tunic and enlarge the inguinal ring. This is best accomplished by incising the proximal tunic on its cranial border, just distal to the external inguinal ring, and continuing the incision cranially through the external abdominal oblique muscle.

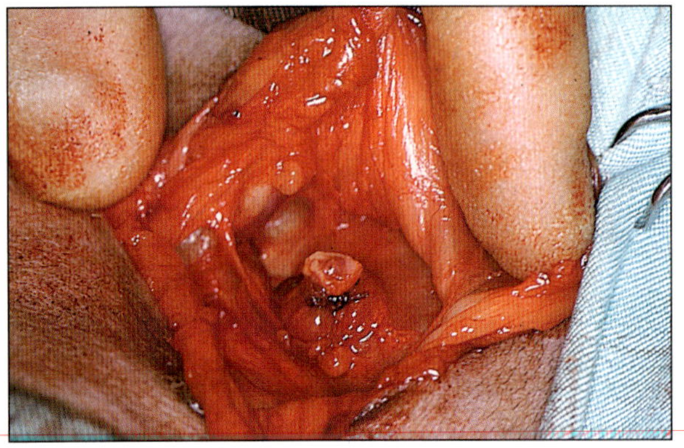

5.58 After reduction of the hernia contents, a closed castration is performed in male animals (see 5.2–5.24). This effectively obliterates the hernia sac. In bitches, the hernia sac is returned intact to the abdomen. The ligated sac remnants are now reduced through the inguinal canal.

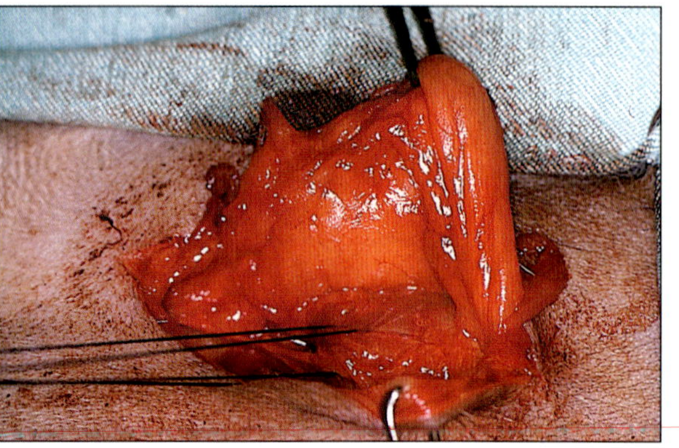

5.59 The external inguinal ring is now closed. Simple interrupted sutures of monofilament nylon or synthetic absorbable suture material are used to appose the edges of the external inguinal ring, formed by the caudal edge of the external abdominal oblique muscle craniomedially and the inguinal ligament caudolaterally. Sutures should be pre-placed, as shown, and a 0.5–1.5 cm space left (depending on the size of the animal) at the caudal end of the ring to avoid strangulation of the external pudendal vessels and lymphatics.

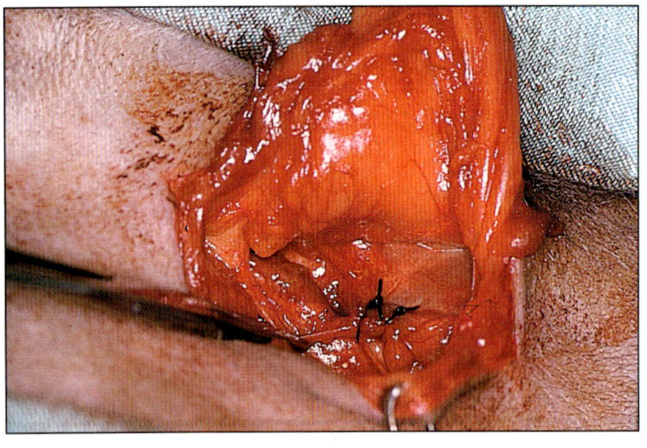

5.60 The sutures are now tied to complete the repair. The gap at the caudal end of the ring is checked to ensure that it is large enough to prevent strangulation of vessels and lymphatics but not to allow prolapse of viscera adjacent to these structures. The subcutaneous fat, fascia and skin are closed routinely. If a large dead space is present, it is prudent to use a Penrose drain for 3–5 days to minimize swelling.

Episiotomy

Indications

Occasionally, episiotomy is indicated in bitches with urological signs. It may be necessary, for example to remove vaginal masses (e.g. tumours, cysts) which are compressing the distal urethra or obstructing the external urethral orifice. In some bitches, particularly those with a narrow vestibule, episiotomy may be required to provide access for procedures on the caudal urethra and external urethral orifice.

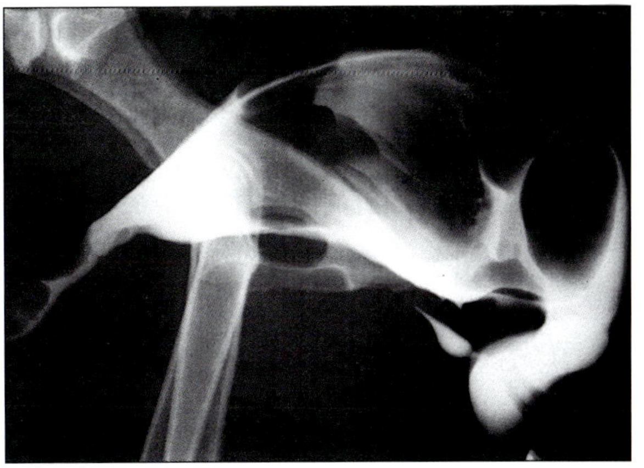

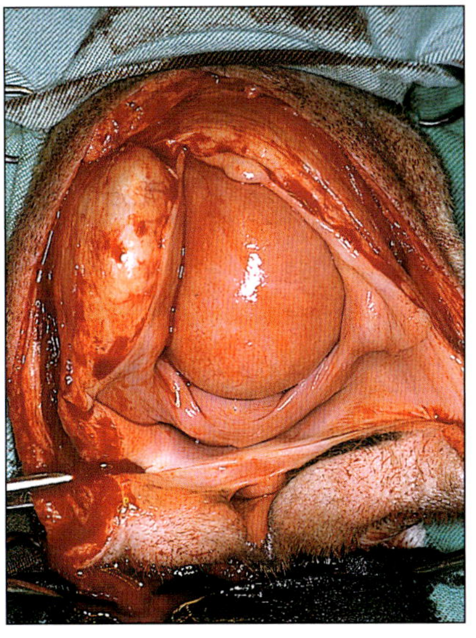

5.61 Vagino-urethrogram (top) of an adult Cocker spaniel bitch presented with perineal swelling and dysuria (see 2.33a). Although the vaginal masses which were compressing the urethra were palpable, their size prevented adequate insertion of a finger or endoscope. The vagino-urethrogram shows the size, location and extent of the masses. The tumours were removed via an episiotomy **(bottom)** and histopathological examinations of the excised tissues revealed that they were benign leiomyomas of the vaginal wall.

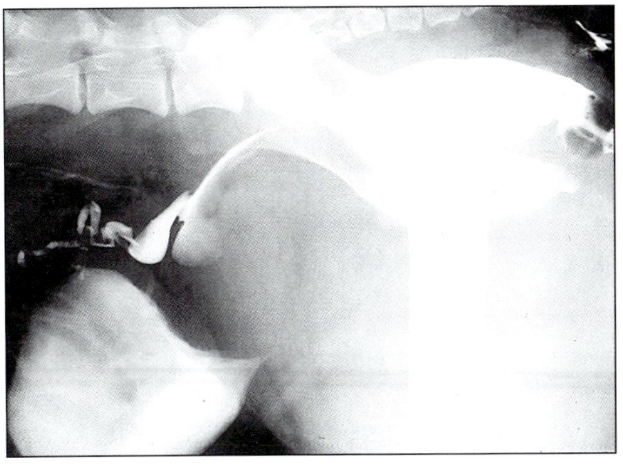

5.62 Vagino-urethrogram (performed shortly after intravenous urography) of an adult Airedale bitch presented with dysuria. A soft-tissue density can be seen in the ventral part of the vaginal lumen, extending cranially and compressing the urethra and bladder neck. Ultrasonography revealed that this was a fluid-filled swelling. Bacteriological and cytological examinations of the fluid confirmed that this was a vaginal wall cyst.

Pre- and peri-operative considerations

If the bitch is dysuric, the bladder should be drained and the metabolic consequences of dysuria (uraemia, acidosis, hyperkalaemia) corrected with fluid/electrolyte therapy before surgery is performed. The nature of the disorder may mean that bladder drainage is best carried out prepubically rather than via a urethral catheter as the latter may be difficult or impossible to introduce if an extensive vaginal lesion is present.

The owners of breeding bitches should be made aware of the possibility that extensive vaginal surgery may result in vaginal stenosis and the bitch may subsequently be unable to mate and/or give birth normally.

Once the animal has been anaesthetized, the anus should be closed with a purse-string suture to prevent faecal contamination.

In the bitch, a mid-line episiotomy is usually suitable but the dorsal extent of the incision should be below the level of the external anal sphincter muscle to avoid the possibility of iatrogenic postoperative faecal incontinence.

Once the episiotomy has been performed, the urethra should be catheterized (if this was not possible preoperatively) to facilitate its identification during subsequent surgical procedures.

Possible surgical/post-surgical complications

There are few complications during or after episiotomy. Iatrogenic urethral trauma is possible during dissections of ventral vaginal lesions. The risk of this can be minimized by the use of a urethral catheter peri-operatively to aid in identification of the urethra.

Haemorrhage from vaginal wall vessels may occur during surgery, particularly if large and/or extensive vaginal tumours are resected. This can usually be controlled by adequate haemostasis but occasionally will persist after surgery. Tampons may be used to pack the vagina and control the haemorrhage but, if haemorrhage is severe, plasma expanders or transfusions of whole blood may be required.

Vaginal stricture may be a long-term sequella of extensive vaginal surgery but is not usually a problem, apart from preventing subsequent mating and parturition. The owners of breeding bitches should therefore be made aware of this potential problem preoperatively.

Technique

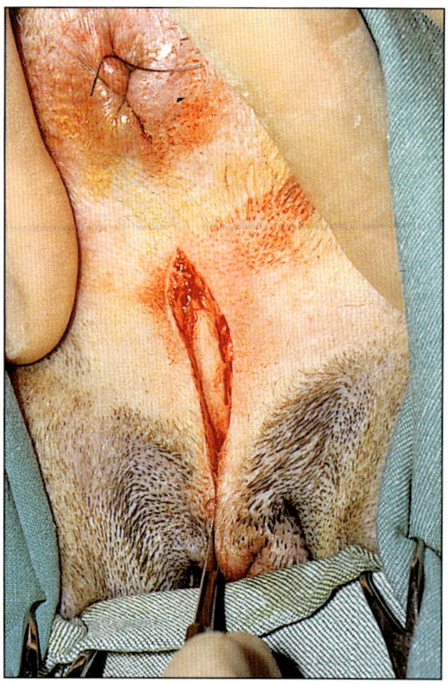

5.63 The bitch is placed in ventral recumbency with the hind quarters raised over a sandbag, as in perineal rupture repair (see 5.40). The tail is elevated and the perineum prepared for aseptic surgery. The anus is closed using a purse-string suture. A vertical skin incision is made, extending from just ventral to the external anal sphincter muscle to the dorsal commissure of the vulval lips.

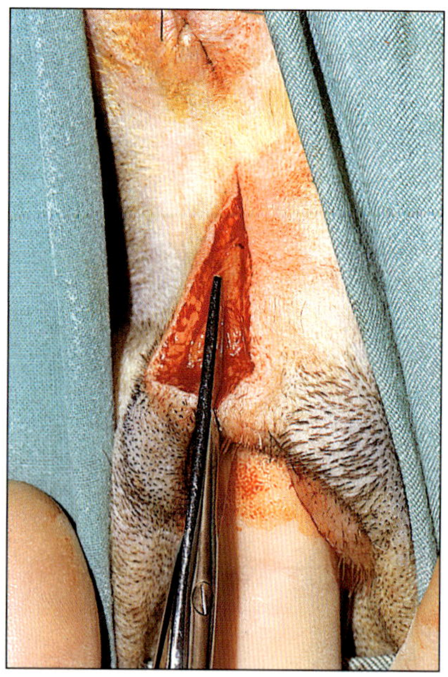

5.64 The incision is continued through the dorsal vaginal wall using scissors.

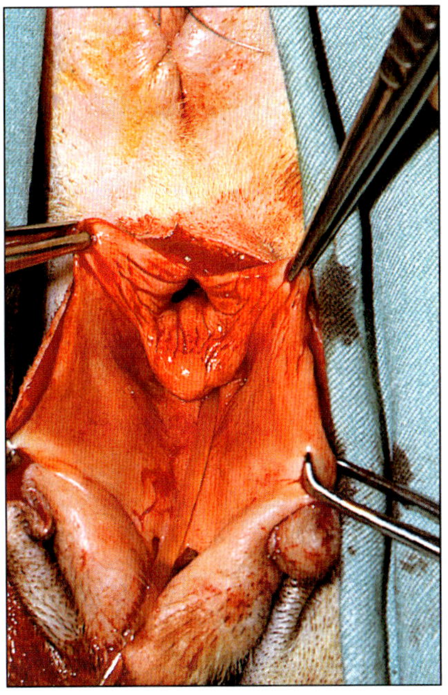

5.65 Separation of the skin/vaginal wall edges provides access to the vestibule, external urethral orifice and caudal vagina. The urethra should be catheterized, if this has not been done already. In this bitch, an episiotomy was performed to attempt excision of a caudal urethral tumour. Part of the tumour can be seen in the vaginal floor, dorsal to the external urethral orifice. Unfortunately, the tumour proved to be inoperable and euthanasia of the bitch was carried out.

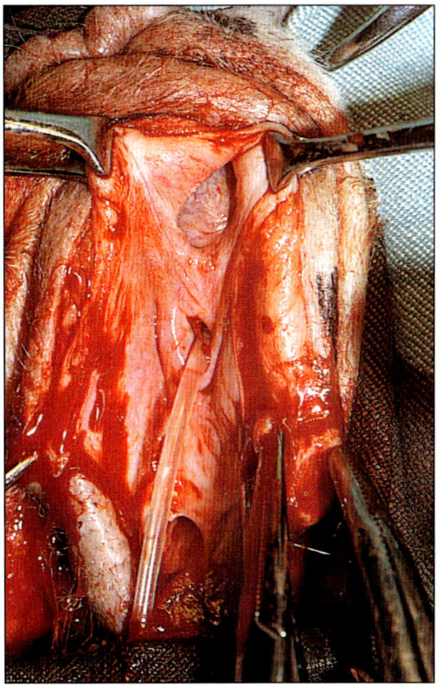

5.66 In this example, an episiotomy was performed on a dysuric Yorkshire terrier bitch to provide access to a vaginal floor cyst. The cyst can be seen bulging in the vagina just cranial to the external urethral orifice.

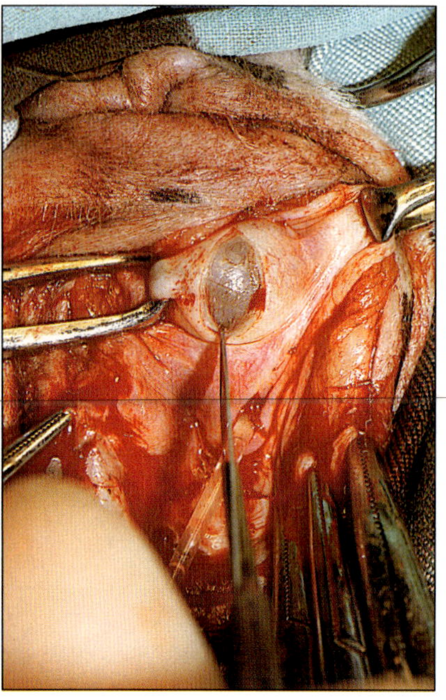

5.67 These cysts can be treated by marsupialization into the vaginal lumen. The vaginal mucosa over the cyst is incised, revealing the cyst wall, as shown. The cyst wall is then incised and the cyst drained.

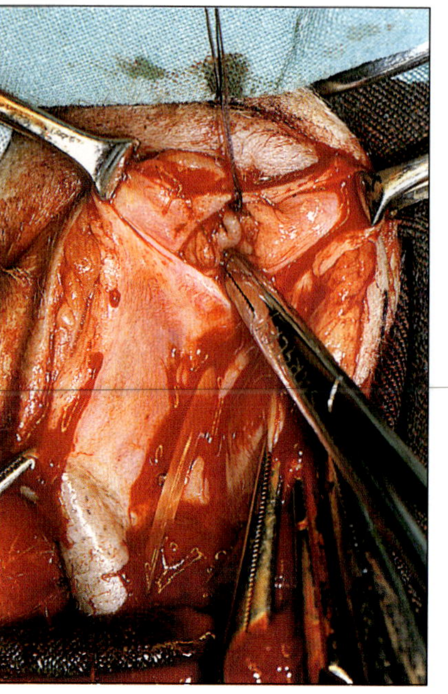

5.68 The cyst and vaginal mucosal incisions are then apposed using a simple continuous pattern of synthetic absorbable suture material, resulting in a stoma between the cyst and vaginal lumina (the tip of Kilner needle holders has been inserted into the stoma). Closure of an episiotomy is routine and involves closure of the dorsal vaginal wall using synthetic absorbable material in a simple continuous pattern followed by simple interrupted sutures of monofilament nylon in the skin. The purse-string suture is then removed from the anus. The urethral catheter is also removed unless there is the possibility of postoperative dysuria resulting from urethral or peri-urethral swelling, in which case it can be sutured *in situ* as an in-dwelling catheter (see **3.4**).

References and Further Reading

The reference list given below is by no means exhaustive. However, the books and articles cited are excellent sources of additional reading material.

General

Binnington, A.G. & Cockshutt, J.R. (Eds) (1988) *Decision Making in Small Animal Soft Tissue Surgery.* B.C. Decker Inc., Toronto.

Bjorling, D.E. & Petersen, S.W. (1990) Surgical techniques for urinary tract diversion and salvage in small animals. *Compendium on Continuing Education for the Practicing Veterinarian* **12,** 1699–1708.

Bradley, R.L. (Ed.) (1989) *Problems in Veterinary Medicine,* Vol. 1 (1). *Urogenital Surgical Conditions.* J.B. Lippincott Co., Philadelphia.

Bush, B. (1992) Lower urinary tract disorders of small animals. *In Practice* **14,** 309–316.

Coats, C. (1988) *Things Your Dad always Told You But You Didn't Want to Hear.* Carolyn Coats' Bestsellers, Orlando, Florida.

Holt, P.E. (1990) Dysuria in the dog. Part 1: management of the dysuric animal. *In Practice* **12,** 121–125.

Holt, P.E. (1990) Dysuria in the dog. Part 2: differential diagnosis of dysuria. *In Practice* **12,** 147–153.

Holt, P.E. (1990) Urinary incontinence in dogs and cats. *Veterinary Record* **127,** 347–350.

Holt, P.E. & Gibbs, C. (1992) Congenital urinary incontinence in cats: a review of 19 cases. *Veterinary Record* **130,** 437–442.

Holt, P.E. (1992) Aspects of feline urology. In *The Veterinary Annual.* 32nd Issue (Eds. M.E. Raw & T.J. Parkinson). Blackwell Scientific Publications, Oxford. pp. 13–28.

Lulich, J.P., Osborne, C.A., Lawler, D.F., O'Brien, T.D., Johnston, G.R. & O'Leary, T.P. (1987) Urologic disorders of immature cats. *Veterinary Clinics of North America: Small Animal Practice* **17**(3), 663–696.

Morgan, R.V. (1982) Urogenital emergencies: part I. *Compendium on Continuing Education for the Practicing Veterinarian* **4,** 908–915.

Osborne, C.A., Low, D.G. & Finco, D.R. (1972) *Canine and Feline Urology.* W.B. Saunders Co., Philadelphia.

Osuna, D.J. (1987) Postoperative management of urinary tract surgical patients. *Compendium on Continuing Education for the Practicing Veterinarian* **9,** 873–881.

Pechman, R.D. Jr. (1982) Urinary trauma in dogs and cats: a review. *Journal of the American Animal Hospital Association* **18,** 33–40.

Sackman, J.E. (1991) Pain. Part II. Control of pain in animals. *Compendium on Continuing Education for the Practicing Veterinarian* **13,** 181–193.

Stone, E.A. & Barsanti, J.A. (1992) *Urologic Surgery of the Dog and Cat.* Lea & Febiger, Philadelphia.

Waterman, A. (1984) Practical fluid therapy for small animals. *In Practice* **6,** 143–150.

Investigation

Barr, F. (1990) *Diagnostic Ultrasound in the Dog and Cat.* Blackwell Scientific Publications, Oxford. pp. 46–77.

Barr, F.J. (1990) Evaluation of ultrasound as a method of assessing renal size in the dog. *Journal of Small Animal Practice* **31,** 174–179.

Barr, F.J., Holt, P.E. & Gibbs, C. (1990) Ultrasonographic measurement of normal renal parameters. *Journal of Small Animal Practice* **31,** 180–184.

Biller, D.S., Kantrowitz, B., Partington, D.P. & Miyabayashi, T. (1990) Diagnostic ultrasound of the urinary bladder. *Journal of the American Animal Hospital Association* **26,** 397–402.

Brearley, M.J., Cooper, J.E. & Wedderburn, N. (1986) Urinary cytology as an adjunct to bacteriology in the laboratory investigation of canine bladder disease. *Journal of Small Animal Practice* **27,** 425–432.

Brearley, M.J. & Cooper, J.E. (1987) The diagnosis of bladder disease in dogs by cystoscopy. *Journal of Small Animal Practice* **28,** 75–85.

Brearley, M.J., Cooper, J.E. & Sullivan, M. (1991) *A Colour Atlas of Small Animal Endoscopy.* Wolfe Publishing Ltd, London. pp. 77–86.

Feeney, D.A., Johnston, G.R., Klausner, J.S., Perman, V., Leininger, J.R. & Tomlinson, M.J. (1987) Canine prostatic disease – comparison of ultrasonographic appearance with morphologic and microbiologic findings: 30 cases (1981–1985). *Journal of the American Veterinary Medical Association* **190,** 1027–1034.

Gregory, S.P. & Holt, P.E. (1993) Comparison of stressed urethral pressure profiles between anesthetized continent and incontinent bitches with urethral sphincter mechanism incompetence. *American Journal of Veterinary Research* **54,** 216–222.

Herrtage, M. & Carr, L. (1986) Urine sampling in the bitch. *In Practice* **8,** 221–224.

Herrtage, M.E. & Dennis, R. (1987) Contrast media and their use in small animal radiology. *Journal of Small Animal Practice* **28,** 1105–1114.

Holt, P.E., Lucke, V.M. & Brown, P.J. (1986) Evaluation of a catheter biopsy technique as a diagnostic aid in lower urinary tract disease. *Veterinary Record* **118,** 681–684.

Holt, P.E. (1988) 'Simultaneous' urethral pressure profilometry: comparisons between continent and incontinent bitches. *Journal of Small Animal Practice* **29,** 761–769.

Holt, P.E. (1989) Positive contrast vagino-urethrography for diagnosis of lower urinary tract disease. In *Current Veterinary Therapy X. Small Animal Practice* (Ed. R.W. Kirk). W.B. Saunders Co., Philadelphia. pp. 1142–1145.

Holt, P.E. (1989) 'Simultaneous' urethral pressure profilometry in the bitch: methodology and reproducibility of the technique. *Research in Veterinary Science* **47,** 110–116.

Holt, P.E., Gibbs, C. & Wathes, C.M. (1990) Simultaneous urethral pressure profilometry using a microtip transducer catheter in the bitch: effects of bitch position and transducer orientation. *Neurourology and Urodynamics* **9,** 281–296.

Holt, P.E. & Gregory, S.P. (1993) Resting urethral pressure profilometry in bitches – artefact or reality? *Compendium on Continuing Education for the Practicing Veterinarian* **15,** 1207–1215.

Johnston, G.R., Stevens, J.B., Jessen, C.R. & Osborne, C.A. (1983) Complications of retrograde contrast urography in dogs and cats. *American Journal of Veterinary Research* **44,** 1248–1256.

Kay, N.D., Ling, G.V., Nyland, T.G., Kennedy, P.C. & Zinkl, J.G. (1989) Cytological diagnosis of canine prostatic disease using a urethral brush technique. *Journal of the American Animal Hospital Association* **25,** 517–526.

Kay, N.D., Ling, G.V. & Johnson, D.L. (1989) A urethral brush technique for the diagnosis of canine bacterial prostatitis. *Journal of the American Animal Hospital Association* **25,** 527–532.

Lappin, M.R. & Barsanti, J.A. (1987) Urinary incontinence secondary to idiopathic detrusor instability: cystometric diagnosis and pharmacologic management in two dogs and a cat. *Journal of the American Veterinary Medical Association* **191,** 1439–1442.

Melhoff, T. & Osborne, C.A. (1977) Catheter biopsy of the urethra, bladder and prostate gland. In *Current Veterinary Therapy VI. Small Animal Practice* (Ed. R.W. Kirk). W.B. Saunders Co. Ltd., Philadelphia. pp. 1173–1175.

Nash, A.S., Boyd, J.S., Minto, A.W. & Wright, N.G. (1983) Renal biopsy in the normal cat: an examination of the effects of a single needle biopsy. *Research in Veterinary Science* **34,** 347–356.

Neuwirth, L., Mahaffey, M., Crowell, W., Selcer, B., Barsanti, J., Cooper, R. & Brown, J. (1993) Comparison of excretory urography and ultrasonography for detection of experimentally induced pyelonephritis in dogs. *American Journal of Veterinary Research* **54,** 660–669.

Sackman, J.E. & Sims, M.H. (1990) Electromyographic evaluation of the external urethral sphincter during cystometry in male cats. *American Journal of Veterinary Research* **51,** 1237–1241.

Sackman, J.E. & Sims, M.H. (1991) Use of fine-wire electrodes for electromyographic evaluation of the external urethral sphincter during urethral pressure profilometry in male cats. *American Journal of Veterinary Research* **52,** 314–316.

Senior, D.F. & Sundstrom, D.A. (1988) Cystoscopy in female dogs. *Compendium on Continuing Education for the Practicing Veterinarian* **10,** 890–895.

Walter, P.A., Johnston, G.R., Feeney, D.A. & O'Brien, T.D. (1988) Application of ultrasonography in the diagnosis of parenchymal renal disease in cats: 24 cases (1981–1986). *Journal of the American Veterinary Medical Association* **192,** 92–98.

Kidney

Holt, P.E., Lucke, V.M. & Pearson, H. (1987) Idiopathic renal haemorrhage in the dog. *Journal of Small Animal Practice* **28,** 253–263.

Klein, M.K., Cockerell, G.L., Harris, C.K., Withrow, S.J., Lulich, J.P., Ogilvie, G.K., Norris, A.M., Harvey, H.J., Richardson, R.F., Fowler, J.D., Tomlinson, J. & Henderson, R.A. (1988) Canine primary renal neoplasms: a retrospective review of 54 cases. *Journal of the American Animal Hospital Association* **24,** 443–452.

Stone, E.A. (1987) Canine nephrotomy. *Compendium on Continuing Education for the Practicing Veterinarian* **9,** 883–888.

Ureter

Dean, P.W. & Constantinescu, G.M. (1988) Canine ectopic ureter. *Compendium on Continuing Education for the Practicing Veterinarian* **10,** 146–158.

Dupree, G.P., Dee, L.G. & Dee, J.F. (1990) Ureterotomies for treatment of ureterolithiasis in two dogs. *Journal of the American Animal Hospital Association* **26,** 500–504.

Holt, P.E. Gibbs, C. & Pearson, H. (1982) Canine ectopic ureter – a review of twenty-nine cases. *Journal of Small Animal Practice* **23,** 195–208.

Mason, L.K., Stone, E.A., Biery, D.N., Robertson, I. & Thrall, D.E. (1990) Surgery of ectopic ureters: pre- and postoperative radiographic morphology. *Journal of the American Animal Hospital Association* **26,** 73–79.

Robins, G.M. & Presnell, K.R. (1974) Uretero-neocystostomy in the dog. *Journal of Small Animal Practice* **15,** 185–188.

Bladder

Bojrab, M.J., Perry, L. & Tamas, S.P. (1986) Transitional cell carcinomas of the canine bladder: diagnosis and management. *Compendium on Continuing Education for the Practicing Veterinarian* **8,** 495–500.

Brearley, M.J., Thatcher, C. & Cooper, J.E. (1986) Three cases of transitional cell carcinoma in the cat and a review of the literature. *Veterinary Record* **118,** 91–94.

Burnie, A.G. & Weaver, A.D. (1983) Urinary bladder neoplasia in the dog; a review of seventy cases. *Journal of Small Animal Practice* **24,** 129–143.

Dhein, C.R., Person, M.W., Leathers, C.W. & Gavin, P.R. (1989) Prepubic (suprapubic) catheterization of the dog. *Journal of the American Animal Hospital Association* **25,** 261–271.

Dhein, C.R. & Person, M.W. (1989) Prepubic (suprapubic) catheterization of eight dogs with lower urinary tract disorders. *Journal of the American Animal Hospital Association* **25,** 272–276.

Finkbeiner, A. & Lapides, J. (1974) Effect of distension on blood flow in dog's urinary bladder. *Investigative Urology* **12,** 210–212.

Osborne, C.A., Kroll, R.A., Lulich, J.P., Johnston, G.R. & Kruger, J.M. (1989) Medical management of vesicourachal diverticula in 15 cats with lower urinary tract disease. *Journal of Small Animal Practice* **30,** 608–612.

Patnaik, A.K., Schwarz, P.D. & Greene, R.W. (1986) A histopathologic study of twenty urinary bladder neoplasms in the cat. *Journal of Small Animal Practice* **27,** 433–445.

Radasch, R.M., Merkley, D.F., Wilson, J.W. & Barstad, R.D. (1990) Cystotomy closure. A comparison of the strength of appositional and inverting suture patterns. *Veterinary Surgery* **19,** 283–288.

White, R.A.S. & Herrtage, M.E. (1986) Bladder retroflexion in the dog. *Journal of Small Animal Practice* **27,** 735–746.

Williams, J.M. & White, R.A.S. (1991) Tube cystostomy in the dog and cat. *Journal of Small Animal Practice* **32,** 598–602.

Urethra

Bilbery, S.A., Birchard, S.J. & Smeak, D.D. (1991) Scrotal urethrostomy: retrospective review of 38 dogs (1973–1988). *Journal of the American Animal Hospital Association* **27,** 560–564.

Davies, J.V. & Read, H.M. (1990) Urethral tumours in dogs. *Journal of Small Animal Practice* **31,** 131–136.

Gaskell, C.J., Denny, H.R., Jackson, O.F. & Weaver, A.D. (1978) Clinical management of the feline urological syndrome. *Journal of Small Animal Practice* **19,** 301–314.

Gregory, C.R. (1987) The effects of perineal urethrostomy on urethral function in male cats. *Compendium on Continuing Education for the Practicing Veterinarian* **9,** 895–899.

Griffiths, D.W. & Gregory, C.R. (1992) Prevalence of bacterial urinary tract infection after perineal urethrostomy in cats. *Journal of the American Veterinary Medical Association* **200,** 681–684.

Holt, P.E. (1985) Urinary incontinence in the bitch due to sphincter mechanism incompetence: prevalence in referred dogs and retrospective analysis of sixty cases. *Journal of Small Animal Practice* **25,** 181–190.

Holt, P.E. (1985) Importance of urethral length, bladder neck position and vestibulo-vaginal stenosis in sphincter mechanism incompetence in the incontinent bitch. *Research in Veterinary Science* **39,** 364–372.

Holt, P.E. (1985) Urinary incontinence in the bitch due to sphincter mechanism incompetence: surgical treatment. *Journal of Small Animal Practice* **26,** 237–246.

Holt, P.E. (1989) Hindlimb skin loss associated with urethral rupture in two cats. *Journal of Small Animal Practice* **30,** 406–409.

Holt, P.E. (1990) Long-term evaluation of colposuspension in the treatment of urinary incontinence due to incompetence of the urethral sphincter mechanism in the bitch. *Veterinary Record* **127,** 537–542.

Holt, P.E. (1993) Surgical management of congential urethral sphincter mechanism incompetence in eight female cats and a bitch. *Veterinary Surgery* **22,** 98–104.

Holt, P.E. & Thrusfield, M.V. (1993) The association between breed, size, neutering, docking and acquired urinary incontinence due to urethral sphincter mechanism in bitches. *Veterinary Record* **133**, 177–180.

Hosgood, G. & Hedlund, C.S. (1992) Perineal urethrostomy in cats. *Compendium on Continuing Education for the Practicing Veterinarian* **14,** 1195–1207.

Layton, C.E., Ferguson, H.R., Cook, J.E. & Guffy, M.M. (1987) Intrapelvic urethral anastomosis. A comparison of three techniques. *Veterinary Surgery* **16,** 175–182.

Milroy, E.J.G., Chapple, C.R., Cooper, J.E., Eldin, A., Wallsten, H., Seddon, A.M. & Rowles, P.M. (1988) A new treatment for urethral strictures. *Lancet* **ii,** 1424–1427.

Moroff, S.D., Brown, B.A., Matthiesen, D.T. & Scott, R.C. (1991) Infiltrative urethral disease in female dogs: 41 cases (1980–1987). *Journal of the American Veterinary Medical Association* **199,** 247–251.

Osborne, C.A., Caywood, D.D., Johnston, G.R., Polzin, D.J., Lulich, J.P. & Kruger, J.M. (1991) Perineal urethrostomy versus dietary management in prevention of recurrent lower urinary tract disease. *Journal of Small Animal Practice* **32,** 296–305.

Piermattei, D.L. & Osborne, C.A. (1977) Urohydropropulsion – non-surgical removal of urethral calculi in male dogs. In *Current Veterinary Therapy VI. Small Animal Practice* (Ed. R.W. Kirk). W.B Saunders Co. Ltd, Philadelphia. pp. 1194–1196.

Sackman, J.E., Sims, M.H. & Krahwinkel, D.J. (1991) Urodynamic evaluation of lower urinary tract function in cats after perineal urethrostomy with minimal and extensive dissection. *Veterinary Surgery* **20,** 55–60.

Waldron, D.R., Hedlund, C.S., Tangner, C.H., Watters, J., Turk, J. & Cox, H.U. (1985) The canine urethra. A comparison of first and second intention healing. *Veterinary Surgery* **14,** 213–217.

White, R.S. & Pomeroy, C.J. (1989) Phenypropanolamine: an α-adrenergic agent for the management of urinary incontinence in the bitch associated with urethral sphincter mechanism incompetence. *Veterinary Record* **125,** 478–480.

Prostate

Basinger, R.R., Rawlings, C.A., Barsanti, J.A. & Oliver, J.E. (1989) Urodynamic alterations associated with clinical prostatic diseases and prostatic surgery in 23 dogs. *Journal of the American Animal Hospital Association* **25,** 385–392.

Bell, F.W., Klausner, J.S., Hayden, D.W., Feeney, D.A. & Johnston, S.D. (1991) Clinical and pathologic features of prostatic adenocarcinoma in sexually intact and castrated dogs; 31 cases (1970–1987). *Journal of the American Veterinary Medical Association* **199,** 1623–1630.

Cowan, L.A., Barsanti, J.A., Crowell, W. & Brown,J. (1991) Effects of castration on chronic bacterial prostatitis in dogs. *Journal of the American Veterinary Medical Association* **199,** 346–350.

Hardie, E.M., Barsanti, J.A. & Rawlings, C.A. (1984) Complications of prostatic surgery. *Journal of the American Animal Hospital Association* **20,** 50–56.

Hardie, E.M., Stone, E.A., Spaulding, K.A. & Cullen, J.M. (1990) Subtotal canine prostatectomy with the neodymium:yttrium–aluminum–garnet laser. *Veterinary Surgery* **19,** 348–355.

Mullen, H.S., Mattiesen, D.T. & Scavelli, T.D. (1990) Results of surgery and postoperative complications in 92 dogs treated for prostatic abscessation by a multiple Penrose drain technique. *Journal of the American Animal Hospital Association* **26,** 369–379.

Newell, S.M., Mahaffey, M.B., Binhazim, A. & Greene, C.E. (1992) Paraprostatic cyst in a cat. *Journal of Small Animal Practice* **33,** 399–401.

White, R.A.S., Herrtage, M.E. & Dennis, R. (1987) The diagnosis and management of paraprostatic and prostatic retention cysts in the dog. *Journal of Small Animal Practice* **28,** 551–574.

Index